PARTNERING WITH PARENTS

Family-Centred Practice in Children's Services

Edited by Barry Trute and Diane Hiebert-Murphy

Internationally recognized as the gold standard in providing services to children with special needs and their family members, family-centred practice has expanded and evolved considerably over the past two decades. However, until now there has not been a basic text geared to professional education and skill building across diverse disciplines and settings. Filling this significant gap, *Partnering with Parents* is a primer on family-centred practice for professionals working in children's health and developmental services.

The material in this practice text covers interdisciplinary training in key child service sectors, particularly child development, child mental health, and children's health. The contributors identify and discuss the main principles of the model as it is practised in Canada, with a focus on working alliances, empowerment methods, and the development of social support resources. Providing examples of the application of family-centred practice in a wide range of service settings, this book will be useful for the social workers, nurses, psychologists, and allied health professionals who work within complex service situations.

BARRY TRUTE is an emeritus professor in the Faculty of Social Work at the University of Calgary and the University of Manitoba.

DIANE HIEBERT-MURPHY is a professor in the Faculty of Social Work at the University of Manitoba.

Partnering with Parents

Family-Centred Practice
in Children's Services

EDITED BY
BARRY TRUTE AND
DIANE HIEBERT-MURPHY

UNIVERSITY OF TORONTO PRESS
Toronto Buffalo London

© University of Toronto Press 2013
Toronto Buffalo London
www.utppublishing.com
Printed in Canada

ISBN 978-1-4426-4122-8 (cloth)
ISBN 978-1-4426-1050-7 (paper)

Library and Archives Canada Cataloguing in Publication

Partnering with parents : family-centred practice in children's services /
edited by Barry Trute and Diane Hiebert-Murphy.

Includes bibliographical references.
ISBN 978-1-4426-4122-8 (bound)   ISBN 978-1-4426-1050-7 (pbk.)

1. Parents of children with disabilities – Services for.   2. Children with
disabilities – Services for.   I. Trute, Barry, 1944–   II. Hiebert-Murphy, E.
Diane (Elizabeth Diane), 1960–

HQ759.913.P37 2013   362.4083   C2012-907034-3

University of Toronto Press acknowledges the financial assistance to its
publishing program of the Canada Council for the Arts and the Ontario
Arts Council.

   Canada Council   Conseil des Arts
for the Arts   du Canada

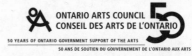

University of Toronto Press acknowledges the financial support of the
Government of Canada through the Canada Book Fund for its publishing
activities.

Contents

Foreword

The information contained in this book will lead to clear and fundamental understanding of family-centred practice. It will help practitioners to employ a respectful, honourable, and effective approach when working with families of children with disabilities.

As outlined in this text, the approach in the field of child health and disability was traditionally "child-focused" and expert-based. It has been a breath of fresh air for me to read and see in print the beliefs of family-centred practice which has emerged as an alternative way of doing business in the field of disability and children's services. This shift in focus acknowledges the following:

- Family is an anchoring centre and a constant in a child's life.
- Helping a child means simultaneously helping the family and vice versa.
- Whenever possible, parents should be considered "senior" partners with professionals in the creation of service plans.
- The family's perceived needs and service priorities are a primary focus of service planning and professional intervention.

Not only do the authors understand the "shoes a parent walks in," the model they espouse is clearly presented by them in this book. The approach they detail is committed to family well-being through *action* – to strengthen and empower parental functioning, and thereby assist the enhancement of the family as a vital resource in the positive development of children.

From a parent's perspective, this model is heartening and helpful; it engenders trust in the service system and helps alleviate the loneliness that accompanies the joys of life when parenting a child with developmental disabilities.

My parenting journey began 35 years ago with a difficult birth and my son Jonathan being severely brain injured. Our family entered a new world of uncertainty, fear, trepidation, and the unknown – including a complex service system for developmental disabilities. Our family's early experiences with the service system at that time involved the traditional practice model, which focused on the child and considered family circumstances as background noise. The beliefs held by these traditional services included the following:

- Professionals are the experts and family has limited information to offer
- Service plans (assessments, resources) should be left entirely to the judgment of professionals
- Children's needs are seen as the sole basis for service decisions, and families' needs are ignored

As I reflect back on those early years, what stands out for me as a parent was my sense of exclusion rather than inclusion (assessments, plans, allocations of scarce service resources). I remember experiencing "a cone of silence," which usually involved the sharing of information only between professionals. There most often was an "us versus them" mentality projected by professionals in the service system that left this parent feeling that she was working at odds with professionals rather than working as a partner. I said to many professionals: "I am your best resource when it comes to understanding my son – we need to work together." However, this suggestion was often ignored, and that left me with a feeling of loneliness and aloneness. We wondered what our family's place was in the planning of the course of our child's life. At times we wondered if the professionals took up more of Jon's life than we did.

Families like ours that have travelled the long road to where we are currently in the child disability field need to learn from our past experiences and move together towards a better future. Most important is the promotion of the family-centred practice model and all that it entails. Families are grateful that we now stand as part of a committed, experienced, and willing service team with professionals, to work together to achieve the greatest benefit for our children with disabilities. From my perspective, as a parent of a son living with a life-disrupting disability, several aspects of the family-centred practice model detailed in this book stood out for me:

- Assessment should include both child and family, and is a tool to record ongoing changes as a child and family evolve.
- Service delivery is about partnerships and the willingness to involve more participants, not fewer.
- Service delivery is a process that includes both professionals and family members.
- Attention must be given to family realities (strengths and weaknesses) to develop family member capacities for the long term (recognizing that parents have a lifetime commitment).
- Fathers as well as mothers are an essential part of the service picture.

Thank you to the contributors, authors, researchers, and supporters of this work. We are humbled and heartened that you chose this field and our families as the basis of your efforts, for the benefit of us all. After reading this book, as a parent I feel that our voices have been heard and our journey has been understood. Our children thank you. Our families thank you.

Doreen M. Draffin
Jonathan's Grateful Mother

Acknowledgments

Our research and clinical practice involving families with children with disabilities has been ongoing for some 25 years. It was first supported by Children's Special Services in the Province of Manitoba through study grants and training contracts. In particular, we wish to acknowledge the dedication, service insights, and inspired thinking of Brian Law and Tracy Moore. In our minds, Manitoba has always been a leader in the design and implementation of family-centred services for children with disabilities in Canada. Alberta has also been a champion of family-centred practice in children's services. It remains the only province in Canada that has legislation that mandates basic government support resources and establishes such services as a right of all Alberta families with children with special needs.

Over the years, the research findings contained in most chapters of this book were supported in part by grants from Children's Special Services of the Province of Manitoba; the Sister Bertha Baumann Research Award, the St. Amant Society, Winnipeg, Manitoba; and the Social Sciences and Humanities Research Council of Canada. Without a publication grant from the Faculty of Social Work at the University of Calgary, this book would have not been possible. We wish to thank deans Gayla Rogers and Jackie Sieppert for their ongoing encouragement and support.

The appendix to this book contains two empirical measures that have emerged from our family studies in Manitoba. These measures, the Family Impact of Childhood Disability Scale and the Parenting Morale Index, have been field tested in Alberta. We wish to acknowledge the important replication studies led by our colleague Dr Karen Benzies in the Faculty of Nursing at the University of Calgary, which was supported by the Alberta Centre for Child, Family, and Community Research. We hope that in some small way these brief assessment and survey tools will be useful to family-centred practitioners and advance their work with parents of children with special needs. We consider these measures to be in the public domain and welcome their future use as aids to practice and to applied family research.

The bulk of the practice knowledge contained in this book is derived from our study and research with hundreds of families in Manitoba and Alberta. Without their generosity in working with us, much of the practice knowledge that is contained in this book would have never been identified and verified. We are deeply grateful to these families for sharing their experiences, their knowledge of family life, and their wisdom. They have taught us much about the joys and challenges of raising children with special needs and about how we, as professionals, can work in partnership with them.

Barry Trute and Diane Hiebert-Murphy
Editors

Contributors

David Este, PhD
Professor
Faculty of Social Work
University of Calgary

Diane Hiebert-Murphy, PhD, CPsych
Professor
Faculty of Social Work and Psychological Service Centre
University of Manitoba

Tricia Klassen, MSW
Therapist
Macdonald Youth Services

Kathryn Levine, PhD
Associate Professor
Faculty of Social Work
University of Manitoba

David B. Nicholas, PhD
Associate Professor
Faculty of Social Work
University of Calgary

Barry Trute, PhD, RMFT
Professor Emeritus
Faculty of Social Work
University of Calgary
and
Professor Emeritus
Faculty of Social Work
University of Manitoba

Alexandra Wright, PhD
Associate Professor
Faculty of Social Work
University of Manitoba

PARTNERING WITH PARENTS

Family-Centred Practice in Children's Services

PART ONE

Introduction

1 Practice Parameters and Definition of Terms

BARRY TRUTE AND DIANE HIEBERT-MURPHY

The Service Context of Family-Centred Practice

Family-centred practice has been internationally recognized over the past several decades as being highly relevant in the design and delivery of children's services. To varying degrees it has been incorporated into programs of service delivery in child developmental disability, child health, child mental health, and child welfare. In many ways the operational definition of family-centred practice has depended on the service context in which it is applied. It can mean different things when applied in community-based family support programs such as child disability services, in highly specialized services such as paediatric surgery departments in hospitals, or in mandated services such as child protection.

A detailed history of the evolution of family-centred practice across the major sectors of children's services (e.g., childhood disability services, paediatric community and hospital care, child welfare) and across the range of professional training programs (e.g., social work, nursing, occupational therapy) is beyond the scope of this text, as each of these contexts of practice warrants a special story of its own. It should be noted that important steps have been taken in each sector towards providing services that are family-centred. For example, for a number of decades several provinces in Canada (including Manitoba and Nova Scotia) have had formal family-centred programs for children with special developmental challenges and complex health care needs. Alberta is the first province to ensure that the provision of specific levels of child and family support resources are anchored in a family-centred model of service delivery. Legislation in the Province of Alberta mandates family-centred services for children and youth with special needs. The Family Support for Children with Disabilities Act (Statutes of Alberta, Chapter F-5.3) was enacted in 2003. It directs family-centred practice with two main components: one based on the support needs of parents and families and another addressing the support needs of a child or youth with disabilities. Through this act, Alberta has become the one provincial jurisdiction in Canada that has legislated the provision of family-centred services, has set specific practice parameters within these services, and has ensured basic support resources for children, youth, and families, support resources which are received as a civil right rather than a service privilege. Within child health, leading children's hospitals in Canada self-identify as being "family-centred facilities," a formal recognition of agreement with family-centred principles. In practice, however, the extent to which family-centred practice has penetrated deeply into child health care services is variable. Family preservation as an approach to family-centred child protection services has been activated on a limited basis in some provinces, but Canadian child welfare services largely retain a "child rescue" stance with a paramount interest in the protection of the child (and with secondary attention given to respecting the integrity and permanence of the child's family). There remains much work to be done to advance family-centred practice in Canadian children's services. Such advancement will need mandated authority from provincial governments, more widely entrenched development of family-centred programs in community settings, and more formalized inclusion of family-centred knowledge and skill development in professional training programs.

Although family-centred practice is widely endorsed in children's services across North America, it seems to have made only modest gains in professional practice and has had minimal impact on service delivery policy (Craft-Rosenberg, Kelley, & Schnoll, 2006; Patterson & Hovey, 2000). Dempsey and Keen (2008) assess the family-centred field in children's disability services as being in an "adolescent phase of development" (p. 43). We hope that this text will serve to contribute to the advancement of the understanding and employment of family-centred practice in children's services in Canada.

Defining Family-Centred Practice

Despite a lack of clarity in the terminology used during the early years of this model (words such as family-centred, family-focused, and

family-based were often interchanged), the use of the term "family-centred" has now become more carefully defined and consistently applied
across service sectors (Allen & Petr, 1996; Johnson, 1990; Trute, 2007;
Walton, Sandau-Beckler, & Mannes, 2001). Allen and Petr (1996) provide a parsimonious and functional definition of family-centred care
that has emerged from the literature:

> Family-centered service delivery, across disciplines and settings, recog-
> nizes the centrality of the family in the lives of individuals. It is guided by
> fully informed choices made by the family and focuses upon the strengths
> and capabilities of these families. (p. 68)

Two themes emerge from this definition of family-centred services:
informed choices and professional practices based on seeking and
building on family strengths. In this book, we consider the strengths-
based perspective, in situational assessment and the planning and execution of service delivery, as a key element of family-centred practice.
The assumptions underlying the strengths perspective include the fundamental recognition that despite life's challenges, all persons and environments possess strengths and resources that can be mobilized to
in some way meet these challenges. It is asserted that when service
providers identify and support people's strengths, this action will create opportunities for those individuals to enhance their environmental
support resources and psychological coping abilities, and will serve to
advance their ability to solve or better cope with life challenges. Further, it is recognized that identifying and activating these strengths and
resources optimally requires a collaborative process between the person and the service provider. Saleebey (1997) offers an overview of the
strengths perspective in a collection of papers that describe the application of this perspective across a wide range of human services. He
states that the strengths perspective honours two things: "the power of
the self to heal and right itself with the help of the environment, and the
need for an alliance with the hope that life might really be otherwise"
(Saleebey, 1996, p. 303). We see the strengths perspective reflected in a
marked shift in service delivery that moves away from primarily "fixing" problems in children, parents, and families to collaborative parent-professional action. It requires a practice lens that goes beyond a
focus on the person to include the social environment, ranging from
the family to the larger society, to allow efforts that optimally augment
strengths and reduce vulnerability. McQuaide and Ehrenreich (1997)

review elements in the assessment of strengths that include cognitive and appraisal skills, cognitive coping mechanisms, temperamental and dispositional factors, interpersonal skills, and proximal and distal social or institutional support (p. 205). The strengths perspective thereby goes beyond focusing on deficiencies in the person or narrowly addressing specific unmet needs in the family to empowering children, youth, parents, and families to obtain greater mastery over their life challenges and stressors, to better define their goals and aspirations, and to develop the skills they need. These skills enable people to obtain the support that they require, whenever they wish to do so and whenever this is feasible and possible.

There are two caveats that we should identify in regard to the embrace of the strengths perspective and empowerment methods. First, we are aware that the strengths-based perspective and empowerment theory can be distorted and misused politically to rationalize neo-liberal or New Right conservative views. That is, these perspectives can be used to argue that government services should be curtailed and families should take care of their own (Gray, 2011). We see the strengths-based perspective as advancing practice theory in the human services and not as a rationale for reducing state support for children's services and offloading the responsibility for caring for children with special needs onto the backs of families. We also believe that the strengths perspective and professional problem solving in service delivery are not always diametrically opposed or dichotomous alternatives. Dangers can be associated with too much emphasis on problem solving in professional practice, including a misplaced emphasis on diagnostic labels, categorizing people according to person-centred symptoms, and missing crucial elements in family and environmental circumstances. Saleebey (1996) offers a detailed comparison and contrast of the pathology and strengths practice approaches, including a listing of common criticisms of the strengths perspective. We believe it is important to acknowledge that attention to client service needs (i.e., problems) and attention to client strengths (i.e., personal, family, and community resources) both come into play at different times in service delivery, and in the service response to different client needs and priorities. McMillen, Morris, and Sherraden (2004) offer a thoughtful consideration of the interplay of the two approaches. They suggest that there can be a capacity-building element in problem-focused frameworks, and that problem-focused and strengths-based approaches need not be mutually exclusive "but need each other and work well together" (p. 323).

We see the identification of client-identified needs and challenges as being the place to start, but that strengths-based approaches are the optimal way to proceed in ongoing collaborative efforts of clients and service providers to address client-identified needs and service priorities. This being said, it is important to give priority attention to client strengths as these can be seen to provide "the fuel and energy" to empowerment methods (Cowger, 1994, p. 263). We believe that empowerment methods are an essential ingredient of family-centred practice; Chapter 6 in this book gives more focused attention to empowerment theory and methods.

Throughout this book we will repeat the importance of "partnership" as a fundamental element of family-centred practice. Working in partnership with families is a defining feature of family-centred practice (Dunst, 2002). Much has been written about the importance of family-professional partnership and collaboration in achieving the desired goals and outcomes of intervention (e.g., Dunst, 2002; Roberts, Rule, & Innocenti, 1998). Dunst, Johanson, Trivette, and Hamby (1991) reviewed family-oriented programs, particularly those involving early intervention children's services, and compared these programs across their foundational principles, service delivery models, and practice elements. This synthesis identified four broad classes of programs, each with a different emphasis on family-professional partnership: professional-centred, family-allied, family-focused, and family-centred. Similarly, four clusters of family-oriented programs were suggested by Pletcher (1995) that distinguished programs across a consistent set of differentiating service characteristics, but with slightly different terminology (i.e., family-involved in place of family-allied). These models exist across a continuum ranging from professional-centred to family-centred. Understanding the differences between these models helps to define family-centred practice and points to the practice elements that make it distinct. It should be noted that these clusters are not independent and mutually exclusive categories, but can overlap as programs develop and as professionals and agencies move towards advancing the family-centred practice emphasis in their services.

Professional-centred services. These services adopt the "traditional" approach to children's services. The professional holds the role as the expert who assesses need for service, determines an intervention plan, and leads the way in ameliorating, fixing, or treating the problem or service need. Families may be seen as the causal agent of the child's difficulties or as being complicit in maintaining a child's problem or service need. Alternatively, family members may be seen as passive victims of child deficits or pathology. The focus of service is usually the child, with secondary attention sometimes given to parents or to families. A linear progression of assessment, diagnosis, and intervention (i.e., the "traditional medical model") guides professional action, which is often offered according to inflexible practice protocols and limited by program resources which professionals hold as their prerogative to allocate as they judge best for the child and her or his family.

Family-allied/family-involved services. Family members are seen as extensions or aids to formal services or professional intervention. Family members are engaged to enhance the professional's service to the child. This can include family members providing prescribed interventions in the home or helping to ensure compliance with treatment regimens or service plans. Families are viewed as having little or no expertise to offer in the determination of service need or in the design of a service plan. Professionals may act as "parents to the parents" to enhance the parents' ability to care for their child. Family members are sometimes asked to approve service plans that professionals determine for a child, particularly if this involves informed consent to child treatment or out-of-home placement.

Family-focused services. Families and professionals collaborate in the determination of service needs for the child and the family. Although professionals remain the experts on what should be done to help the child, the family is seen as a valuable source of information to facilitate professional practice. Professionals acknowledge the importance of the family in the development and well-being of the child. Professionals seek to inform the family regarding helpful and important allied service resources and will assist families in securing the resources that the professional feels are most appropriate in the local community network of human services. The primary intent of services is problem resolution or achievement of the service goal that is consistent with the service mandate of the professional or agency (which usually sees service to the child as its paramount mission).

Family-centred services. Unlike the previous orientations to service delivery, within family-centred services, partnership is the defining feature of the relationship between family members and professionals. If capable and willing, parents are "senior partners" with professionals in determining the service plans for themselves and their children. Professionals do engage in problem solving and service strategizing with family members, but with family capacity building as a fundamental goal. A strengths-based approach to professional practice is interwoven into the exploration of service need and into the service plans that are mutually determined by the family and professional. Careful attention is given to the identification, mobilization, and/or building of community resources available to the family, both from informal (e.g., family, friends) and formal (e.g., governmental programs, non-governmental agencies) sources of child and family support. Information provision is seen as central in family empowerment efforts. Family capacity building to support, educate, and protect children is a key element of professional practice. Throughout all intervention efforts, a strong working alliance is maintained between the professional and the family.

Defining Family in Family-Centred Practice

Hartman and Laird (1983, p. 30) offer a phenomenological definition of a family that includes

- when two or more individuals have decided they are a family
- when, in the intimate here-and-now environment in which they gather, there is a sharing of emotional needs for closeness and of those roles and tasks necessary for meeting the biological, social, and psychological requirements of the individuals involved.

This definition of family is a functional one that sets broad and flexible service boundaries for family-centred practice. In some service situations, organizations will have formal definitions of what can constitute a "family case" when opening new service files. However, in terms of operational practice definitions that may be applied in family-centred services, family can be defined by those receiving service as including those individuals who they identify as being members of their family. It is the proximal emotional ties and mutual support that are the most salient aspects of family life for the family-centred practitioner.

As we will discuss more fully in Chapter 2, in family-centred children's services, a key consideration when identifying the constituent elements of a family is "who is doing the parenting." Parents provide the executive authority in a family and serve as the "hub in the wheel of family life." This function may be done by many different and alternative parenting units including, for example, a single parent mother, a mother-father dyad, or a mother-grandmother team. We know that many single mothers are strong, resilient parents who take excellent care of their child with special needs (Levine, 2009). However, we also know that in situations involving a child with a serious, complex disability, a parenting team is often required, as the time and effort demands can be too much for one person to adequately manage on her or his own. When tragedies occur and a child is abandoned, abused, or killed, it is not just the overwrought parent who holds responsibility, but a social support system that has collapsed or has not been available to support the family. In these situations, it is often an entire service and social support network that has failed the child. From the viewpoint of family-centred practice, it is important to assess, understand, and assist children as they are nested in families and families as they are nested in communities.

In this book we will use the term "parent" to refer to any configuration of one or more individuals who hold responsibility for providing the ongoing guidance, nurturance, and support as caretakers in a family unit that is "the home" for a child with special needs. This may include many caretakers of children such as a mother, father, grandparent, aunt, uncle, adoptive parent, or foster parent.

Clarifying the Term "Service Provider"

In Chapter 3 we differentiate between levels of professional expertise and practice parameters in family-centred services that can span such distinct practice elements as facilitative counselling, family therapy, or service coordination. We use the term *service provider* to be interchangeable across these separate categories of intervention objectives and skills. We also use the terms *professional* and *service provider* to be applicable across distinct disciplines such as social work, nursing, psychology, medicine, and allied health professions (e.g., occupational therapy and speech-language pathology). In our view, family-centred practice is a way of thinking and relating that supplements and advances the special practice abilities that social workers, nurses, primary care physicians, and other disciplines working in children's services bring based on their training and experience. Some disciplines will more directly and extensively use family-centred practice in their work (such as social workers serving as service coordinators to families with children with serious and chronic health challenges). Other service providers will be counted on to provide highly technical interventions that require specialized knowledge and competencies (such as paediatric neurologists assisting children with neuromuscular or neuromotor challenges). The key to enhancing the family-centredness of children's services, that transcends the wide range of professionals that can be. engaged with children and their families, is that all professionals understand and endorse the principles of family-centred practice. Some professionals will employ the practice elements of this service delivery strategy (e.g., empowerment practice, social support mobilization) more directly and fully than others. However, all will work together to ensure that parents act as partners with professionals in the planning of services and in the long-term support of children with special needs.

All professionals engaged in providing family-centred services to a particular child and his or her family will work with respect for each other and with the understanding that different components of care can best be delivered by their colleagues who hold the necessary expertise. That is, there will be different service roles across disciplines and professional groups that will be differentially required through phases of child treatment and family service delivery. For example, in many geographic locales in Canada, paediatricians are a scarce commodity in children's health care services. It would not make sense for them to act as formal service coordinators for children with complex and chronic health care needs, as it would be an inefficient use of the time and skills of these physicians. However, it is important that they have the knowledge and capability to conduct their medical practice from a family-centred perspective so that they can cooperatively support other professionals, such as social workers or public health nurses, who have the service role and expertise to act as family service coordinators. In turn, as part of service coordination, it is important that the social workers and public health nurses have the understanding and capability to collaborate with the child's paediatrician whenever this becomes necessary for the maximum well-being of the child and his or her family.

Foundational Beliefs for Family-Centred Practice

One of us (BT) offered a public presentation on family-centred health services and was approached afterwards by a young lawyer who was a member of the board of a local community agency. This person commented that family-centred practice seemed logical and was basically common sense. The "expert" on family-centred services had to agree with him. This recognition that following the principles of family-centred practice is "common sense" shows us how illogical many programs in children's services have become over the years. It brings to consciousness the reality of many existing children's services. That is, they are not organized in a way that is logical or makes sense from the family's point of view. They are organized to be convenient to the professional and to make sure that things are done expediently for the benefit of the professional. When you step back, you can see why this is often the case in contemporary children's services. Professionals have become so overloaded in their work that they look to streamline and expedite things for themselves. Unfortunately, in the process, professionals lose sight of what families need and what makes sense to them. They do not realize that, to streamline and expedite the services they are employed to deliver, they would be much wiser to involve parents (and other concerned family members) as partners in service planning.

Several decades ago, most professionals working with families with children with serious developmental, cognitive, or emotional disabilities believed that having a child with serious disability de facto meant family pathology. If a mother expressed sadness and exhaustion, she was often labelled and treated as clinically depressed or anxious. If she stated that things were stressful but she was doing well, she was identified as in denial. It was a no-win situation for parents. There were terms such as "chronic sorrow" that professionals took as a common and persistent parent state (Olshansky, 1962). However, "chronic sorrow" is not a constant state for parents of children with serious disability, but is experienced periodically by some (Teel, 1991). It was believed that having a child with a serious disability was like having a death in the family, and Kubler-Ross's well-known stages of death and dying (Kubler-Ross, 1969) were transplanted to the child disability field. Research suggests that professional beliefs regarding chronic sorrow were inaccurate (Dunning, 1999). One can describe professional beliefs and theories at the time as being narrow, negativistic, and pathology-oriented. Unfortunately, these skewed beliefs supported a "fix it" mentality that regarded parents as deficient, often stripped them of their dignity, and set professionals up as "the experts" that were there to direct parents and families in their coping with stress and loss.

By the 1980s, research evidence began to emerge that indicated that parents of children with disability were essentially normal (e.g., Tavormina, Boll, Dunn, Luscomb, & Taylor, 1981) and that most of these families were coping adequately (e.g., Longo & Bond, 1984). In Manitoba, we completed one of the first research projects that had been done internationally on resilient families with special needs children (Trute

& Hauch, 1988a, 1988b). We studied strong families to learn what other families with special needs children could learn from them. This initial research led to several longitudinal tracking studies that followed the same random, cross-sectional or "average" sample of families as their children with disabilities grew older. What we found was that these families had times of sadness and times of joy. We found that these families could best be described as typical families with special children.

Our research and other related studies taught us that there were what could be called "transformational experiences" in which the challenge of childhood disability led to growth and enhanced personal strength in the parents and siblings of children with serious disability. We have learned that as children with special needs grow older, parenting stress does increase substantially, but that most parents do not suffer psychopathology or pervasive chronic sorrow; it seems that most parents adequately cope with the increased stress over time. Contemporary family-centred practice in children's services is based on this view of parents as having strengths and resources to cope with the challenges that they encounter when caring for a child with special needs. Building on these strengths, family-centred practice seeks to establish partnerships with parents and solidarity in mutual effort and is not simply out in search of pathology to fix.

Family-centred practice is essentially a "compassion-based" method of delivering human services. As Dr James Orbinski, past international president of Médecins Sans Frontières, Doctors Without Borders, has noted: "When we relate to others with compassion we are capable of seeing 'sameness of self' in the 'being of other.'" Compassion leads professionals to relate to their clients with *solidarity*. That is the key word: solidarity – not working with pity, not with paternalism, but with solidarity. Solidarity leads us to engage with youth, parents, and family members with unity or agreement of action as much as is appropriate and possible.

Overview of the Book

Through the chapters of this book it will emerge that family-centred practice can be considered to be basically "CCC Practice." That is, it is professional practice that seeks to incorporate three major themes: context, collaboration, and capacity building. First, practice must consider human behaviour and beliefs to be anchored in social context (i.e., person-in-situation). In this book, we consider the family to be the most profound and enduring social context in the development and well-being of children. Second, practice must seek partnerships with parents and family members when designing and delivering support to children with special needs. Third, practice must hold as paramount the goal of increasing service satisfaction, parent self-efficacy, and coping resources of family members caring for children and youth with special needs.

Building on these general themes, the book is organized into five parts. In the first part, the service parameters and fundamental elements of family-centred practice are discussed. The basic concepts relevant to understanding family-centred practice are described. In the second part, the ways in which family-centred practice is distinct from family therapy and case coordination is explained. Key practice elements are then explored: establishing a relationship with families, conducting a family assessment, empowering families, and working with social networks. The chapters in the third part illustrate how families are invited to take part in service planning and how service provider practice elements are integrated into a family-centred support plan. In the fourth part, special themes relating to the application of family-centred practice are explored. In the fifth and final part, supervision and administrative issues in family-centred services are considered.

This book seeks to assist professionals to understand the fundamentals of family-centred services and to advance their skill in relational and participatory practices. Further, it is our hope that this book will assist in the implementation and development of children's services that are congruent with family-centred principles. Such services will seek to strengthen partnerships with parents and create the best possible developmental opportunities for children with special needs.

REFERENCES

Allen, R.I., & Petr, C.G. (1996). Toward developing standards and measurements for family-centered practice in family support programs. In G. Singer, L. Powers, & A. Olson (Eds.), *Family support policy and America's caregiving families: Innovations in public-private partnerships* (pp. 57–86). Baltimore, MD: Brookes.
Cowger, C.D. (1994, May). Assessing client strengths: Clinical assessment for client empowerment. *Social Work, 39*(3), 262–8. Medline:8209288

Craft-Rosenberg, M., Kelley, P., & Schnoll, L. (2006). Family-centered care: Practice and preparation. *Families in Society, 87*, 17–25.

Dempsey, I., & Keen, D. (2008). A review of the processes and outcomes in family-centered services for children with a disability. *Topics in Early Childhood Special Education, 28*(1), 42–52. http://dx.doi.org/10.1177/0271121408316699

Dunning, E.J. (1999). *Construct validation of chronic sorrow in mothers of children with chronic illness.* Unpublished doctoral dissertation, University of Pittsburgh, Pittsburgh, PA.

Dunst, C.J. (2002). Family-centered practices: Birth through high school. *Journal of Special Education, 36*(3), 141–7. http://dx.doi.org/10.1177/00224669020360030401

Dunst, C.J., Johanson, C., Trivette, C.M., & Hamby, D. (1991, October-November). Family-oriented early intervention policies and practices: Family-centered or not? *Exceptional Children, 58*(2), 115–26. Medline:1836180

Gray, M. (2011). Back to basics: A critique of the strengths perspective in social work. *Families in Society, 92*, 1–7.

Hartman, A., & Laird, J. (1983). *Family-centered social work practice.* New York, NY: Free Press.

Johnson, B. H. (1990). The changing role of families in health care. *Children's Health Care, 19*, 234–41.

Kubler-Ross, E. (1969). *On death and dying.* New York, NY: MacMillan.

Levine, K.A. (2009). Against all odds: Resilience in single mothers of children with disabilities. *Social Work in Health Care, 48*(4), 402–19. http://dx.doi.org/10.1080/00981380802605781 Medline:19396709

Longo, D.C., & Bond, L. (1984). Families of the handicapped child: Research and practice. *Family Relations, 33*(1), 57–65. http://dx.doi.org/10.2307/584590

McMillen, J.C., Morris, L., & Sherraden, M. (2004). Ending social work's grudge match: Problems versus strengths. *Families in Society, 85*, 317–25.

McQuaide, S., & Ehrenreich, J.H. (1997). Assessing client strengths. *Families in Society, 78*, 201–12.

Olshansky, S. (1962). Chronic sorrow: A response to having a mentally defective child. *Social Casework, 43*, 190–3.

Patterson, J.M., & Hovey, D.L. (2000). Family-centred care for children with special health needs: Rhetoric or reality. *Families, Systems & Health, 18*(2), 237–51. http://dx.doi.org/10.1037/h0091849

Pletcher, L.C. (1995). *Family-centered practices: A training guide.* Chapel Hill, NC: ARCH National Resource Center.

Roberts, R.N., Rule, S., & Innocenti, M.S. (1998). *Strengthening the family-professional partnership in services for young children.* Baltimore, MD: Brookes.

Saleebey, D. (1996, May). The strengths perspective in social work practice: Extensions and cautions. *Social Work, 41*(3), 296–305. Medline:8936085

Saleebey, D. (Ed.). (1997). *The strengths perspective in social work practice* (2nd ed.). New York: Longman.

Tavormina, J.B., Boll, T.J., Dunn, N.J., Luscomb, R.L., & Taylor, J.R. (1981, March). Psychosocial effects on parents of raising a physically handicapped child. *Journal of Abnormal Child Psychology, 9*(1), 121–31. http://dx.doi.org/10.1007/BF00917862 Medline:6452472

Teel, C.S. (1991, November). Chronic sorrow: Analysis of the concept. *Journal of Advanced Nursing, 16*(11), 1311–19. http://dx.doi.org/10.1111/j.1365-2648.1991.tb01559.x Medline:1753027

Trute, B. (2007). Service coordination in family-centered childhood disability services: Quality assessment from the family perspective. *Families in Society, 88*, 283–91.

Trute, B., & Hauch, C. (1988a). Building on family strength: A study of families with positive adjustment to the birth of a developmentally disabled child. *Journal of Marital and Family Therapy, 14*(2), 185–93. http://dx.doi.org/10.1111/j.1752-0606.1988.tb00734.x

Trute, B., & Hauch, C. (1988b). Social network attributes of families with positive adaptation to the birth of a developmentally disabled child. *Canadian Journal of Community Mental Health, 7*(1), 5–16.

Walton, E., Sandau-Beckler, P., & Mannes, M. (Eds.). (2001). *Balancing family-centered services and child well-being*. New York, NY: Columbia University Press.

2   Basic Family-Centred Practice Concepts and Principles

BARRY TRUTE

Key Beliefs That Guide Family-Centred Services

There is consensus (Dunst, Trivette, & Deal, 1994; Rosenbaum, King, Law, King, & Evans, 1998; Shelton, Jeppson, & Johnson, 1987; Trute, 2007) that key beliefs underlying a family-centred practice model across children's services include

1 the family is a constant in a child's life (not the professional), and the family holds essential child expertise and knowledge to inform service planning and delivery;
2 you cannot help a child without simultaneously helping a family (and often working with the community within which the family is embedded);
3 whenever possible, parents should be "senior" partners with professionals in the creation of service plans; and
4 the family's perceived needs and service priorities should be a primary focus of service planning and professional intervention.

Parent as expert. For most children, their "parent" or primary caretaker (whether biological, adoptive, or foster) is a consistent presence in their lives, while professionals assisting the child and family come and go as the need arises. For children with serious health challenges or developmental disabilities, professionals tend to enter their lives at times of crisis or transition, whereas their parents are there during these stressful periods and, as well, at all times between these sporadic occasions of intensive professional involvement. In some special circumstances, such as admission to a paediatric intensive care unit in hospital or when a child is apprehended by a child welfare agency following a disclosure of child abuse, professionals will "take over" as surrogate parents in that the professionals will hold temporary responsibility for the well-being of the child and will make decisions regarding childcare and child management while the child is held under their authority. However, these special circumstances are usually seen as temporary or transitional events in the life of a child, with permanency in a family home being the natural and preferred place for a child.

Since a parent is the most consistent person in the life of a child, usually sees the child daily, and relates to the child in what can be considered the child's "normal" life circumstances, the parent holds a wide range of child information, observations, and experience. In terms of knowledge of the life history, everyday behaviours, and psychosocial needs of their children, parents are usually greater "experts" on their children than are professionals. Family-centred practice is delivered with the understanding that it is folly to ignore or underestimate the value of the expertise that a parent brings to the ongoing process of child assessment and service planning.

Helping a child means helping a family. In the past, most children's services maintained a central focus on the child. For example, if one looks back at patterns of service in child psychiatry in prior decades in North America, it would not be uncommon to see seriously troubled children admitted to in-patient treatment units with minimal attention given to including parents in treatment planning or delivery. In such traditional service delivery models, parents provided the intake history that preceded treatment, with subsequent intervention focused almost entirely on the child. Children were admitted to in-patient treatment and often responded well to that treatment while in hospital. However, professionals were frequently surprised and perplexed when the child reverted back to old, familiar patterns of behaviour within days (or in some cases within hours) of leaving in-patient treatment settings. What was happening in these circumstances was a clash of situational contexts. The child learned to function more positively within the ward environment, but behavioural changes that were achieved could not be maintained within the home setting when the family was left uninvolved and uninformed by providers of child treatment. The lesson to be learned was that, in dealing with complex behavioural issues, both the child and the child's intimate or immediate home environment need to be simultaneously involved in service delivery to ensure permanency of change. When the child was discharged to home after in-patient treatment, family members often did not fully appreciate what was accomplished with the child, did not understand how this was achieved, and often were unconvinced that something would actually be different with the child, or did not trust that this difference would endure. In most of these instances, children were discharged back to their home environment without adequate preparation of their families. The result was that new patterns of child behaviour tended not to be recognized or reinforced at home.

Parents as partners in intervention. For many years there was ongoing debate in child psychiatry as to whether families were causal agents in a child's psychopathology or were actually victims of that psychopathology. If a parent or family is viewed as being the causal agent in the aetiology of psychopathology in a child, then it logically flows that the parent or family cannot be seen as a trusted partner in that child's treatment. This service pattern, in which professionals were blind to the importance of parents as valid service partners in their efforts to assist a child with special needs, was commonplace in the past across major service areas such as child welfare, child mental health, and juvenile corrections.

Within the family-centred practice model, parents must optimally be first viewed, and initially engaged, as valid partners with professionals in the child intervention process and supported as participants in the long-term enhancement of their child's well-being. Viewing the family as the "cause" or the "victim" of child behavioural disorders may fit in some family situations. However, professionals should relate to all parents as potential partners in planning services for their children and proceed with this assumption until it is proven to be wrong by deleterious parent actions (or lack of action). It should be noted that, in some situations, "unhelpful" parent behaviours may signal that there is a problem in the service delivery process (e.g., that the parent does not trust or have faith in the professional) rather than indicate that the parent is somehow complicit in the distress or maladaptation of the child.

It should also be clarified that partnership does not mean that responsibility for intervention is passed onto parents. For example, in "traditional" child mental health settings, when parents are involved in treatment planning and service delivery to address the needs of children with behavioural difficulties, they are often engaged as "therapeutic agents" operating on behalf of professionals. Such can be the case in intensive behavioural interventions for children with a diagnosis of pervasive developmental delay or within the autism spectrum of disorders when parents are trained as therapists of their children to deliver services within their own homes. Parents who find themselves in these situations often welcome the specialized and intensive treatment for their child, but do not want to alter their role as mother or father and take on the role of therapist. Sometimes the parent is not adequately prepared, or does not have sufficient time or resources at their disposal, to maintain what can be quite rigorous and demanding treatment protocols. Avenues of treatment inadequacy include when the parent provides intensive interventions at home and does not adequately understand protocols or procedures, when home-based treatment is not collaboratively planned with a parent, and when parents are not appropriately consulted and supported by professionals. In these circumstances, home-based treatment is doomed to fail. In these less-than-optimal instances, such in-home treatment services could be considered family-involved but not family-centred.

Perhaps one of the most contentious beliefs in family-centred practice is that parents should be "senior" (Dunst et al., 1994) or "equal" (Allen & Petr, 1996) partners in service planning whenever this is possible. This runs counter to the traditional training and practice experiences of most professionals, particularly those employed in child health care settings. Most professionals have been trained to see themselves as needing to take control and to "fix" things that are brought to their attention. In family-centred practice, parents are optimally seen as being as strong a partner as they wish to be and are capable of being in service planning. This does not mean that parents and professionals can replace each other in terms of the special expertise each brings to the delivery of child and family services, but that they respect each other's roles, knowledge, and competencies.

Partnerships between professionals and parents do not always need to be equal partnerships in terms of importance of voice or decision-making power. It is understood that in many situations a parent will need the expertise of the professional to guide service planning and intervention. In psychosocial crises and in circumstances requiring acute or emergency health care services for children, family members often need professionals to take control of the situation and provide their special expertise to treat and stabilize a child. Parents know full well that there are times that they need professionals to "take over" and deliver direct aid to their child. However, when addressing long-term needs associated with repeated or chronic conditions, parents become key actors in the ongoing situational assessment and treatment of their child. There are many chronic conditions that are faced by children and their families which cannot be "cured" by professional intervention and that call for accommodation and adjustment. In these situations parents should, whenever possible, be the pivotal "team leaders" in service priority setting and planning.

There will be times when parents want to have a strong voice in service planning for their children and times when those same parents wish a professional would provide direction and leadership. Family-centred practice means that parents have the option to be as directive and involved in services for their children as they wish to be, and have the opportunity to change their level of authority in the planning of services when they feel adequately knowledgeable and capable. Great care must be exercised not to usurp the normal place parents hold as the ultimate caretakers of their children. When the professional takes the lead in service provision, it is always with a view to inviting the parent to assume a more active role in service planning when the parent is ready and willing to assume a leadership role.

Partnership makes sense when one recognizes that parents are the experts regarding the child in her or his everyday environments, such as in the home and within the child's extended network of family and friends. It is important to recognize that parents know what interventions will be reasonable in the life of the family and understand the limits of what can be achieved within their home settings. What may seem like a logical treatment plan to a professional (such as frequent appointments in a hospital setting) may be impractical and unachievable from the parent's perspective (such as a single parent mother on income assistance, with several preschool aged children, who lives at a distance from the hospital). In order for the service plan to be effective in meeting a family's identified needs and priorities, the family should have a voice in determining what services are provided. What one family might determine would make sense to them, in terms of their level of participation in a service network assisting their child, might not make sense to other families in similar situations.

Professionals often lose sight of the fact that parents of children with serious disabilities or special needs can have many professionals in the life of their child and in the life of their family. For example, in our experience, it is not uncommon for young children who are seriously challenged with cerebral palsy to have 40 to 50 professionals involved in the planning and delivery of services to them and their family members at any one time. Each professional entering the life of these children often operates as if s/he is the "sun around which the child and family orbits, rather than recognizing that the family needs to contend with many such suns" (Rosenbaum, 2005). In fact, the parent is the centre of the child's service universe, and professionals must recognize and respect this fact. Unfortunately, most human services for children and their families proceed to plan and schedule appointments and interventions which are at their convenience, without consideration to what is reasonable, practical, and relevant from a family's perspective. When service delivery does not go smoothly, many professionals blame parents for being "resistant" or "non-compliant," rather than appreciating that their plan of treatment or service intervention may not be possible to achieve given the ongoing life realities of the child, parent, or family.

It must be recognized that this aspect of family-centred practice, namely acknowledging the importance of the parent voice in service planning, is superseded by the paramount importance of the safety of the child and professional ethical directives in this regard. When the child is not safe in her or his home because of circumstances of neglect or abuse, then offending parents have a restricted role in child and family service planning and processes of service delivery while the child is vulnerable. That is, professionals cannot ignore, condone, or collude in parent choices and behaviours that are illegal or unethical (Allen & Petr, 1996). In extreme service situations such as child abuse or neglect, the best interests and safety of the child must be paramount and precede the best interests of a parent or family. Child welfare workers are mandated to ensure stability and safety for each child who comes to their attention. However, even in situations of abuse or presenting a high probability of abuse, family-centred practice can be activated when the time is right (i.e., when child safety is assured), as most parents have the capacity and commitment to be the kind of parents they want to be, if given the right support and assistance in ways that are sensitive to their capabilities and life circumstances.

Family-Centred Practice: Relational and Participatory Elements

Dunst and Trivette (1996) identify two core components of family-centred practice: relational and participatory. The relational component includes generic skills known to be essential for effective practice in counselling (e.g., empathy, active listening, respect). Most professionals are aware of the importance of a trust-based, empathic, and hopeful relationship with those they seek to assist and are adequately skilled in developing and maintaining this important element in their work. Several chapters in this volume (Chapters 4, 6, and 8) address the development and maintenance of positive relations between family members and professionals, between professionals seeking to assist a child and her or his family, and between families themselves as they collaborate to help their children and other families like their own. The participatory component of family-centred practice is more challenging and less understood. This component includes practices that are individualized and responsive to unique family needs and that provide opportunities for families to be actively involved in service planning decisions and service choices. Participatory experiences include collaborative transactions that strengthen existing client competencies and promote the acquisition of new competencies. This component of practice is key to capacity-building efforts to promote and advance family empowerment. Although parent and family empowerment is widely embraced in children's services, it is among the most poorly understood aspects of how to deliver programs that are committed to family-centred practice.

Working alliance and the relational component of family-centred practice. A key element in family-centred practice is a professional's capacity and skill to build positive working relationships with youth, parents, and family members (Trute & Hiebert-Murphy, 2007). Family-centred practice has been seen to require, at the most foundational level, the establishment of a functional relationship between family members and professionals that is characterized by mutual trust and respect, collaborative rapport, and clear communication (Beckman, 1996). Beckman, Newcomb, Frank, and Brown (1996) suggest that four professional attributes serve as basic building blocks for positive family-centred practice:

- respect for the importance and competence of the family in taking leadership in a child's life;
- being non-judgmental and respectful of the family members' wish to do the best for their child;
- having empathetic understanding of family members' beliefs and feelings; and
- possessing the capability to communicate that respect, understanding, and empathy to family members.

These basic competencies facilitate positive and productive working relations, leave family members feeling respected and understood by the professional, and build hope in parents that services can be trusted to be helpful to the family and the child with special needs.

Empowerment and the participatory component of family-centred practice. We have noted that core beliefs in family-centred practice include acknowledgment that parents are the constant in a child's life and the executive authority in the family. Further, the family is recognized as the most important social-environmental context for the positive development of young children. Therefore, it follows that a primary goal of family-centred practice is to strengthen and empower parental functioning and to assist in the enhancement of the family as a vital resource in the positive development of children. Dunst, Trivette, and Deal (1988) define empowerment as including (a) access and control over needed resources, (b) decision-making and problem-solving abilities, and (c) acquisition of instrumental behaviour needed to interact effectively with others to procure resources (p. 3). That is, empowerment involves knowing what is available, knowing what will best help your child and family from what is available, and knowing how to obtain it. Empowerment for self-agency is one of the most essential aspects of family-centred practice, yet one of the most challenging to adequately understand and execute in ongoing practice.

The Practice Context of Family-Centred Care

There is not a prescribed and specific set of practice steps in the delivery of family-centred child health and children's social services. It has been our contention that practice patterns are strongly anchored in service context and service setting. For example, there are distinct differences between how family-centred practice is conceived and employed within hospitals compared to community settings. There are differences within hospital settings between acute care wards and programs that address chronic health issues. There are differences between chronic care programs that deal with life threatening illnesses (e.g., paediatric oncology) and those addressing life-disrupting health challenges (e.g., asthma). Background literature on family-centred practice differs markedly across child health, child mental health, child development, early intervention, and child welfare. These service domains operate as practice "information silos" with little cross-sector information exchange, synergistic development of service strategies, or integration of terms. What is the difference in how professionals practice when comparisons are made between "family-centred, child focused" paediatric

developmental services and "child-centred, family focused" child welfare services? The semantic differences seem to be more responsive to
the politics or service culture of the practice setting than to conceptual
or substantive meaning.

Another factor influencing family-centred practice has to do with the
beliefs and service cultures of the professional disciplines that take a
leading role in a particular service context, be it social work, medicine,
nursing, occupational therapy, or primary school education. Some key
allied health care disciplines have been largely trained to operate out
of institutions such as hospitals or clinics. Many human service professionals have been taught to "fix" children and have been given little
background education on working with families. Professional disciplines vary dramatically in how well prepared they are to assume collaborative problem-solving roles and to build capacity in a child, youth,
or family, rather than moving immediately to fix the problem that the
child presents for service. Many human service professionals believe
that they are family-centred in their practice when they include conversations with a parent or family member in their everyday process
of service delivery. In this sense, it is a rare social worker, paediatric
nurse, or paediatrician who does not see herself or himself as being
"family-centred." However, most human service professionals are still
trained to seek out deficits, weaknesses, or abnormalities that they are
to repair or ameliorate, rather than to understand how to expeditiously
assess and mobilize personal strengths and informal social support resources to enhance independent and self-sufficient family coping and
problem solving. As I have already noted, when it comes to capacity
building, many human service professionals do not know how much
they do not know about this key component of family-centred practice.

In some service contexts involving an emergency response or crisis
care, families want and expect professionals to move in quickly, to provide leadership, and to assist them with a situation that is out of their
control and that exceeds their coping or management skills. They do
not expect to take on the role of "senior partners" or to closely collaborate in treatment or service planning in situations calling for a high
level of professional competency and technical skill. However, even in
these situations, there are opportunities for a family-centred response.
For example, parents do not expect or want to be consulted in how paediatric surgery should be conducted. However, there are many ways in
which anaesthesia and surgical procedures can be enhanced through
parent involvement in the induction and in the recovery process that

immediately precedes and follows surgery. For example, parents' knowledge of how to interpret their young child's crying behaviour can be helpful in managing that child in the recovery room. When children have communication disorders, crying can represent pain or anxiety or a need to be held or touched. Sometimes it is significant when a child does not cry. Research and practical experience have shown that parent expertise and support in the surgery recovery room can lead to better child post-operative recovery and also to improved nursing staff morale in the surgery workplace (Fina, Lopas, Stagnone, & Santucci, 1997; Smykowski & Rodriguez, 2003).

Child welfare protection service is another challenging context for family-centred practice. In these situations, children are often removed from their biological families because they are at risk of maltreatment or have been abused or neglected. In this situation, the timing and logistics of family-centred practice needs to be skilfully managed and delivered. However, when this is done by staff skilled in family-centred practice methods, who operate with adequate service resources, family reunification is facilitated and longer-term stability can be achieved for children who have been in the care of a child welfare authority (Walton, Sandau-Beckler, & Mannes, 2001).

It is important to emphasize that some human service settings do require a high level of professional expertise and leadership, and that parents are not expecting or wanting to be partners in circumstances that require such specialized practice skill. This includes the need to conduct assessments, diagnose, and identify treatments that are currently understood to be most effective. In these situations, parents gratefully accept the important assistance the professional is giving their child and family, and often ask little more than to be well informed through the process of care. As the intervention moves into more long-term family care, or involves deeper emotional and behavioural understanding of the child, or requires the parent to take on a nursing or teaching role with the child, or involves a choice among treatment options, parent expectations are heightened that they will have a voice in decision-making and service planning.

I am not suggesting here that in some service situations family-centred practice will be inappropriate. I am suggesting that family-centred practice will have different ways of being "packaged" depending on the service setting and nature of the care. For example, even in critical and emergency health care, it is important to develop treatment approaches that are consistent with the family-centred model. Baren

(2001) identifies the importance of family-centred care in emergency medicine, and Henneman and Cardin (2002) describe how the model can be better applied and advanced in this highly technical and intense treatment environment. Van Riper (2001) has carefully studied family-professional relationships in neonatal intensive care units that assist parents and their newborn children with serious medical challenges. Her study shows that positive family-centred relationships lead to higher parent satisfaction with care and higher levels of parent psychological well-being in these hospital environments that are highly stressful for both parents and health care professionals.

There will be a number of factors that influence the professional-family partnership in family-centred services, particularly in terms of the sharing of responsibility for decision-making. The adaptive practice model (Feldman, Ploof, & Cohen, 1999) suggests that compassionate and effective practice by paediatricians can involve a range of approaches from practitioner as expert to service recipient as determiner of strategy of care. This model views family-centred practice as bringing a flexible approach to the control of service planning and delivery that depends on the service situation and on the family. As we have noted, the family will need professional leadership in the provision of care such as when sophisticated technology or complex interventions are required. There also will be variability in service recipients' "knowledge, experience, motivation, psychological state, culture and style" (Feldman et al., 1999, p. 112). These family variables will not be static and may change and evolve over the course of service delivery. Essentially, the professional must be sensitive to these issues and be capable of inviting whatever level of leadership the family is willing and able to exercise.

There are types of special knowledge that parents will expect professionals to routinely bring when planning for the care of their child. This includes knowledge of existing services that may be activated to help their child and family, knowledge of which services can be the most helpful in achieving specific service goals, and knowledge about families like their own with children with the same type of service needs. Parents of children with special needs are typically information hungry. They expect professionals to help them understand their options and to assist them in locating and acquiring the resources their child and family requires. At times, a parent may want the professional to take the lead in selecting and securing needed service resources. At other times, the same parent may want to be well informed by the professional, but left to decide on the timing and sequencing of the services that will be sought for their child and their family.

It is also important to acknowledge that some professional disciplines, working in some service settings, will take on a more active role in the provision of family-centred practice than will other disciplines. Much will depend on the expertise and availability of each discipline for family practice. Some professionals fear that if they become too deeply involved in the emotions and needs of families, it will overwhelm them and restrict their availability to work with children. There is some truth underlying this fear. For example, in many locales there is a marked shortage of paediatricians and speech therapists, and it would not make sense to have these specialists using large blocks of their time coordinating community support resources for individual children with complex health care needs. Necessary case coordination tasks can be best done by an empowered and well-supported parent, or by a social worker or community nurse who has the mandate and skills to function as a service coordinator for a number of families who are high service users. In such a situation, it would be important for a paediatrician or speech therapist directly involved with the family to be well acquainted with family-centred practice principles, such that she or he could maintain a practice that was consistent with the model and, at the same time, support case coordination duties that are conducted by other members of the health care team or community care system.

Trute, Adkins, and MacDonald (1994) describe an integrated intersectoral application of family-centred practice in child sexual abuse services. In these special children's services that deal with extreme family circumstances, it is important to delineate distinct professional roles that are activated across all the components of service delivery (child welfare, health, mental health, criminal justice). It is not possible for social workers and police responsible for abuse investigation and child protection to immediately engage in a collaborative partnership with family members who may be found responsible or complicit in a sexual assault of a child. However, other interdisciplinary team members may immediately, at the time of the disclosure of abuse, build a family-centred relationship with non-offending parents and siblings of the victim to ensure their positive coping with the disclosure of sexual abuse, a disclosure that can create a crisis for all family members. Trute and his associates describe early intervention services that are based on a model of family-centred practice that helps non-offending parents resolve their pressing family challenges and dilemmas, helps them be a resource to the other children in the family, and helps prevent the family from quickly closing ranks like an "emotional fortress" in its own defence (and thereby blocking future counselling or mental health services while the lawyers and courts dominate the situation).

The lesson here is that family-centred practice may translate as the functioning of a professional team or a network of services rather than be the purview of only the individual practitioner or one service delivery system. In such circumstances, different professionals representing different disciplines may play different roles in the execution of a service plan. Some professionals may feel that their "real work" is with the child. This may be true for some professional disciplines practicing in some service contexts. However, they still should have a basic understanding of family-centred practice principles so that they can understand, respect, and support other professionals who work in concert with them to provide care that extends beyond the child to include her or his family and community.

Partnership in Practice

Family-centred practice is a two-sided coin in that it requires not only knowledge and expertise in professionals, but also requires the involvement of informed and activated youth and parents. It is important that families understand their rights and responsibilities under the scope of this model. It is important that parents can take on as active a service planning and delivery partnership as they want and that makes sense to them in the specific service situation in which they and their children are involved. As we noted earlier in this chapter, at times parents may want a direct voice in the planning of services for their children, at times they may not be available to make such decisions, and at times they may wish to turn to professionals to temporarily take over for them as the best decision-makers in providing needed care for their children.

There are no simple steps or basic recipes for the delivery of family-centred services. Much depends on service context, professional capability, family capacity, administrative support, and availability of formal and informal community support resources for children and families. In order to participate in family-centred practice, parents need to know what "normal expectations" they should hold about the services they receive and, as well, what responsibilities are theirs as partners in the positive application of this model of service delivery. In this

regard, parent education is just as important as professional education for the advancement of family-centred practice so that parents can
make informed decisions and can participate to the extent that they
chose and feel capable. Family-centred practice does not simply mean
downloading of responsibilities for care for a child onto the family. It
does not mean reducing the state's support (e.g., provincial government) for children with special needs and their family members. It fundamentally means greater participation of parents in the assessment
of service need, and in decision-making for the care of their children,
within an adequately resourced service system.

Family-Centred Practice and the Involuntary Client

Families that seek health or social services usually recognize that they
cannot provide the care that is required by their children with a disability or special needs and know that they need information, support
resources, or skilled assistance. Those that become involved in manda-
tory services, such as child welfare or juvenile corrections, sometimes
do not recognize the limitations in their capabilities to raise their children, may resent when services are required that they do not want,
and may be fearful of losing their children through court directed apprehension and out-of-home placement (McCroskey & Meezan, 1998).

   Many of the families coming to the attention of a social service agency,
particularly families living in poverty, may have had negative service
experiences in the past and will not trust or have faith that professionals can make life better for them and their children. In a sense, the problem in these situations is not necessarily the immediate needs of the
child and family, but the service history that the family has endured
and carries with it. That is, for many involuntary or distrusting families
the primary service issue may not be the presenting problem or need
of the child, but may be all the attempted solutions that have failed in
the past when professionals have engaged with the family (Watzlawick,
Weakland, & Fisch, 1974).

   Working in a setting in which families are involuntary or distrusting does not mean that family-centred practice will be inappropriate
or ineffective. It does mean that special attention must be given to the
development of a working alliance between the family and the professional before any further interventions can be initiated. Studies of
family preservation programs in child welfare have suggested that
the working alliance between the parent and social worker is more

important to service outcome than is length or intensity of services or worker caseload (Jones, Neuman, & Shyne, 1976; McCroskey & Meezan, 1997). Needless to say, however, if you do not have a consistent person working with the family, who has ongoing contact with the family in a timely manner, then there will be family dissatisfaction and an inadequate working alliance (Chapman, Gibbons, Barth, McCrae, & NSCAW Research Group, 2003).

Just because there has been an allegation or disclosure of child abuse or neglect in a family does not mean that the family cannot be immediately, or over time, assisted by workers practicing from a family-centred model. As an extreme example, consider the child welfare response to incest. Much depends on the circumstances of the "child in family in community." Maddock and Larson (1995) have identified a number of "incest ecologies" with differing circumstances in regard to child vulnerability, perpetrator motivation, family culture, and parenting resources. The family typologies that they present assist in the assessment and planning of interventions to stop the assaults on the child and strengthen the family as a place of safety and developmental well-being for the child victim. Whenever child safety is reasonably assured, and an adequate working alliance can be maintained with family members, the door is open to family-centred practice.

Common Misconceptions of Family-Centred Practice

Understanding what "family-centred" means and its implications for practice. We suggested earlier in this chapter that the term "family-centred practice" has meant many different things to many different groups of professionals. Many university faculty in nursing believe that their profession has been doing family-centred practice for decades, even though family-centred practice often moves well beyond what has been incorporated into existing programs of training in family nursing. Many paediatricians believe that they are family-centred in their practice, even if this simply translates in their mind to the fact that they talk with parents when treating a child. Similarly, many social workers confuse family-centred practice with family therapy, even though the two can be significantly different in how the professional relates to families and the extent to which the service partnership theme is employed in practice. There is a marked difference between "facilitative family counselling" and "family therapy" (this difference is considered more fully in Chapter 3 of this book). Often, the profound nature of the shift in practice patterns is not appreciated by front-line social workers. It is not understood that family-centred practice requires a major change in service culture from professional as expert to professional as partner. As Epps and Jackson (2000, p. 88) note, family-centred practice involves a change in the culture of service delivery that moves from "paternalism to enablement" and from "judgmental to supportive stances."

The professional practice that has historically been most closely consistent with the family-centred practice model, which first began breaking new ground identifying "the person with family" as client and developing methods in empowerment practice, is social work (Allen & Petr, 1996; Bula Wise, 2005). Social casework has traditionally identified "capacity building" as a fundamental aspect of problem solving with clients (Hepworth, Rooney, Dewberry Rooney, Strom-Gottfried, & Larsen, 2006). Family-centred social work has been more extensively advanced through the central place of systems theory in the practice model, and the employment of ecological thinking in professional training (Hartman & Laird, 1983). The development of strengths-based social work methods (Saleebey, 1997) runs in close concert with family-centred practice principles. However, child welfare agencies, along with child health, child mental health, and child development services, still do not have the model well entrenched in their daily practices. Research that we have conducted in the provinces of Manitoba and Alberta in Canada suggests that, for the most part, working alliances are well achieved in child disability services, in that clients show high satisfaction with the working relationships that they have with the professionals who are assisting them. However, it was found that challenges presently remain in (a) activating self-agency or empowerment experiences in service delivery, (b) identifying and mobilizing client strengths in the resolution of needs and concerns of children and their family members, and (c) securing adequate administrative understanding of family-centred practice so that administrators act in concert with staff delivering services.

Our experience has taught us that professionals working in children's services are, for the most part, capable of creating positive working alliances. Where they stumble is when they move to the intervention phases of family-centred practice, which involve creating and maintaining functional service partnerships with parents and other key family members, activating intervention strategies that are based on capacity building in clients, and coordinating family-centred service delivery with other professionals and allied agencies.

The importance of capacity building and enhancing social support. There is a widespread misconception that family-centred practice involves the use of traditional practice methods in new ways, namely, that family-centred practice simply gives greater emphasis to what has traditionally been considered "interpersonal communications skills" and "family treatment." This underplays the increased importance of "capacity building" and "social resource mobilization" practice elements that are inherent in this model of practice. Many professionals have not had adequate training in these practice elements and, further, have had little background preparation (through training and supervision) in family assessment and family interviewing. This misconception leaves the definition and delivery of family-centred practice to intuition rather than actual knowledge and skill and results in professionals being highly vulnerable to misunderstanding family-centred practice. Furthermore, it results in practice being implemented at a low level of "integrity of treatment" or fidelity with the foundational principles of family-centred practice.

Ignoring the community in family-centred practice. Another misconception is that the model means just putting more emphasis on the family when treating children and youth, and not appreciating community implications or higher-level political concerns. This misconception involves identification of the "child with the immediate family" as the sole focus of care. This view does not appreciate the conceptual importance of ecological theory (Bronfenbrenner, 1979) to family-centred practice, which identifies a range of social systems or "ecological niches" within which the child is nested, all of which can directly or indirectly influence child development and well-being. In the family-centred practice literature, priority attention is given to the importance of social support resources in child, parent, and family well-being, be it from informal networks of support (extended family, friends, parent self-help groups, etc.) or formal networks of support (hospital staff, community care staff, clergy, etc.). However, family-centred practice does acknowledge that the most salient source of social support for the child most often is the family. The "child with family" therefore is the place to start as a beginning focus of services. This not disqualify or diminish the important work that must be done to address key community support issues (such as fragmentation of support provided by community agencies, or inadequate psychosocial family support resources) that in their own right can profoundly affect the well-being of a child and his/her family.

Ignoring the child in family-centred practice. Another key misconception is that family-centred practice ignores the centrality of the child in children's services and gives first priority to the family. The well-being of the child is a first priority in family-centred children's services, and that is why careful attention is given to the family in which that child lives and grows. It is taken as a given that you cannot help a child without helping a family. Part of the confusion about allegedly ignoring the child in the service of the family may be based in part in the many alternative interpretations of what constitutes "the family." Family-centred practice does not always mean that all members of a family-of-origin (e.g., biological mothers and fathers) or of an extended family (e.g., grandparents, aunts) are included in the process of care. The determination of what constitutes "family" in services for a child can vary dramatically depending on the service issues being addressed, the age and emotional needs of the child or youth, and the membership and resources available in the family. In many families entering children's health services, the mother may serve as the formal representative of the family, with other family members seeing her as the conduit of information and acting as the family spokesperson. This child-mother configuration may be the focus of care in many instances of family-centred services if that seems the most logical to the professionals and most appropriate to the family. In some situations, the child's "family" in service provision may be a mother-grandmother team that works together to care for a child with special needs. Flexibility needs to be exercised in terms of what constitutes the definition of family in family-centred practice. Further, what constitutes "family" during the course of services may change as the service responds to the priority needs that emerge and evolve over time.

There will be occasions in children's services when preliminary attention must be focused on the child, with family involvement considered with caution in the early stages of service delivery. Family violence can create such a service situation. In this case, the safety of the child must be paramount, and the family or members of the family may need to be excluded from the direct service being offered to the child. In these situations, the other family members will optimally be assisted by other professionals working in coordination with the care that the child receives. Earlier we described family-centred services in situations of child sexual abuse, in which child welfare and child mental health professionals work in concert to protect victims, yet at the same time keep families from "closing down as emotional fortresses" as legal charges and judicial proceedings are activated. Attention is given to empowering non-offending parents and assisting them to deal with their own anger, confusion, and emotional crises, to deal with the impact of the disclosure of sexual abuse on the victim and victim's siblings, and to plan next steps in the life of the family. In some family situations with youth, great care needs to be exercised so that the youth has a voice in decisions involving the extent to which her or his family members will be involved in the services the youth receives. This may take on even greater salience in situations such as family violence (e.g., sibling incest) or in issues of sexual health (e.g., teen pregnancy). In these circumstances, the issue is not if the family will be involved, but how and when to include family members in ongoing assessments, treatment planning, and service delivery.

Family-Centred Practice: A Review of Essential Components

In this chapter a number of elements that can influence family-centred practice have been identified. Figure 2.1 summarizes the most basic of these to assist in the conceptual understanding of this model of service delivery in children's health and disability services.

The outside box on this schematic, entitled "Structural Issues in Community and Cultural Context of Care," represents the social and administrative context that frames family-centred practice. When working from a family-centred perspective, attention is given to the broad social context in which families are situated and the ways in which forces in this larger context impact their lives. An awareness of how structural factors (such as class, race, attitudes towards disability, gender, etc.) influence the experiences of families is critical to understanding their experiences, their definition of need, and their willingness/ability to engage in partnership with professionals. In addition, the context includes two major elements that define or regulate service delivery and thereby influence the terms and limits of practice. The first is the service setting (i.e., agency, program, or department) which directs the scope of practice through administrative terms of reference, the allocation of budgetary resources, and enforcement of service policy. Support resources (e.g., financial aid, respite assistance, staff time) that are available to children and families are directly related to this element. It is not possible to deliver family-centred practice with integrity (that is, closely adhering to its fundamental practice elements and processes) when carrying a large caseload and only having infrequent contact

Figure 2.1. Family-Centred Practice in Childhood Health and Disability Services

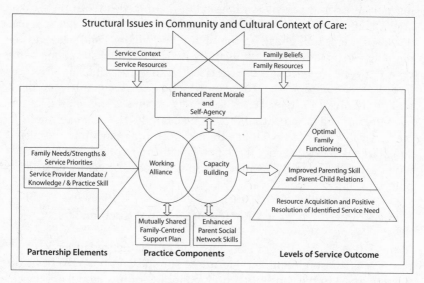

with children and family members. (The administrative context is considered in Chapters 13 and 14.) The second situational context that is of major importance has to do with family beliefs and childcare resources within the family. Some families have an aversion to the intrusion of governmental staff or hospital outreach programs into the life of the family, or are confused about their rights in regard to these services (e.g., recent immigrants from oppressive governmental regimes, families with negative past experiences with social services). Some families may hold beliefs that it is a sign of great personal and family weakness to rely on help from "outsiders" (e.g., self-reliant farm families, highly religious families that believe they should rely primarily on the support of their church or mosque). (These issues related to family beliefs and culture are considered in Chapter 12.) Given stereotypes about the roles of women and men in families, it is not surprising that many service providers are more comfortable when dealing with mothers than with fathers. Many families send mothers to be the liaison between the family and the service system. It may be helpful to families to challenge gender stereotypes and engage fathers in family-centred service planning and implementation of support plans. (This issue is reviewed in Chapter 11.)

In our teaching and research related to family-centred practice, we have found it helpful to employ a more parsimonious and narrow definition of the "relational" component of practice, operationally defining it as "working alliance." Similarly, we have focused the "participatory" component of practice on "capacity building." (More detailed attention to working alliance is provided in Chapter 4 and to capacity building in Chapter 6.)

In this text we consider the basic "partnership elements" of family-centred practice to be closely tied to working alliance, that is, the quality of the collaborative relationship that is built and maintained between family members and the professionals involved in the life of a child with special needs. To achieve an adequate and lasting working alliance, we suggest that service providers must start their work with the family by focusing on family-determined or endorsed service priorities. Further, we assert that the quality of the working alliance will depend in part on (a) the service providers' skill in securing a strong alliance in their work; (b) the mandate service providers carry into the life of the family as a counsellor, therapist, or service coordinator; and (c) the scope of information that service providers can offer that is of importance to family members (e.g., information related to presently available community services, services that their child may need in the future, information related to the challenges for which their child has been diagnosed or formally assessed).

The achievement of a positive working alliance opens the way to the creation of a Family-Centred Support Plan. To facilitate the collaborative planning process that is required in the drafting of a child and family support plan, it is necessary to gather information that is of relevance to the service situation. This will often encompass immediate and necessary information at the level of the child, parent, family, and community. (Assessment theory and procedures are detailed in Chapter 5, and steps in constructing a family support plan are outlined in Chapter 9.)

An important aspect in creating and executing the family support plan is the provision of "capacity building" as a paramount aspect of the plan and the steps taken to achieve this plan. Within the process of capacity building in parents and families, we identify two commonly occurring goals: the first is related to cognitive coping resources of enhanced parenting morale and self-agency, and the second is related to enhancing skill in accessing and using social network support. (The knowledge and skills required in this important aspect of family-centred practice is explicated in Chapter 6. Further, skills required for social network building, mobilization, and utilization are outlined in Chapter 7.)

It is important to note that these components of family-centred practice are not rigidly sequential, nor are they mutually exclusive. Working alliance is an ongoing aspect of the collaborative efforts that fuel and maintain a continuous process of child and family assessment, adjustments to the family support plan, differing targets and intensity of capacity building in family members, and the setting and achieving of goals to advance the well-being of the child and the resiliency of the family. Further, the partnership approach to practice requires knowledgeable and skilful parents as well as professionals, so both can share understandings of how services should be delivered and both appreciate their role in the helping process. (This partnership issue is more fully addressed in Chapter 8.)

In Figure 2.1 we identify a hierarchy of service goals that can be addressed in family-centred practice in children's services. The most common cluster of service goals has to do with resource acquisition and positive resolution of identified service need. These are usually the straightforward, specific, and concrete needs that are identified to facilitate positive family support for a child with special needs. This is what has been traditionally identified as "practical help," direct "problem solving," or "facilitative counselling." A smaller number of service plans will be more complex and involve activities that lead to improved parenting skill and parent-child relations. These will bring service outcomes into the realm of psycho-education and therapy. An ultimate service achievement of family-centred practice is "optimal family functioning." This is characterized by parents and their children responding to life challenges with self-agency and enduring resiliency that is consistent with their personal capabilities and coping resources. The level of service impact or service achievement will depend on baseline risk (i.e., pre-service level of functioning), as stronger intervention effects will generally be found with children and families at higher risk at baseline (Kuhlthau et al., 2011).

Several recent outcome reviews (Dempsey & Keen, 2008) and meta-analyses (Dunst, Trivette, & Hamby, 2007; Kuhlthau et al., 2011) of family-centred practice in children's services have highlighted outcomes that are most congruent and consistent with this model of practice.

In overview, these studies suggest that family-centred practice is directly and positively related to service outcomes such as higher satisfaction with services, access to care, and communication; parent outcomes such as locus of control (or self-agency) and self-efficacy; and family outcomes such as family impact/cost and family functioning. Family-centred practice appears to be indirectly related (as a mediating variable) to parenting outcomes (such as parenting stress, parenting capabilities, and judgments of their child's behaviour). Similarly, child development achievements appear to be mediated through positive changes in parent beliefs and childcare practices. Although most studies reviewed measured only several variables, and some had mixed degrees of association, only a few showed insignificant or negative findings. The positive outcomes of family-centred practice appear to be valid across many cultural backgrounds and demographic differences.

There is growing research evidence that unless family-centred practice is delivered with high integrity, or close consistency with the model, the positive service outcomes are reduced (Walton et al., 2001; Washington State Institute for Public Policy, 2006). The chapters that follow in this book are intended to help service providers better understand the principles and knowledge required for competent practice that is in close fidelity with the family-centred model.

REFERENCES

Allen, R.I., & Petr, C.G. (1996). Toward developing standards and measurements for family-centered practice in family support programs. In G. Singer, L. Powers, & A. Olson (Eds.), *Family support policy and America's caregiving families: Innovations in public-private partnerships* (pp. 57–86). Baltimore, MD: Brookes.

Baren, J.M. (2001, December). Rising to the challenge of family-centered care in emergency medicine. *Academic Emergency Medicine, 8*(12), 1182–5. http://dx.doi.org/10.1111/j.1553-2712.2001.tb01138.x Medline:11733299

Beckman, P.J. (Ed.). (1996). *Strategies for working with families of young children with disabilities.* Baltimore, MD: Brookes.

Beckman, P.J., Newcomb, S., Frank, N., & Brown, L. (1996). Evolution of working relationships with families. In P.J. Beckman (Ed.), *Strategies for working with families of young children with disabilities* (pp. 17–30). Baltimore, MD: Brookes.

Bronfenbrenner, U. (1979). *The ecology of human development: Experiments by nature and design.* Cambridge, MA: Harvard University Press.

Bula Wise, J. (2005). *Empowerment practice with families in distress.* New York, NY: Columbia University Press.

Chapman, M.V., Gibbons, C.B., Barth, R.P., McCrae, J.S., & NSCAW Research Group. (2003, September-October). Parental views of in-home services: What predicts satisfaction with child welfare workers? *Child Welfare, 82*(5), 571–96. Medline:14524426

Cole, E.S. (1995). Becoming family centered: Child welfare's challenge. *Families in Society, 76,* 163–72.

Dempsey, I., & Keen, D. (2008). A review of processes and outcomes in family-centered services for children with a disability. *Topics in Early Childhood Special Education, 28*(1), 42–52. http://dx.doi.org/10.1177/0271121408316699

Dunst, C.J., & Trivette, C.M. (1996, July-August). Empowerment, effective helpgiving practices and family-centered care. *Pediatric Nursing, 22*(4), 334–7, 343. Medline:8852113

Dunst, C.J., Trivette, C.M., & Deal, A.G. (1988). *Enabling and empowering families: Principles & guidelines for practice.* Cambridge, MA: Brookline Books.

Dunst, C.J., Trivette, C.M., & Deal, A.G. (Eds.). (1994). *Supporting and strengthening families.* Cambridge, MA: Brookline Books.

Dunst, C.J., Trivette, C.M., & Hamby, D.W. (2007). Meta-analysis of family-centered helpgiving practices research. *Mental Retardation and Developmental Disabilities Research Reviews, 13*(4), 370–8. http://dx.doi.org/10.1002/mrdd.20176 Medline:17979208

Epps, S., & Jackson, B.J. (Eds.). (2000). *Empowered families, successful children: Early intervention programs that work.* Washington, DC: American Psychological Association. http://dx.doi.org/10.1037/10354-000

Feldman, H.M., Ploof, D., & Cohen, W.I. (1999, April). Physician-family partnerships: The adaptive practice model. *Journal of Developmental & Behavioral Pediatrics, 20*(2), 111–16. http://dx.doi.org/10.1097/00004703-199904000-00007 Medline:10219690

Fina, D.K., Lopas, L.J., Stagnone, J.H., & Santucci, P.R. (1997, June). Parent participation in the postanesthesia care unit: Fourteen years of progress at one hospital. *Journal of Perianesthesia Nursing, 12*(3), 152–62. http://dx.doi.org/10.1016/S1089-9472(97)80033-0 Medline:9214939

Hanson, M.J., & Lynch, E.W. (2004). *Understanding families: Approaches to diversity, disability, and risk.* Baltimore, MD: Brookes.

Hartman, A., & Laird, J. (1983). *Family-centered social work practice.* New York, NY: Free Press.

Henneman, E.A., & Cardin, S. (2002, December). Family-centered critical care: A practical approach to making it happen. *Critical Care Nurse, 22*(6), 12–19. Medline:12518563

Hepworth, D.H., Rooney, R.H., Dewberry Rooney, G., Strom-Gottfried, K., & Larsen, J. (2006). *Direct social work practice: Theory and skills* (7th ed.). Toronto, ON: Thomson Nelson.

Jones, M.A., Neuman, R., & Shyne, A. (1976). *A second chance for families: Evaluation of a program to reduce foster care*. New York, NY: Child Welfare League of America.

King, S., Teplicky, R., King, G., & Rosenbaum, P. (2004, March). Family-centered service for children with cerebral palsy and their families: A review of the literature. *Seminars in Pediatric Neurology, 11*(1), 78–86. http://dx.doi. org/10.1016/j.spen.2004.01.009 Medline:15132256

Kuhlthau, K.A., Bloom, S., Van Cleave, J., Knapp, A.A., Romm, D., Klatka, K., …, & Perrin, J.M. (2011, March-April). Evidence for family-centered care for children with special health care needs: A systematic review. *Academic Pediatrics, 11*(2), 136–43.e8. http://dx.doi.org/10.1016/j.acap.2010.12.014 Medline:21396616

Maddock, J.W., & Larson, N.R. (1995). *Incestuous families: An ecological approach to understanding and treatment*. New York, NY: W.W. Norton.

McCroskey, J., & Meezan, W. (1997). *Family preservation and family functioning*. Washington, DC: Child Welfare League of America.

McCroskey, J., & Meezan, W. (1998). Family-centred services: Approaches and effectiveness. *Protecting Children from Abuse & Neglect, 8*, 54–71.

Nelso, K.E., & Landsman, M.J. (1990). Three models of family-centered placement prevention services. *Child Welfare, 69*, 3–21.

Pletcher, L.C. (1995). *Family-centered practices: A training guide*. Chapel Hill, NC: ARCH National Resource Center.

Rosenbaum, P. (2005). Keynote speaker at the Family Supports for Children with Disabilities Research Symposium, Alberta Centre for Child, Family & Community Research, Edmonton, AB.

Rosenbaum, P., King, S., Law, M., King, G., & Evans, J. (1998). Family-centered service: A conceptual framework and research review. *Physical & Occupational Therapy in Pediatrics, 18*, 1–20. http://dx.doi.org/10.1080/ J006v18n01_01

Saleebey, D. (Ed.). (1997). *The strengths perspective in social work practice* (2nd ed.). White Plains, NY: Longman.

Shelton, T.L., Jeppson, E.S., & Johnson, B.H. (1987). *Family-centered care for children with special healthcare needs*. Bethesda, MD: Association for the Care of Children's Health.

Smykowski, L., & Rodriguez, W. (2003, January-March). The post anesthesia care unit experience: A family-centered approach. *Journal of Nursing Care Quality, 18*(1), 5–15. http://dx.doi.org/10.1097/00001786-200301000-00002 Medline:12518833

Trute, B. (2007). Service coordination in family-centered childhood disability services: Quality assessment from the family perspective. *Families in Society, 88,* 283–91.

Trute, B., Adkins, E., & MacDonald, G. (1994). *Coordinating child sexual abuse services in rural communities.* Toronto, ON: University of Toronto Press.

Trute, B., & Hiebert-Murphy, D. (2007). The implications of "working alliance" for the measurement and evaluation of family-centered practice in childhood disability services. *Infants and Young Children, 20*(2), 109–19. http://dx.doi.org/10.1097/01.IYC.0000264479.50817.4b

Van Riper, M. (2001, January-February). Family-provider relationships and well-being in families with preterm infants in the NICU. *Heart & Lung: The Journal of Critical Care, 30*(1), 74–84. http://dx.doi.org/10.1067/mhl.2001.110625 Medline:11174370

Walton, E., Sandau-Beckler, P., & Mannes, M. (Eds.). (2001). *Balancing family-centered services and child well-being.* New York, NY: Columbia University Press.

Washington State Institute for Public Policy. (2006). Intensive family preservation programs: Program fidelity influences effectiveness. Retrieved from http://www.wsipp.wa.gov

Watzlawick, P., Weakland, J., & Fisch, R. (1974). *Change: Principles of problem formulation and problem resolution.* New York, NY: W.W. Norton.

Weston, W.W. (2005). Patient-centered medicine: A guide to the biopsychosocial model. *Families, Systems & Health, 23*(4), 387–92. http://dx.doi.org/10.1037/1091-7527.23.4.387

PART TWO

Practice Fundamentals

3 Family-Centred Counselling, Family Therapy, and Service Coordination

BARRY TRUTE

Introduction

It is not uncommon for human service professionals to confuse service delivery duties and competencies when the differences between family-centred counselling, family therapy, and family service coordination are considered. Although there can be overlap between these three spheres of service delivery, each of these distinct practice domains has its own cluster of intervention goals and level of required practice skill. In some basic ways these three practice domains overlap, and in some important ways they differ. The intent of this chapter is to define and describe these three practice domains, all of which can fall under the aegis of family-centred children's services.

In family-centred practice, family-centred counselling usually begins in early engagement with families with an anticipation of family "normality" and proceeds with this assumption until adequate exposure and experience with family members proves otherwise. Family therapy, which may be activated as part of an individualized family support plan, engages with families with the expectation that a family may be "stuck" in its response to a life challenge or crisis, and in some ways brings intervention concerns that involve the necessity of family reorganization or the amelioration of serious relationship concerns or psychosocial need in family members.

Service coordination has its roots in traditional "case management" practice. It is seen as a fundamental aspect of family-centred children's services, particularly for those families with children with serious or chronic developmental challenges or health issues who receive care from multiple service providers. Family-centred service coordination focuses on family-identified needs and priorities, and the securing of resources to meet these needs and priorities. The service coordination function can be conducted by family members or by professionals depending on the complexities of the service network involved in the life of the family and on the wishes and capabilities of the members of the family. In many locales, "dedicated" service coordinators (or "key workers" or "primary case managers") provide ongoing and long-term counselling along with support for the service coordination function as it arises (whether conducted by the parent or the professional herself/himself). A skilled service coordinator will understand how her/his involvement with a family needs to adhere to family-centred practice principles while s/he works with a family and the many individuals, agencies, and organizations that play a role in the support of a child with special needs and her/his family.

Of the three practice domains (counselling, therapy, and coordination), family therapy is the most specialized and, in children's services, is often time-limited. When provided in concert with family-centred principles, family therapy will be strengths-based, competency building, and solution focused. Human service professionals who are family-centred (be they in front-line practice in child development, child health, child welfare, or child mental health) will understand the key components of family-centred service delivery (such as working alliance, empowerment practice, family capacity building, etc.) and will be competent in the execution of these elements. Some will also be capable family service coordinators, but few will have the specialized knowledge and intervention skill that family therapy requires. As a bottom line, family-centred practice requires an understanding of when and how a practitioner in children's services (and their family partners) can adequately meet a family's service needs on their own, and when a referral should be made for the involvement of "child with family" treatment specialists.

Basic differences can be identified between family-centred counselling, family therapy, and service coordination, as they start at a different point in terms of basic working assumptions, addressing a different type of client need or service goal, and requiring a different level of interventionist skill.

Counselling in Family-Centred Services

Laborde and Seligman (1991) suggest that the counselling process can include three main functions: educative counselling, facilitative counselling, and personal advocacy counselling.

Educative counselling. Educative counselling is an important element of information provision. It often is the first step in family-centred practice. That is, open and full provision of information is often a fundamental step in the development of a positive working alliance between family members and the professional. Although educative counselling is usually considered as the professional offering family members useful information, there often is a reciprocal element to information provision. That is, the family will educate the professional about its special circumstances, be these important child nuances, cultural values, or special family circumstances. This reciprocal information flow serves to strengthen the family-professional partnership. In most situations, parents will appreciate new and needed information that the professional can provide. This may include information about child development or health conditions, basic guidance in regard to child behaviour management, or the local availability and routine steps in accessing services and resources. The counsellor may act as a guide to help family members find sources of information, be it formally or informally distributed by community agencies and organizations. For many parents, having a child with a disability or developmental challenge represents a circumstance of novelty or one of "not knowing" as they will have had little life experience to prepare them for the special needs of their child. Educative counselling serves to strengthen their understanding and advance their knowledge to bolster their parenting skill, confidence, and coping, and to reduce parenting confusion, insecurity, and stress.

Facilitative counselling. Facilitative counselling moves beyond information provision to address emotions and beliefs. At its core is the provision of emotional support and enabling interventions. We do know that it is not unusual for parents of children with special needs to experience both positive and negative reactions to being a mother or father of a child who is not "normal" and who does not conform to their idealized beliefs about the son or daughter they hoped to have. Many will question through the early months and years of their child with special needs whether they can handle the stress that child disability can bring to family life, and whether they can be the mother or father they want to be. For some, there may be guilt associated with self-blame for their child's disability or for letting down or disappointing their spouse or the child's grandparents. Facilitative counselling involves the provision of empathy, understanding, and support to gently explore parents' negative beliefs and feelings such as sadness and remorse, while opening the emotional acceptance of the positive aspects of a parent's love of her/his child, the unique personhood of the child, and the personal strengths they have for parenting. In family-centred practice, central attention is given in facilitative counselling to enhancing parents' sense of mastery in their role of mother or father, to strengthening parents' psychological and social support resources in advancing their own and their family's coping, and to improving their capacity as parents to provide support, guidance, and nurturing to their children. It involves providing emotional support to parents while motivating and coaching. Facilitative counselling does not mean taking action on behalf of clients but encouraging clients to take actions for themselves. In some special situations, such as times of parent crisis, the counsellor will need to be proactive and intervene directly to meet a pressing need or solve a problem. However, the central intent of facilitative counselling is to empower and maximize client directed actions for themselves and their family members. Facilitative counselling may be provided by human service professionals, or by other parents in similar family circumstances, or by spiritual advisors and guides.

Facilitative counselling may include the following practice objectives:

- Stress reduction: The goal of this effort is to bring child, family, and community stressors, and responses to these stressors, to open awareness and to expand the repertoire of emotional and situational resources that can be mobilized to enhance coping with the stressors.
- Time management coaching: It is not unusual for parents of children with serious health or developmental needs to have many service providers in their life. These situations call for careful coordination of appointments and meetings that often require skilled time management on the part of parents. Many parents can feel that their childcare duty has close similarities to an air traffic controller, who coordinates aircraft takeoffs and landings in busy airports, in terms of keeping on top of a wide range of professionals, programs, and agencies.
- Morale support: These efforts seek to strengthen or maintain a mother's or father's morale (i.e., energy, commitment, and psychological strength) to meet and positively respond to parenting challenges.
- Social involvement coaching and social support mobilization: Families with children with chronic health and developmental disabilities tend to be socially isolated. Often the time demands of caring

for a child with special needs leaves parents with little time to maintain social contacts or to take part in social events. To maintain positive parent adjustment and coping, focused attention sometimes needs to be given to a parent's social life and recreational activities outside of the family. In some instances this constitutes a preventative action to bolster or maintain positive parent coping.

- Problem solving or solution seeking collaboration: A central goal of family-centred practice in children's health and social services is to meet family identified priorities and needs in the care and well-being of children. Facilitative counselling goes beyond the activation of strategies to directly meet identified needs for child and family support resources from informal sources (e.g., family and friends) and formal providers (e.g., professionals, programs, and agencies). It also assists in the development of "internal" or psychological coping resources such as positive parenting self-esteem and morale. It is important for professionals to normalize feelings of anger and occasional sadness related to the disability or challenge that shapes the life of the child. It is important that parents are helped to understand and deal with the shame that may be imposed on them because of their child's "differentness" or with the rejection their child suffers from adults in the community, from extended family members, or from their child's schoolmates or neighbourhood friends. Occasional bouts of denial of their child's challenges can be thoughtfully, gently, and collaboratively explored with the understanding that at times denial can be hazardous to the well-being of their child, and at times a little denial can be a positive coping strategy.

Personal advocacy counselling. Laborde and Seligman (1991) identify that the primary goal of personal advocacy counselling "is to help parents to experience a sense of control over events in their own lives and their children's lives" (p. 237). Service providers have a responsibility to go beyond working directly with clients to seek to advance more efficient coordination of resources in the community network of services. Their responsibility includes acting to ensure that families are not suffering service inaccessibility because of barriers that are unjust, that are confrontational or coercive, or that reflect systemic oppression of families disadvantaged by conditions such as poverty, racism, or stigma related to social attitudes such as beliefs about single parenthood.

In our experience, it is not always the families that have the greatest need that receive their fair share of family support resources from governmental agencies or community groups. Often people who live in poverty and those with limited formal education feel uncomfortable with professionals and find their relationships with professionals to be difficult. These parents do know what they need, but not how to get it. They often do not know what services are available nor the ways to access these services. Unfortunately, scarce child and family support resources are not always allocated in ways that are equitable, fair, and according to level of need. Personal advocacy counselling aims to strengthen parents' ability to "work the systems" and to access resources they need for their children and their families.

Personal advocacy counselling can be done by self-help groups and non-governmental agencies, as well as by human service professionals. It is clear that over the past several decades major developments in services for children with special needs have come about largely through the initiative and advocacy of parents. Empowerment of parents does not just include personal or psychological empowerment (as is addressed in facilitative counselling), but more broadly includes empowerment in advancing a stronger parent voice in the local availability of community resources, and in the enhancement of societal understanding and governmental response to children with special needs. Advocacy counselling assists parents to better understand how they may more strategically gain access to programs and support resources for their children, families, and themselves. When such services are limited or non-existent in their home communities, advocacy counselling in family-centred practice can encourage and support political entrepreneurship on the part of parents to work collectively to advance the quality of children's services for themselves and for families that face similar challenges to their own.

Family-Centred Counselling and Family Therapy: Different Service Contracts

There is a different service contract in family-centred counselling than in family therapy. In family-centred counselling, clients fundamentally see service as a help in obtaining needed information and resources, which are of high priority to them. The family turns to the family-centred service provider for assistance in resource acquisition and, in complex multi-service situations, for assistance with service coordination. Often, service providers need to be active on behalf of the family, while modelling alternative tactics to locate, secure, and utilize needed community and social resources. The intent is to assist family members to build their competency so that, when they are ready and willing, they can then turn to their natural social support networks and be their own service coordinators and service advocates.

The family therapist needs a higher level of service mandate or "client permission." That is, the family therapist provides more than collaborative problem solving and facilitative counselling and must obtain client permission to enter the emotional life of the family. This requires a more profound level of family trust and worker skill.

Parenting stress levels in families with children with special needs are significantly higher than in other families with children who do not have serious health or developmental challenges. Further, it seems that as children with special needs grow older, levels of parenting stress increase. However, even though the parenting stress in families with children with serious developmental or health challenges can be significant, and tends to increase over time, this does not mean that the parents or families will become "pathological" and show conditions that are clinically significant such as depression or anxiety. It does not mean that divorce is likely, or that serious family maladjustment is an inevitable consequence. In households where parenting stress increases as children with special needs grow older, it seems that parents largely find ways to meet these challenges and cope with them. For the most part the parents directly address the parenting stressors, ably deal with them, and manage to maintain "ordinary" family life. It is a common error on the part of professionals to assume that there is a direct relationship between level of parenting stress and level of family pathology. There is not a direct and significant relationship between life stress and psychopathology in individuals or families (Aldwin, 1994; Seligman & Darling, 1997).

I have argued (in Chapter 2 of this book) that it makes more sense for professionals to assume family normality and to proceed with this assumption until their observations and experiences with the family prove otherwise. That being said, it is important to recognize that some parents and families will show behaviours that signal parent or family distress and that go beyond the reach of facilitative counselling. There is no clear demarcation that helps professionals define the different practice purview of facilitative counselling and psychotherapy. Therapy tends to be appropriate in situations involving severe emotional and behavioural challenges or disorders. It tends to be more long-term and address challenges and disorders in greater depth. Counselling tends to be more appropriate when dealing with or attempting to ameliorate situationally anchored problems or needs. When conditions are such that they appear to exceed what can be addressed by family-focused facilitative counselling, or when counselling seems to not be helpful or effective, a referral should be made to a professional with the necessary knowledge and skill in couple and family therapy. Family therapy differs from other psychotherapeutic approaches in that the focus is on working with clinical issues as problems of a family or couple rather than a person. Even if only one member of the family is seen in therapy, the treatment can be considered family therapy as long as attention is given to relationships in the family, to dynamics of family interaction, or to issues in family organization and functioning. The intent of family therapy is to not simply change individuals but, further, to ensure that individual change occurs in concert with family change.

Constantine (1986) differentiates between "enabled" and "disabled" family systems. He builds on Kantor and Lehr's (1975) definition:

An enabled family system is one in which: (1) on the average, is able to meet most of its collective or jointly defined needs and goals; (2) on the average, enables most of its members to meet most of their individual needs and individually defined goals; (3) does not consistently and systematically disable any particular member(s) from meeting individual needs and goals. (p. 26)

I have slightly altered these terms to "enabling" and "disabling" to reflect that these conditions are transitory and reflect a contextual aspect of family life rather than a static or fixed identity of a family. I see enabling families as being capable of balancing family needs as a working unit, while simultaneously operating in the best interests of all members of the family. It is what Kerr and Bowen (1988) identify as a key dynamic in all families, which involves each family member finding the right balance between meeting her/his own individual needs, while maintaining loyalty or mutuality as a member of the family. In enabling families, there is the freedom "to be your own person" while meeting your obligations to support the well-being of other family members as best you can. Enabling families show resiliency in that they are able to invent and apply methods to adjust to family stressors or challenges while adequately satisfying the sometimes competing interests of members of the family.

Disabling family systems become stuck in rigid or chaotic patterns when under stress and are prone to family conflict, relationship distress, stereotyping or devaluing of family members (e.g., scapegoating), or imposing unfair or inequitable distribution of family duties or responsibilities (e.g., a "parentified" child). Disabling families often have limited repertoires of problem solving. When their favoured approach to problem solving does not work, they tend to just do more of it or increase the intensity of their favoured solutions that are not working to resolve their difficulties. For example, if a child is behaving poorly and punishment is not changing the child's behaviour, then their tendency would be to simply increase the punishment. It is what Watzlawick, Weakland, and Fisch (1974) call the "more of the same impasse." When disabling families become highly stressed, they tend to become "stuck"; that is, they lack adaptability in their coping strategies. In some situations the family distress may have been in place before the child with special needs entered the life of the family, and the new and intense parenting stressors serve to exacerbate existing, but sometimes dormant, patterns of family distress or disorganization.

There are some patterns of family malfunctioning that are often observed when a referral is made to family therapy for families with children with developmental or cognitive disabilities or serious health challenges. My intent is not to offer a comprehensive listing of family circumstances that need family therapy, but to identify examples of situations in which family needs exceed the limits of facilitative counselling and enter the realm of family therapy.

Acceptance of initial diagnosis and implications of disability. For some parents, it may be difficult to come to terms with, or be at peace with, their child's diagnosis or assessment of disability. The meaning made of the disability by a parent has implications for the parent's expectations for the development and future of her/his child, and acceptance of treatment or service goals for the child. If there is high reactivity and long-term non-acceptance of what has been confirmed through professional assessment (and verified by observations in the home, daycare facility or school, health clinic, etc.), then more careful dialogue is required between the professional and the parent to gently explore the emotional meaning and background family context that holds inappropriate levels of denial in place. I suggested earlier in this chapter that at times a little denial can go a long way in supporting positive coping. However, unrealistic and persistent denial can block avenues of positive coping and adjustment. The directness of engagement and speed of the therapeutic discussions, relating to the use and utility of denial as a personal and family defence, can best be conducted by a skilled family therapist. In such situations it is important for parents to be able to move forward with a thoughtful understanding of their child's strengths and challenges to ensure their positive contribution to the optimal well-being of their child with special needs. For example, early intervention can be important for many children with cognitive or developmental disabilities, and it is important that parents and professionals work in partnership to heighten the probability that early intervention services can be activated as quickly as is feasible and appropriate.

Resolution of serious and persistent conjugal distress. Couple distress is often based on fundamental disagreements on important relationship issues. In situations of childhood disability, this can be based on parents' differing views about the limitations facing their child or of the positive and negative family impacts of their child's disability. Resilient couples create shared meanings of key life events that often involves respecting and weaving together each other's life narratives, dreams, and values. In the best of circumstances, a parent not only shares a common view of family life with her/his conjugal partner, but further, acts as a member of a coordinated working team with her/his partner to share childcare duties in a practical, equitable, and mutually satisfactory manner. It should be noted that at times this "parenting team" may involve a mother and grandmother, mother and aunts, or some other child-caring unit, and will not always be the traditional mother-father configuration. In households with two parents sharing the parenting duties, a serious lack of consensus between them on what constitutes the fair distribution of parenting tasks, both within and outside of the family, can be a sign of a distressed family. Resentment will increase over time and erode basic commitment and cohesion in the parenting unit, the conjugal relationship, and the well-being of the family and the children it contains.

Emotional extremes in a parent. A parent whose "emotional tank" has run out of "psychological gas," and who is suffering low parenting morale, will often show emotional volatility such as episodes of rage or clinical depression. Others will signal psychological suffering through emotional withdrawal and cutoffs from intimate relations. In couples or family units there can be reciprocity of emotions in which an entire family can be wrapped in a mantle of depression, feelings of defeat and incompetence, or anger and hostility. In these situations, parents are in high need of therapeutic intervention, and the encouragement and support of facilitative counselling will not help move them from their negativity, isolation, anger, or despair. When these situations of mal-adjustment in a parent go to the extreme, terrible things can happen to children in the family, such as abuse or child death. It is important that counsellors recognize the signals of serious emotional distress and fa-cilitate the securing of therapeutic assistance that can go "deeper" with parents and more effectively help parents cope with and adjust to their challenging life demands.

Dysfunctional family communication. Communication quality in couples is a key sign of couple stability and a predictor of divorce (Gott-man, 1994) and is a key element in the assessment of family functioning (Nichols & Schwartz, 2001). Communication serves both emotional and functional purposes in relationships. It is the central means of achiev-ing a sense of intimacy and closeness. It facilitates shared coping with the tasks and challenges of family life. Unconscious or not openly dis-closed expectations, non-discussed disagreements, emotional defen-siveness, or misguided projections or interpretations can make the achievement of seemingly simple communication tasks difficult at best and impossible at worst. Further, some family members may have a rigid and non-productive communication style that reflects a lack of basic skill in listening and exchanging information. The costs of poor communication can build over time to result in relationship confusion, frustration, disappointment, and tension. Poor communication skills in family members can usually be identified and improved through facili-tative counselling. However, when it becomes clear that it is not simply a matter of advancing communication skills in family exchanges but that deep emotions and complex personal histories are blocking open communication, this is a signal that family therapy may be needed to help family members better communicate and understand each other. If communication is not working, then the family cannot adequately function as a "task accomplishing unit," which is a fundamental pur-pose of a family.

Dysfunctional division of parent roles. Families with young chil-dren with serious disabilities are busy places. There are often compli-cated and time-consuming childcare duties to be done along with all home-care tasks. Many couples, even those that were egalitarian in the assignment of household duties before the entry of the child with a disability into family life, can be drawn to a more traditional, patriarchal pattern of parenting. That is, the mother often is drawn into being a full-time homemaker, while the father often is drawn into being the primary family wage earner. It is not uncommon in Canadian surveys of families with young children with disabilities to find that approximately 50% of mothers do not work outside of the home (and that those who do have part-time employment) while almost all fathers are employed full-time outside of the home (unemployment of fathers is rare in these families). Most single parent mothers have little choice but to remain largely as full-time homemakers. In two parent families, mothers and fathers are pulled into assuming traditional gender roles to cope with highly demanding family tasks, to clarify task responsibility, and to share duties in a way that optimizes family benefits. This can become problematic if mothers are overburdened with family responsibilities at all times, and fathers drift away from activities within the home and become marginalized in terms of their parenting responsibilities and roles. While each parent fulfils her/his duty to the family as s/he sees it, the cost to overall family well-being and to spousal well-being can seriously deteriorate in time. Parents living in these circumstances may become locked into their roles and disheartened about their options given their family situation. Facilitative counselling will not break the well-entrenched allocation of family duties, or the belief parents have that they are just doing what they need to do and have no alternative. However, without the help of a family therapist, the danger is heightened that mothers will build a growing reserve of resentment, while the fathers drift away from their emotional attachments as fathers and conjugal partners.

Disorganization in family processes. Families are fundamentally social systems that require clear but flexible boundaries (or rules) to govern and regulate individual's assumptions and behaviours (Minuchin, 1974). Distressed families are disorganized (or under-organized). There are some common patterns of family disorganization that can occur in disabling families with children with special needs. Resilient families will often speak about their child with special needs as "just one of our children" or "just part of the family." In disabling families, the child with special needs often becomes the "centre of the family." That is, family life revolves around the special needs and concerns of that child. This can play out as "boundary issues" when other children in the family feel largely ignored or as "second-class citizens" in the family. In this situation, parents have unfairly focused on one child at the cost of others in the family. Parents in these circumstances can forget that the "spousal subsystem" requires attention and nurturing in the same way as the "child subsystem." That is, by giving total attention to the child with special needs and by not attending to their needs as spousal partners (e.g., for time-outs from parenting, for recreation and fun as a couple, and to maintain important social relations with extended family and friends), they leave themselves vulnerable to fatigue and burnout. At issue is couple vitality that is based on mutual relations that are loving, stimulating, and enriching. Vitality is a core element in family resilience. When parents lose sight of the fact that they are also spousal partners, it can leave them feeling emotionally drained, alienated, and on "automatic pilot" in conjugal relations (Karpel, 1994). Facilitative counselling may adequately deal with the issue of looking out for the needs of the spousal subsystem. However, if the parents remain fervently dedicated to their child with special needs while not attending to their own personal needs, this may be an indicator that more intensive involvement of family therapy is needed to explore and resolve this circumstance. It may be the consequence of a deeper emotional issue or lack of spousal maturity and not simply one of time management as a couple. Another family "boundary concern" is the involvement of siblings in the care and parenting duties of their brother or sister with special needs. It is not uncommon for an older sibling to be recruited as a "surrogate parent" occasionally and temporarily when this is needed. There is no question that being a sibling of a brother or sister with serious developmental disabilities or chronic health concerns can enhance the personal development of that sibling. Such experiences can teach older children many valuable lessons about life and about living with intimate others. These are not pathological situations but family circumstances in which the expertise and maturity of siblings can be appreciated and celebrated. However, when a sibling becomes a major caretaker of her/his brother or sister and fulfils parenting duties on a regular basis at the cost of her/his own personal freedom and developmental needs, it is an indicator that the family and parental subsystem may be disabling. At times, sibling relations and sibling responsibilities become a contentious issue in the family, or can become a burden and exact a serious emotional cost to some of the children in the family. At these times, family therapy is indicated.

Persistent and intense grieving related to child disability. There is confusion in mental health services in regard to what constitutes normal grieving and what should be identified as pathological (Wortman & Silver, 1989). It is not clear what degree, duration, or consequences of grieving justify its identification as abnormal or requiring psychotherapy. It is evident that some parents will show minimal distress following the birth or diagnosis of a child with a serious disability, and some will show a range of reactions that range from occasional dysphoria to clinical depression. Some practitioners anticipate that all parents will inevitably have grief reactions to disability in their child and will see the absence of evidence of "chronic sorrow" (Olshansky, 1962; Wikler, Wasow, & Hatfield, 1981) as a sign of denial and masked suffering. In our experience, parental reaction to diagnosis of disability can range from persistent depression to relief (i.e., that finally what they knew to be true was confirmed, and plans were finally underway to help their child). It seems clear that parents have both times of sadness and times of joy simultaneously, in terms of their emotional adjustment to their child's health challenges or disability (Trute, Hiebert-Murphy, & Levine, 2007). Distinct and sequential stages of grief (e.g., see Kubler-Ross, 1969) are not often evident, and it is more common to have occasional episodes of grief that are linked to transitions or special times in the life of the family. Positive adaptation to the loss that childhood disability or illness represents to a parent does not equate with acceptance or resolution of the situation, but rather it "involves finding ways to put the loss in perspective and to move on with life" (Walsh & McGoldrick, 1995, p. 9). When it is evident that a parent shows signs of serious emotional reactivity to their child's challenges (such as a parent suffering persistent cognitive intrusiveness of thoughts about the disability or illness, or emotional avoidance of the stressful child or family implications of the disability or illness) or shows signs of clinical depression (such as marked disruption of regular life routines at home and at work because of a grief reaction), these are indicators that therapy is necessary.

Parents of children with developmental, cognitive, or health challenges often come to couple and family therapy when all else has failed. They usually make heroic efforts to cope with parenting challenges and turn to informal sources of support such as extended family and friends as their first option in seeking help. They are used to solving their own problems, even when the solutions only partially address their concerns or pressing needs. For some, a referral to therapy is a sign of their failure as parents or as conjugal partners. In our family therapy practice, it has not been uncommon to receive referrals that represent a "last resort" for parents of children with special needs and to the professionals who have been working with them. It is often at a point of crisis involving a pending decision to divorce or to surrender their child to child welfare authorities. This delayed access to therapy is an unfortunate situation, as earlier interventions have a greater probability of successful impact on couple and family functioning. At times, when therapy is delayed and the issues in the family become deeply entrenched and resentment and anger are deeply set in family relations, the probability of salvaging hope and mutual commitment in family members becomes a more difficult job. In these situations, the intensity and duration of therapy will depend on the family's overall level of functioning; the social support available to the family from members of the extended family, friends, and spiritual or cultural community; and the expectations and motivation of those entering therapy.

Service Coordination in Children's Services

Service coordination in childhood disability, child health, and child mental health services has a recent history in North America (Caires & Weil, 1985; Friesen & Poertner, 1995), although a wide variety of terms have been used interchangeably in this regard (e.g., care coordination, therapeutic case management, intensive case management, therapeutic case advocacy; Stroul, 1995). Case management has traditionally incorporated two broad purposes: (a) providing information, advice, and counselling; and (b) linking service recipients with needed resources and services in helping networks (Rothman, 1991). Case management appears to be the best organizational technology to assist allied human service organizations to meet the needs of consumers with complex needs and the most effective strategy for assisting and empowering consumers as they negotiate multiple service delivery systems (Moore, 1992).

Although case management is deeply anchored in a literature that goes back to the early 1900s in social work, there is a preference in contemporary child health and disability service literatures for the use of the term *service coordination* rather than *case management*. One of the incentives for this has been rejection by parents of the notion that they are cases to be managed (Illback & Neill, 1995). Duwa, Wells, and Lalinde (1993) differentiate between service coordination and case management in the manner in which success is achieved. In their view, service coordination "involves facilitating a family's decision-making process while case management helps a family pick the right plan or goal from a predetermined list" (p. 117). In Canada, the service coordinator function is similar to that of a "key worker," a role recently identified in childhood health and disability services in the United Kingdom (Dale, 1996; Greco & Sloper, 2004). In North America, the term *dedicated service coordinator* (Stepanek, Newcomb, & Kettler, 1996) refers to professionals who enter the life of the family when service files are opened and remain with the family as the child with disabilities grows older and meets key life transitions (e.g., the entry to the school system). Service coordination is a fundamental component of family-centred practice. It can be seen as the hub in the network of care involved in family-centred children's services. Service coordination is a pivotal aspect of family-centred practice in that this model of service delivery requires that the needed services for the child and the family must be delivered in an integrated and coordinated manner (Dunst, 1997). Duwa et al. (1993) note that, for many, the term "service coordination" is synonymous with the family-centred approach to service delivery.

Service coordination can include the following practice roles:

Service broker. This is one of the most common activities of a service coordinator, as it essentially involves assisting families with referrals to support the parents' efforts to find and secure the resources and supports needed by their child and family. The service brokerage function seeks to assist parents to better articulate their service needs, to understand their rights within the existing network of children's services, and to closely link the identification of their needs with the resources that are available to them. At times, parents require, as a first step in the brokerage function, assistance to identify and clarify their specific service needs and priorities. Sometimes they are not sure what to expect from the formal network of programs and agencies that are in place to help families like their own. Some families require encouragement as they may be fatigued or discouraged by their past lack of access to scarce community resources and frustration with potential service providers. Essentially the job entails assisting families in their need to link with appropriate service agencies and ensuring that this linkage is a positive and productive one.

Service mediator. Mediation seeks to improve existing connections and relations between families and the professionals or agencies that serve them. Often, families with children with special service needs have a wide constellation of agencies and professionals in their lives. At times, these families can be caught in a service maze that is marked by service provider disregard for other providers' priorities in the care they deliver, and the multiple time and effort requirements that are placed on the family. Sometimes, well-meaning agencies and professionals can be duplicating services or working at cross purposes. The mediator's efforts are directed at facilitating positive communication so that resolution of conflict and agreement on service provision can be maintained. This role is important even when the mediator has an ongoing service relationship with the family that may include such activities as facilitative counselling. However, in these situations, the mediator should be seen as a professional in the service network that respects and values the important contributions of the other professionals and agencies in the family's network of services. The mediator does not judge service access, delivery, or quality as a family advocate. Ideally, the mediator is seen by all parties as working in the best interests of the family, while maintaining a place of neutrality in the network of services the family receives.

Resource developer. Some families face community situations in which there is low integration of sparsely available child and family care resources. Moore (1992) identifies these circumstances as calling for the resource developer role in service coordinators. That is, the job requires developing or patching together needed community resources. It requires a detailed understanding of the scope and history of existing services, as well as the capability to convince existing agencies or professionals to divert resources to roles that are different from their usual one. It may call for the new or creative use of existing community resources to comply with unmet family needs (such as the use of a church basement for a parent self-help initiative). It may vary from mobilizing local cooperative efforts, such as in the provision of family shared respite or transportation pools, to inter-agency investment in the collaborative securing of needed but unavailable treatment resources, such as speech therapy or kidney dialysis equipment. Moore (1992) cautions that having resource development as a large component of a service coordinator's job description is an impossible situation for practitioners who are not burnout resistant.

Advocacy counsellor. Advocacy does not imply neutrality in the service network; it involves the service coordinator acting as a champion of the family, being a person who takes a partisan stance on the family's behalf. It may involve ensuring that families receive the services they have a right to receive through agency mandate or governmental legislation. It may involve adversarial tactics that place the service coordinator as an ally with family members who find themselves in a challenging or aggressive relationship with another service provider. This may be a situation of advocacy within the agency in which the advocate is employed. Or it may involve an action that targets an external agency which can exercise less immediate sanctions against the advocate and family. The ethics of advocacy require that actions initiated will not ultimately hurt the family or limit their access to needed services, and that all advocacy actions have the informed consent and collaborative involvement of the family.

Generic Elements of Family-Centred Practice

Whether a professional is delivering *family-centred* counselling, therapy, or service coordination, there are key practice elements that are consistently applied. Dunst, Trivette, and Deal (1988) were the first to identify empowerment-enhancing methods or participatory components to be a fundamental aspect of family-centred practice. They also suggest that a relational component is central to, and a prerequisite of, family-centred services and is largely demonstrated by effective, respectful communications and positive professional attitudes about family wisdom and competencies. Similarly, King, Rosenbaum, and King (1996) clustered interpersonal aspects of family-centred care into three general themes: information exchange, respectful and supportive care, and partnership enabling. Although recognition has been given to the importance of relational skills in the delivery of family-centred practice (Dinnebeil, Hale, & Rule, 1996; Turnbull & Turnbull, 1985), it can be argued that the essence of family-centred practice is the family-professional partnership (Roberts, Rule, & Innocenti, 1998), and that this partnership should be fundamentally focused on capacity building (Dunst, Boyd, Trivette, & Hamby, 2002; Dunst, Trivette, & Deal, 1994). Capacity building in children's services means enhancing a family's ability to provide a positive developmental environment for the child and advancing the family's preferred level of self-agency in securing needed child and family support resources. Whether the family-centred practitioner is offering counselling services, family therapy, or service coordination, these overarching practice elements will frame service delivery.

REFERENCES

Aldwin, C.M. (1994). *Stress, coping, and development: An integrative perspective.* New York, NY: Guildford Press.

Caires, K.B., & Weil, M. (1985). Developmentally disabled persons and their families. In M. Weil, J.M. Karls, & Associates (Eds.), *Case management in human service practice* (pp. 233–74). San Francisco, CA: Jossey-Bass.

Constantine, L.L. (1986). *Family paradigms: The practice of theory in family therapy.* New York, NY: Guilford Press.

Dale, N. (1996). *Working with families of children with special needs: Partnership and practice.* London, UK: Routledge. http://dx.doi.org/10.4324/9780203296028

Dinnebeil, L.A., Hale, L.M., & Rule, S. (1996). A qualitative analysis of parents' and service coordinators' descriptions of variables that influence collaborative relationships. *Topics in Early Childhood Special Education, 16*(3), 322–47. http://dx.doi.org/10.1177/027112149601600305

Dunst, C.J. (1997). Conceptual and empirical foundations of family-centered practice. In R. Illback, C. Cobb, & H. Joseph, Jr (Eds.), *Integrated services for children and families: Opportunities for psychological practice* (pp. 75–91). Washington, DC: American Psychological Association. http://dx.doi.org/10.1037/10236-004

Dunst, C.J., Boyd, K., Trivette, C.M., & Hamby, D.W. (2002). Family oriented models and professional helpgiving practices. *Family Relations, 51*(3), 221–9. http://dx.doi.org/10.1111/j.1741-3729.2002.00221.x

Dunst, C.J., Trivette, C.M., & Deal, A.G. (Eds.). (1988). *Enabling & empowering families: Principles & guidelines for practice.* Cambridge, MA: Brookline Books.

Dunst, C.J., Trivette, C.M., & Deal, A.G. (Eds.). (1994). *Supporting and strengthening families.* Cambridge, MA: Brookline Books.

Duwa, S.M., Wells, C., & Lalinde, P. (1993). Creating family-centered programs and policies. In D.M. Bryant & M.A. Graham (Eds.), *Implementing early intervention: From research to effective practice* (pp. 92–123). New York, NY: Guilford Press.

Friesen, B.J., & Poertner, J. (Eds.). (1995). *From case management to service coordination for children with emotional, behavioral, or mental disorders: Building on family strengths.* Baltimore, MD: Paul H. Brookes.

Gottman, J.M. (1994). *What predicts divorce? The relationship between marital processes and marital outcome.* Hillsdale, NJ: Erlbaum.

Greco, V., & Sloper, P. (2004, January). Care co-ordination and key worker schemes for disabled children: Results of a UK-wide survey. *Child: Care, Health and Development, 30*(1), 13–20. http://dx.doi.org/10.1111/j.1365-2214.2004.00381.x Medline:14678307

Illback, R.J., & Neill, T.K. (1995, Winter). Service coordination in mental health systems for children, youth, and families: Progress, problems, prospects. *Journal of Mental Health Administration, 22*(1), 17–28. http://dx.doi. org/10.1007/BF02519194 Medline:10141267

Kantor, D., & Lehr, W. (1975). *Inside the family.* San Francisco, CA: Jossey-Bass.

Karpel, M.A. (1994). *Evaluating couples: A handbook for practitioners.* New York, NY: W.W. Norton.

Kerr, M.E., & Bowen, M. (1988). *Family evaluation.* New York, NY: Norton.

King, S.M., Rosenbaum, P.L., & King, G.A. (1996, September). Parents' perceptions of caregiving: Development and validation of a measure of processes. *Developmental Medicine and Child Neurology, 38*(9), 757–72. http://dx.doi. org/10.1111/j.1469-8749.1996.tb15110.x Medline:8810707

Kubler-Ross, E. (1969). *On death and dying.* New York, NY: Macmillan.

Laborde, P.R., & Seligman, M. (1991). Counseling parents with children with disabilities. In M. Seligman (Ed.), *The family with a handicapped child* (2nd ed., pp. 337–69). Boston, MA: Allyn & Bacon.

Minuchin, S. (1974). *Families and family therapy.* Cambridge, MA: Harvard University Press.

Moore, S. (1992). Case management and the integration of services: How service delivery systems shape case management. *Social Work, 37,* 418–23.

Nichols, M.P., & Schwartz, R.C. (2001). *Family therapy concepts and methods* (5th ed.). Boston, MA: Allyn and Bacon.

Olshansky, S. (1962). Chronic sorrow: A response to having a mentally defective child. *Social Casework, 43,* 190–3.

Roberts, R.N., Rule, S., & Innocenti, M.S. (1998). *Strengthening the family-professional partnership in services for young children.* Baltimore, MD: Brookes.

Rothman, J. (1991, November). A model of case management: Toward empirically based practice. *Social Work, 36*(6), 520–8. Medline:1754929

Seligman, M., & Darling, R.B. (1997). *Ordinary families, special children* (2nd ed.). New York, NY: Guilford Press.

Stepanek, J.S., Newcomb, S., & Kettler, K. (1996). Coordinating services and identifying family priorities, resources, and concerns. In P.J. Beckman (Ed.), *Strategies for working with families of young children with disabilities* (pp. 69–89). Baltimore, MD: Brookes.

Stroul, B.A. (1995). Case management in a system of care. In B.J. Friesen & J. Poertner (Eds.), *From case management to service coordination for children with emotional, behavioral, or mental disorders: Building on family strengths* (pp. 3–25). Baltimore, MD: Paul H. Brookes.

Trute, B., Hiebert-Murphy, D., & Levine, K. (2007, March). Parental appraisal of the family impact of childhood developmental disability: Times of sadness and times of joy. *Journal of Intellectual & Developmental Disability, 32*(1), 1–9. http://dx.doi.org/10.1080/13668250601146753 Medline:17365362

Turnbull, A.P., & Turnbull, H.R. (1985). *Parents speak out: Then and now*. Columbus, OH: Charles E. Merrill.

Walsh, F., & McGoldrick, M. (1995). Loss and the family: A systemic perspective. In F. Walsh & M. McGoldrick (Eds.), *Living beyond loss: Death in the family* (pp. 3–26). New York, NY: W.W. Norton.

Watzlawick, P., Weakland, J., & Fisch, R. (1974). *Change: Principles of problem formulation and problem resolution*. New York, NY: Norton.

Wikler, L., Wasow, M., & Hatfield, E. (1981, January). Chronic sorrow revisited: Parent vs. professional depiction of the adjustment of parents of mentally retarded children. *American Journal of Orthopsychiatry, 51*(1), 63–70. http://dx.doi.org/10.1111/j.1939-0025.1981.tb01348.x Medline:7212030

Wortman, C.B., & Silver, R.C. (1989, June). The myths of coping with loss. *Journal of Consulting and Clinical Psychology, 57*(3), 349–57. http://dx.doi.org/10.1037/0022-006X.57.3.349 Medline:2661609

4   Fundamentals of Working Alliance

BARRY TRUTE AND DIANE HIEBERT-MURPHY

Working Alliance as a Generic Practice Theme

No matter what the service context, practice setting, or professional discipline, family-centred practice at the most fundamental level requires that professionals are capable of building and maintaining positive working alliances. The working alliance is based on a goal-driven collaboration between the service provider and service recipient. Family-centred practice requires as a foundational element the establishment of a positive working alliance between parents and professionals that is characterized by mutual trust and respect, cooperative rapport, and clear communication (Beckman, 1996; Dunst, Trivette, & Deal, 1994). Since parents represent the executive authority in the family, and optimally can serve as the hub of a family's activities, professionals must be able to communicate openly and clearly with parents, build confidence in the parents that the professional can be trusted to be helpful to their child, and build hope that assistance provided by the professional will make things better and not worse in the life of the family. This applies across children's services whether interventions are largely focused on the child, or more widely on the child in the family situation.

Beckman, Newcomb, Frank, and Brown (1996) suggest that three professional attributes serve as basic building blocks for positive family-centred practice:

- respect for the importance and competence of the family in taking leadership in a child's life;
- being non-judgmental and respectful of the family's wish to do the best for their child; and

- having empathetic understanding of family members' beliefs and feelings, and possessing the capability to communicate that understanding to family members.

These core competencies facilitate positive and productive relations, leave family members feeling respected and understood by the professional, and build hope that services can be trusted and will be of help.

Dunst, Trivette, and Deal (1988) suggest that the "relational" component is basic to family-centred practice and is largely demonstrated by effective, respectful communications and positive professional attitudes about family wisdom and competencies. Although emphasis is given to the importance of relational skills in the delivery of family-centred service (Dinnebeil, Hale, & Rule, 1996; Turnbull & Turnbull, 1985), what has emerged through studies of service outcome is the recognition that the essence of the relational component is the family-professional partnership (Roberts, Rule, & Innocenti, 1998). Working alliance is seen as being a first step in the formation of a family-professional partnership; that is, the establishment of a positive working alliance appears to set the stage for collaborative problem solving between the professional and parent. A positive working alliance appears to facilitate the other essential family-centred practice elements of parent empowerment and capacity building. Without an adequate working alliance, a partnership cannot be developed and maintained. In turn, it is the parent-professional partnership that serves as the foundation for the ongoing development of empowerment and capacity-building practices.

It is our experience that many professionals understand that the concept of working alliance is critical to their practice with children and their families. However, some do not appreciate that this concept should also apply to their collaborations and service coordination efforts with other human service professionals. The same principles of mutual trust and respect, cooperative rapport, and clear communication should prevail in inter-professional relations. That is, it is not appropriate to be authoritarian or loud and aggressive with professional colleagues any more than it is with family members. In hospital settings, nurses and social workers sometimes assert that it is difficult for them to be family-centred and empowering with families when they themselves feel disempowered by what has been traditionally a "military model" of professional and administrative decision-making. In other words, family-centred practice must be system-wide. Its principles are not only relevant to professional-family relations but also to how professionals relate to each other and to how human service agencies, hospitals, and community programs are managed and administered. Working alliance takes on a profound meaning when considered at all levels of professional activity in the design and delivery of human services.

Respect for the Family: A Prerequisite for a Positive Family-Professional Working Alliance

Negative professional stereotypes in health and social services relating to parents of children with special needs have been pervasive and enduring. The literature on stress and coping has only limited, recent consideration of the positive or life-enhancement aspects in family sequelae of the entry of a child with intellectual or developmental disability into the life of a family (Ferguson, 2002; Trute, Hiebert-Murphy, & Levine, 2007). A belief that still seems to persist is that parents of children with developmental disabilities will often be "unreasonably reactive" to professionals and, therefore, that it is difficult to work in partnership with these parents. This creates the anticipation that parents of children with disabilities will be hostile to professional advice and guidance that challenges parental beliefs, and this promotes negative interpretation of parent behaviours that are not closely compliant with the advice and views of professionals. One example of this is the professional complaint about the "shopping around" phenomenon. When parents seek confirmation of their child's diagnosis across several independent professionals, it is often seen as indicative of "dissatisfied and hypercritical" behaviour that shows a lack of acceptance of their child's disability, rather than prudent coping behaviour on the parents' part (Seligman & Seligman, 1980). Many professionals do not realize the "shopping around" may be a function of the "community service maze" which confuses parents and triggers a search for the most appropriate and best services (Rubin & Quinn-Curran, 1983).

Parents' hesitation to label their children with specific diagnoses, which will have powerful implications for their child's future life, may not be seen by some professionals as a responsible thing to do, but will be interpreted as "resistance" or "denial." A belief seems to persist in many professionals that "denial" is common in parents and blocks recognition of their child's deficiencies and limitations. Although persistent and extreme denial is a serious service concern, many professionals do not seem to understand that often some modest degree of denial can go a long way in helping parents adjust and cope to new and upsetting life circumstances. That is, denial can sometimes serve as a positive coping mechanism rather than a pathological response to a challenging life circumstance. The place of denial in overall family coping and resilience is not well understood in research or in practice. We do know that mothers and fathers in the same family can vary dramatically in their complementary and often functional use of optimism, pessimism, hope, and despair. We do know that people need to deal with important life adjustments in a series of steps and at a speed that is congruent with their gender, cultural beliefs, and social resources.

Further, parents have been pathologized in the practice literature as being vulnerable to suffering long-term "chronic sorrow" (Olshansky, 1962) and as facing ongoing childcare circumstances that many professionals see as grim and unbearably complex. This perspective, which dwells on the burdens and deficits associated with serious childhood disability, can be described as distal, value-laden, and pathology-oriented (Longo & Bond, 1984). There are well established theories in the professional literature that suggest that parents of children with disabilities often employ psychological defence mechanisms to cope with their guilt and grief. Many normal parental reactions are taken out of social context, labelled, and pathologized. For example, consider the notion that many parents are overprotective of their children because of the guilt they feel. Many professionals still do not appreciate that for many parents it makes common sense for them to try their best to protect their children against stigma and potential societal abuse, circumstances that they know their children may face in their local community (Seligman & Seligman, 1980).

It is not uncommon for parents to acknowledge feelings of anger, denial, and guilt. However, how persistent and incapacitating these feelings are across all parents of children with disabilities is unclear, as is the process of these adverse emotional reactions over the early years in the life of their child. It does seem that strong negative reactions (such as shock, grief, and depression) are usually short-lived (Darling, 1983; Trute, 1990). However, many professionals still hold a negative view of parents' coping abilities and tend to believe that a child with a serious disability will always cause problems in family functioning and adjustment (Sloper & Turner, 1991). Although this negative anticipation of family maladjustment to disability appears to persist in the field, research evidence suggests that families with young children with disabilities are no different than any other cross-section of families in the community (Dyson, 1991; O'Sullivan, Mahoney, & Robinson, 1992; Reddon, McDonald, & Kysela, 1992; Seligman & Darling, 1997; Trute, 1990; Whitehead, Deiner, & Toccafondi, 1990). It does seem that contact with service providers that is experienced by parents as reflective of negative expectancies or biases on the part of the professional will exacerbate rather than relieve stress in some parents (Burden & Thomas, 1986). In these situations parents, feel misunderstood and unfairly judged.

Building a Working Alliance: Effective, Respectful Communications

Listening skills serve as the basis for effective communication. We have yet to meet a professional who did not think that s/he had strong listening skills, even those who in our view were dismal listeners. Brems (2001) identifies key roadblocks to effective listening, and these are listed in Table 4.1.

Effective listening requires that these "roadblocks" be mindfully avoided. To overcome these roadblocks, there are several caveats or practice warnings that can be considered. These are based on the understanding that all communication has information content, emotional components, and implications for relational power. First, to be an effective listener, one must be calm, patient, and remain focused on what is being said. This is to ensure that adequate attention is given to communication content and details of information. A trap that many professionals see themselves as being caught in is the "time trap." Because of large caseloads or highly structured service schedules, there is pressure to move expeditiously and focus on what is seen as the facts of the situation that seem to be of immediate relevance. This leads one to jump to conclusions and move to decisions without adequate information. It also leads to the inappropriate filtering of information to reinforce premature conclusions. Signs of this are professionals rushing to complete sentences for youth or family members, or frequently misinterpreting what is said because of false assumptions and misjudgments based on sparse information. We would assert that rather than saving time, this leads to service failures and intervention inadequacies that ultimately burn up more of the professional's time. Additional time is required later in subsequent relational repair and restoration or alternative and corrected actions, which need to be re-initiated and based on new or more complete information gathering.

A second consideration for effective communication is the recognition that all communications can carry an emotional component. The

Table 4.1. Key Roadblocks to Effective Listening

- Inadequate listening, in which the professional is "inattentive or preoccupied with personal worries or need states"
- Evaluative listening, in which the professional "makes judgments about what is heard" and loses the ability to collect and understand the full scope of information being communicated
- Filtered or selective listening, in which a professional only hears "what they expect or want to hear based on preconceived notions"
- Fact-centred listening, in which a professional only attends to verbal information and misses non-verbal communications
- Rehearsing-while-listening, in which the professional "is preoccupied with how to respond to the client" and is busy considering what next to say to the client rather than attending to what the client is actually communicating
- Sympathetic listening in which the professional over-identifies with the client and "gets caught up in the client's story" and immersed in the emotional power of the story, rather than the content of the communication.

(Adapted from Brems, 2001, p. 121. Used with permission.)

trap for professionals in this regard is asking questions too quickly or too directly that have emotional meaning to the service recipient, and which the service recipient is not yet ready to discuss with the professional. In Chapter 3 of this book, we clarified that family-centred counselling in children's services is not family therapy. Unless the professional is invited to address highly charged emotional issues, it is not appropriate to go too deeply into the emotional life of the family, as this can appear to be insensitive and disrespectful. On the other hand, ignoring the details of parenting stress or family conflict may block effective service planning. The skills involved in resolving this dilemma include the ability to ask respectful, minimally intrusive questions that can open the conversation to more specific enquiries and, at all times, to follow the family member's lead in addressing issues when and if the issues emerge during an interview as a service concern and a priority of the family.

Research on paediatricians' interviewing style and parents' disclosures of child behavioural or emotional symptoms has been informative. In their study of mothers coming to paediatricians' offices, Hickson, Altemeier, and O'Connor (1983) found that fewer than one third of the mothers discussed psychological or emotional concerns, even when that concern was the mother's single greatest worry. Many mothers appeared to believe that the paediatrician was unqualified, disinterested, or too busy to attend to these concerns, while others felt that such a discussion would be too embarrassing. Parent disclosure of psychosocial issues is facilitated when paediatricians ask directly about family and parent concerns, show empathy, and listen attentively and sympathetically (Wissow, Roter, & Wilson, 1994). A related finding was that when physicians communicated directly and empathetically, it also led to more parent initiated discussions of child issues such as aggressive behaviour and the use of punishments in parenting.

It is important for human service professionals to show parents that they have interest in discussing the parents' concerns with issues related to psychosocial support (Hickson et al., 1983) so that parents understand that it is appropriate to ask for help with family support issues related to their distress. The implication of these findings is that professionals should not be passive and wait for parents to bring psychosocial issues to their attention. It calls for interviewing skill that facilitates discussion relating to uncomfortable or embarrassing topics. It calls for the creation of a working environment in which a parent feels safe, has trust in the sensitivity and understanding of the person assisting her/him, and feels respected as a person and as a mother or father. If a person is distressed, angry, or in shock or crisis, such emotional states will inhibit or constrict her/his ability to communicate, for it is difficult to express inner thoughts and feelings when overwhelmed by strong emotions. It is important to deal with emotional states of clients when these are evident in the interview as a preliminary step in information gathering to ensure that communication is open, thoughtful, and clear. The first intent of the professional should be to relax and calm the parent or youth, rather than to jump into information gathering and assessment procedures.

It is important that professionals are mindful of topics or situations that can trigger an emotional reaction on their own part in their professional practice. This can be anchored in the content of what is said, the manner in which it is said, or in a personal characteristic of a family member. For example, consider the case of an angry father who yells at a health care professional for making the family wait for 2 hours before being seen in an outpatient clinic. The professional may have an emotional reaction to people being impatient and blaming her/him for the delay, may have difficulty processing information in any kind of hostile situations, or may not be able to control her/his own feeling when dealing with "angry fathers" (because of her/his own family history and experiences). Fatigued, emotionally burned out, or chronically bored professionals have seriously diminished abilities to listen and comprehend. They may be too preoccupied with their own needs and priorities to fully attend to the needs and priorities of others. The "emotional field" surrounding any set of interpersonal communications can restrict people's willingness to speak openly and honestly and can limit the listener's capability to hear and understand. This is equally true for family members and professionals.

We do know that level of maternal education is related to the success of parent–service provider communication. In their review of the literature, Nobile and Drotar (2003) cite a number of studies that found that mothers with higher education were given more support, more positive affect, and more partnership-type relationships by physicians. In our experience in studying childhood disability services in several Canadian provinces, higher educated and articulate mothers do appear to access more psychosocial support resources for their children and families. Our speculation is that mothers with higher levels of education can "talk the talk" (i.e., they comprehend and are comfortable with professional jargon and language), can relate in a more attentive and respectful manner (i.e., positive affect), and can help professionals feel comfortable in their presence. This can lead to unfair distribution of scarce resources such as agency-funded parenting respite, in that less educated, less articulate parents who are more likely to be living in poverty have a more difficult time accessing needed psychosocial support resources.

However, it is the professional's job to recognize and navigate these communication hurdles as they negatively impact their practice. This should not be the service recipient's job. A children's hospital in Canada recently encouraged a parents' self-help group to prepare a set of teaching videotapes that taught fellow parents "how to talk with professionals." The intent of these teaching videotapes is to develop skills in parents to deal with emotional reactivity in the professionals that are being paid to serve them. That is, they teach parents to be sensitive to tired, frustrated, reactive professionals in a manner that helps parents relax the professional and communicate with that professional in a manner that will advance the quality of the health care that their child is receiving. This is a sad commentary on the frequency with which parents face professionals who are incompetent communicators. Although it is a noble intent (to improve parents' communication skills), it inappropriately places the onus on the parent to maintain clear, non-threatening, and effective communications rather than keeping this as primarily the responsibility of a professional, and it is insensitive to the personal crises many parents experience when their child is hospitalized.

We are not suggesting that parents hold no responsibility for maintaining respectful and clear communications in their relationships with the professionals who assist them. Family-centred practice does not mean that family members have a right to be rude or abusive. Family-centred practice requires understanding and competence on the part of both family members and professionals. It is best if both sides of the family member–professional partnership understand the rights and expectations of their role and their responsibilities in family-centred practice, so that they may participate in a way that is consistent with the principles of the model. Family-centred practice is a "two-sided coin"; there are basic expectations and participatory competencies inherent in the partnership model, whether a person is involved as a family member or as a professional in the delivery of health and social services.

A consideration for effective communication is the power dimension in any exchange of information. Immediate to this concern is a professional's sensitivity to the reluctance of a service recipient to disclose information when the service recipient lacks confidence that her/his information will not be used in a punitive or damaging way. This is particularly important when dealing with people who have had negative experiences in their past dealings with health care or social service agencies. Unfortunately, this is not an uncommon occurrence with people who have experienced racial, religious, homophobic, or cultural bias, who are recent immigrants from oppressive environments, or who live in poverty. Open communication is blocked when there is fear that the disclosure and discussion of information will create a shameful or demeaning relationship with the professional. At issue is whether the professional is seen as being safe and trustworthy. This trust comes as the service recipient experiences the professional to be respectful, sensitive to community and cultural nuances, and understanding of the life situation of the service recipient.

In health and social services, many child and family programs are "categorical" in terms of rigidly delineating who can or cannot qualify for service resources. This can create a power problem between the professional in control of resources and the person in need. In child welfare, a social worker can apply legal sanctions removing a child from the home or limiting access of a parent to a child. This can importantly hinder open and frank communication, as the parent wishes to be perceived positively and not risk loss of access to her/his child. It is important in situations such as these that service recipients feel understood and trust that there will be fair consideration of their family situation.

Fear of critical judgment and feelings of social distance and powerlessness will impede communication and the development of a positive working alliance.

In summary, effective communication is characterized by a belief that one's voice is heard, that there is empathetic understanding of the information that is transmitted, that there is a basic acceptance and respect between those exchanging information, and that trust and safety are assured when disclosing and processing sensitive information.

Active Listening: Giving Feedback That Information Is Heard and Understood

It is not enough for professionals to believe that they have accurately understood the information they have heard and have empathy for the service recipient's life situation. It is important that the service recipient also shares these beliefs. Active listening comprises techniques that facilitate mutual confidence in the communications that have transpired. These skills are routinely taught in programs of professional education and are worth repeating here as a reminder for those who understand the techniques at a conceptual level but have not yet integrated them into their everyday practice. It is of concern that one of the most frequent complaints made by service recipients is that professionals do not listen to them.

Core techniques of active listening include summarizing, paraphrasing, and questioning. Occasionally, summarizing what has been communicated serves to confirm to a person that the information s/he has given has been clearly heard and empathically understood. It is a way for the professional to validate the information with its source. It confirms that essential content and key themes have emerged from the discourse. Paraphrasing, or repeating back what has been heard in a brief statement, explicitly confirms salient aspects of a conversation and serves as an ongoing clarity check of the detail and context of communications.

Questioning is a vital part of an interview. A smooth and gentle process of inquiry is more skilful than interrupting the conversation with frequent professional insights and opinions. Questioning should not be applied in a stilted, fast, and mechanistic manner. The danger is that any question is then perceived to be part of an interrogation, rather than as a way of seeking clarification and advancing understanding. Reflective questioning at times serves as an invitation for persons involved in the interview to think together, to probe for additional relevant details, to consider alternative interpretations, to gently explore what is left unsaid, and to reach mutual understandings.

Active listening signals that a person is being heard and understood, builds trust in the competency of the interviewer, increases feelings of psychological and situational safety, and serves to enhance the working alliance between the professional and service recipient. Because the interview is a two-way exchange (when it involves two people), listening on the part of all participants is a dynamic, reciprocal process. It is optimal for all participants in an interview process to be encouraged to use active listening, and assisted to do so. At times, the professional will need to help family members frame and ask questions or need to paraphrase what they hear and understand, to ensure that all parties involved carry away similar information and understandings.

Working in Concert with the Family Circumstances and Situational Needs

There are times when a professional can move quickly to establish a collaborative process with parents and times when they can expeditiously and calmly work together with parents in the identification of child and family service needs. However, in times of family crisis and parental emotional distress, the psychological volatility may impede immediate service planning and call for a careful and deliberate response from the professional. At these times, the family-centred practitioner must first recognize and deal with the emotional state of family members. This is a preliminary and necessary step when embarking on the development of a working alliance. It is important for the professional to be able to identify when family members are in crisis, acknowledge the crisis situation with them, seek to assist them to deal with the emotional upheaval, and not rush to begin a child and family assessment for the formal planning of children's services. At a minimum, the professional should keep her/his communications simple, focus on the family members' immediate emotional needs, and postpone conversations related to planning for childcare and family psychosocial supports in the longer term. At these times, it is best to show the family that the professional is sensitive, compassionate, and understanding, and is a person who respects family members and can respond in ways that are appropriate and timely to their practical and emotional needs.

Working Alliance as a Precursor to Capacity Building and Empowerment Practice

Dunst et al. (1988) identify the "relational" component as basic to family-centred practice and see it as being demonstrated by effective, respectful communications and positive professional attitudes about family wisdom and competencies. Working alliance is at the heart of this relational component and is a prerequisite in the formation of a functional family-professional partnership. The establishment of a positive working alliance sets the stage for collaborative efforts between the professional and parent. Further, a positive working alliance appears to facilitate the other essential family-centred practice elements of parent empowerment and capacity building (Dempsey & Dunst, 2004) and is not sufficient in itself for "either strengthening family competence or promoting new capabilities" (Dunst, 2000, p. 101). That is, family-centred practice involves much more than just a positive working relationship. Once a positive working relationship is achieved, then it is important to move on to the more challenging practice elements of mutual problem solving, capacity building, and empowerment.

Adequate Service Contact and Information Exchange: Dynamically Intertwined with Working Alliance

In children's health and social services, information exchange with parents and family members is a basic aspect of service delivery. Access to needed information about childhood challenges, and information in regard to the availability of programs that respond to these challenges, has consistently been shown in parent surveys to be the most fundamental family need that is of highest priority (Westling, 1996). In childhood disability services, families must find and understand an enormous amount of information related to their child's health and developmental concerns (Guralnick, 2000). Information needs do not diminish as the child ages, but change over time. That is, information needs are fluid. They are altered by increasing parent knowledge, changing child circumstances, and shifting service priorities. Parents often identify the lack of information and "not knowing," whether this involves their child's circumstances or service options, as their number one stressor.

In our view, there are two preliminary requirements that need to be in place for a positive working alliance to be developed and maintained. First, there has to be a minimum level of contact between the parent and professional. When family members believe that ongoing contact is too infrequent or fragmented to allow trusted communication with a professional to be maintained, then the relational component of family-centred practice is not possible. Further, when adequate and helpful information is seen as being provided, this fuels and supports the working alliance between the parent and professional. This is a reciprocal process in which professionals need to provide relevant and accurate information, and parents need to feel that they can be open and candid in their disclosure of child and family information (Dinnebeil & Rule, 1994).

The provision of accessible and relevant information is an important precursor to empowerment practice (Mitchell & Sloper, 2002), as informed choice is a key aspect of empowerment. In Chapter 6, focused attention is given to empowerment practice and its roots in strengths-based interventions in children's services. However, before attending to intervention strategies, we will turn our attention in the next chapter to information gathering by the professional, that is, to basic protocols of assessment in family-centred children's services.

REFERENCES

Beckman, P.J. (1996). *Strategies for working with young families of young children with disabilities*. Baltimore, MD: Brookes.

Beckman, P.J., Newcomb, S., Frank, N., & Brown, L. (1996). Evolution of working relationships with families. In P.J. Beckman (Ed.), *Strategies for working with families of young children with disabilities* (pp. 17–30). Baltimore, MD: Brookes.

Brems, C. (2001). *Basic skills in psychotherapy and counseling*. Belmont, CA: Wadsworth.

Burden, R., & Thomas, D. (1986). A further perspective on parental reaction to handicap. *Exceptional Children, 33*(2), 140–5. http://dx.doi.org/10.1080/0156655860330207

Darling, R.B. (1983). The birth defective child and the crisis of parenthood: Redefining the situation. In E. Callahan & K. McClusky (Eds.), *Lifespan developmental psychology: Nonnormative life events* (pp. 115–43). New York, NY: Academic Press.

Dempsey, I., & Dunst, C.J. (2004). Helpgiving styles and parent empowerment in families with young children with a disability. *Journal of Intellectual & Developmental Disability, 29*(1), 40–51. http://dx.doi.org/10.1080/1366825041000 1662874

Dinnebeil, L.A., Hale, L.M., & Rule, S. (1996). A qualitative analysis of parents' and service coordinators' descriptions of variables that influence collaborative relationships. *Topics in Early Childhood Special Education, 16*(3), 322–47. http://dx.doi.org/10.1177/027112149601600305

Dinnebeil, L.A., & Rule, S. (1994). Variables that influence collaboration between parents and service coordinators. *Journal of Early Intervention, 18*(4), 349–61. http://dx.doi.org/10.1177/105381519401800405

Dunst, C.J. (2000). Revisiting "rethinking early intervention." *Topics in Early Childhood Special Education, 20*(2), 95–104. http://dx.doi.org/10.1177/027112140002000205

Dunst, C.J., Trivette, C.M., & Deal, A.G. (1988). *Enabling and empowering families: Principles & guidelines for practice*. Cambridge, MA: Brookline Books.

Dunst, C.J., Trivette, C.M., & Deal, A.G. (Eds.). (1994). *Supporting and strengthening families*. Cambridge, MA: Brookline Books.

Dyson, L.L. (1991, May). Families of young children with handicaps: Parental stress and family functioning. *American Journal of Mental Retardation, 95*(6), 623–9. Medline:1829374

Ferguson, P.M. (2002). A place in the family: An historical interpretation of research on parental reactions to having a child with a disability. *Journal of Special Education, 36*(3), 124–31. http://dx.doi.org/10.1177/00224669020360030201

Guralnick, M.J. (2000). Early childhood intervention: Evolution of a system. *Focus on Autism and Other Developmental Disabilities, 15*(2), 68–79. http://dx.doi.org/10.1177/108835760001500202

Hickson, G.B., Altemeier, W.A., & O'Connor, S. (1983, November). Concerns of mothers seeking care in private pediatric offices: Opportunities for expanding services. *Pediatrics, 72*(5), 619–24. Medline:6634264

Longo, D.C., & Bond, L. (1984). Families of the handicapped child: Research and practice. *Family Relations, 33*(1), 57–65. http://dx.doi.org/10.2307/584590

Mitchell, W., & Sloper, P. (2002, March). Information that informs rather than alienates families with disabled children: Developing a model of good practice. *Health & Social Care in the Community, 10*(2), 74–81. http://dx.doi.org/10.1046/j.1365-2524.2002.00344.x Medline:12121265

Nobile, C., & Drotar, D. (2003, August). Research on the quality of parent-provider communication in pediatric care: Implications and recommendations. *Journal of Developmental and Behavioral Pediatrics, 24*(4), 279–90. http://dx.doi.org/10.1097/00004703-200308000-00010 Medline:12915801

Olshansky, S. (1962). Chronic sorrow: A response to having a mentally defective child. *Social Casework, 43*, 190–3.

O'Sullivan, P., Mahoney, G., & Robinson, C. (1992, December). Perceptions of pediatricians' helpfulness: A national study of mothers of young disabled children. *Developmental Medicine and Child Neurology, 34*(12), 1064–71. http://dx.doi.org/10.1111/j.1469-8749.1992.tb11418.x Medline:1451935

Reddon, J.E., McDonald, L., & Kysela, G.M. (1992). Parental coping and family stress I: Resources for and functioning of families with a preschool child having a developmental disability. *Early Child Development and Care, 83*(1), 1–26. http://dx.doi.org/10.1080/0300443920830101

Roberts, R.N., Rule, S., & Innocenti, M.S. (1998). *Strengthening the family-professional partnership in services for young children*. Baltimore, MD: Brookes.

Rubin, S., & Quinn-Curran, N. (1983). Lost, then found: Parent's journey through the community service maze. In M. Seligman (Ed.), *The family with a handicapped child: Understanding and treatment* (pp. 63–94). Orlando, FL: Grune & Stratton.

Seligman, M., & Darling, R.B. (1997). *Ordinary families, special children: A systems approach to childhood disability* (2nd ed.). New York, NY: Guilford Press.

Seligman, M., & Seligman, P.A. (1980). The professional's dilemma: Learning to work with parents. *Exceptional Parent, 10*, 511–13.

Sloper, P., & Turner, S. (1991). Parental and professional view of the needs of families with a child with severe physical disability. *Counselling Psychology Quarterly, 4*(4), 323–30. http://dx.doi.org/10.1080/09515079108254440

Trute, B. (1990). Child and parent predictors of family adjustment in households containing young developmentally disabled children. *Family Relations, 39*(3), 292–7. http://dx.doi.org/10.2307/584874

Trute, B., Hiebert-Murphy, D., & Levine, K. (2007, March). Parental appraisal of the family impact of childhood developmental disability: Times of sadness and times of joy. *Journal of Intellectual & Developmental Disability, 32*(1), 1–9. http://dx.doi.org/10.1080/13668250601146753 Medline:17365362

Turnbull, A.P., & Turnbull, H.R. (1985). *Parents speak out: Then and now*. Columbus, OH: Charles E. Merrill.

Westling, D.L. (1996). What do parents of children with moderate and severe mental disabilities want? *Education and Training in Mental Retardation and Developmental Disabilities, 31*, 86–114.

Whitehead, L.C., Deiner, P.L., & Toccafondi, S. (1990). Family assessment: Parent and professional evaluation. *Topics in Early Childhood Special Education, 10*(1), 63–77. http://dx.doi.org/10.1177/027112149001000106

Wissow, L.S., Roter, D.L., & Wilson, M.E.H. (1994, February). Pediatrician interview style and mothers' disclosure of psychosocial issues. *Pediatrics, 93*(2), 289–95. Medline:8121743

5 Family Assessment Theory and Information Gathering Processes in Family-Centred Practice

BARRY TRUTE

Expanding the Scope of Assessment to Encompass Child in Family in Community

Family-centred practice in children's services requires a widening of the traditional child assessment lens. The practitioner's focus of interest must move beyond the well-being of an individual child to the well-being of the child while nested in a family. That is, it is understood that family beliefs, family coping resources, and perceived service needs must be considered when working to advance the well-being of a child. Further, consideration needs to be given to the support resources that are available to the child from within the immediate family as well as beyond the family boundary, from friends, extended family members, and community networks. We must move from a perspective that largely focuses on assessment of the individual child to a more careful consideration of the child in family (proximal social support) and of child and family in community (distal social support).

Assumptions of Family-Centred Information Gathering

In family-centred practice, assessment is not seen as a first step or preliminary phase that precedes intervention (as is the case in traditional practice models in human services that prescribe a linear process involving assessment, then diagnosis, and then treatment). In family-centred practice, assessment is recognized as a process that is initiated at service intake, but that continues through the course of service delivery as an interwoven and continuous aspect of biopsychosocial treatment (Borrell-Carrió, Suchman, & Epstein, 2004; Weston, 2005). This assessment process often evolves over time as it responds to new information gathered and responds to gains and failures in service delivery.

Basic tasks in the assessment process. Assessment in family-centred children's services addresses two basic tasks: (a) establishing and maintaining a working alliance, and (b) information gathering with analysis. At the most fundamental level, assessment contributes to the building of a positive working alliance between a professional and family. It is important that a parent believes that the professional who is entering the life of her or his family and assisting with the well-being of his or her child is a person who can be trusted to be competent and respectful, and not a person who will further complicate or worsen the situation for which he or she needs help. Assessments that are practical, that are focused on parental concerns, and that assure families that the professional "knows their story" and understands their situation will facilitate the development of a positive working alliance.

A second major purpose of "child with family" information gathering in family-centred services involves the preparation of a Family-Centred Support Plan (FCSP). The purpose of the FCSP is to identify the family's needs and priorities and to create a plan to address those priorities in a way that is direct, clear, achievable, and congruent with the family's values and preferences. Although the FCSP is best thought of as a process rather than an end product in its own right, professionals will consult with parents in the early phases of service delivery to create an initial FCSP. (The dynamics and mechanics of the preparation of an FCSP are reviewed in Chapter 9.) At times, family need for child and family services will be complex and require the gathering of extensive assessment information while, at other times, the child and family service need will be immediate and specific and require only a sparse collection of background information. In that respect, family-centred practice does not follow an assessment template, or a fixed set of steps, in a routine service protocol, but is responsive to the unique capabilities, needs, and preferences of each family.

Assumption of family normality in initial information gathering. It is best to begin the process of assessment in family-centred practice with the assumption that the family is "normal" in its organization and functioning. Further, it is best if the professional starts with the assumption that parenting stress will likely exceed normal limits, but that there will not be a direct relationship between the level of stress that a parent of a child with a serious disability or health or psychosocial challenge experiences in her/his daily life and that parent's emotional or psychological state (e.g., clinical depression) or that parent's over-all family adjustment (e.g., marital conflict). Finally, the professional should start with the assumption that parent-perceived support needs and service priorities are practical, focused, and relevant to the imme-diate needs and realities of the parents' children and families. That is, it is best not to assume that family service needs for instrumental or physical care resources will be complex in scope or that family needs for emotional support will be profound and unavoidable. If a practi-tioner starts with a perspective that anticipates parent and family nor-mality, s/he will begin in a manner that is in tune with the situation of most families and will avoid going too deeply into the emotional life of the family when it is not necessary, or before the family is ready to ad-dress any of their more sensitive emotional matters. The family should guide the assessment; it is best if practitioners trust the family's wis-dom and priorities. In this sense, the family practitioner should "lead by following" (Minuchin & Fishman, 1981). That is, practitioners should be sensitive to each family's speed of disclosure of personal and sensi-tive information, and comply with this in a curious and respectful way. They should ensure that the family's priorities for service are under-stood, validated, and inasmuch as possible, can be directly achieved.

Components of Family-Centred Assessment

Three information domains are addressed in family-centred service assessment:

- family needs and priorities,
- family functioning and resiliency, and
- family internal (psychological) and external (social network) coping support resources.

Not all families will require comprehensive information gather-ing to respond to their need for support. Most families entering child health and child developmental services will only have immediate and straightforward needs for service or support. For example, a common request is solely for respite support. Some families need to know that such support is available, especially during times of emergency or cri-sis, even if they do not always make use of ongoing respite relief. It is a comfort to them to know that respite is there if they need it. The recom-mended course of action in information gathering is to begin with the family's priorities and perceived needs and, depending on the issues identified by the family, progress from there with the depth and scope in the assessment appropriate to the family's situation.

Use of empirical assessment tools to explore needs and resources. The exploration of family service needs is a primary component in the development of an initial support plan. This is typically completed through interviews with family members. The focus and duration of these interviews is contingent on the scope and complexity of the family's need for support. Although the interview is the primary method of information gathering, we have found that the use of brief, empirical measures can greatly facilitate and supplement the interview process.

The use of empirical assessment tools remains a contentious topic in family-centred practice. Slentz and Bricker (1992) offer a thoughtful critique of the use and misuse of empirical assessment tools, and identify key reasons why they are problematic in initial family service assessments. It has been suggested, however, that a majority of parents will prefer a combination of empirical self-report measures and a personal interview in the preparation of a support plan (Davis & Gettinger, 1995). That has been our experience. We have found that although at first parents will tend to be ambivalent about what they believe will be the potential value of empirical assessment tools, after completing them, most parents find that the measures help them explain their situation and identify the needs of their child and family. Much depends on when and how these empirical assessment tools are introduced in the assessment process. I shall return to this timing issue later in the chapter.

There are many empirical assessment tools available for use in family-centred practice in children's services. One that we have found consistently useful in the beginning stages of the preparation of a support plan is the Family Needs Survey (FNS; Bailey & Simeonsson, 1988). The FNS is a 35-item instrument that identifies needs in families with young children with disabilities within seven general clusters of service categories. It is a widely adopted assessment tool in childhood disability services (Krauss, 2000) and also has been used in chronic health care of children (e.g., Pit-ten Cate, Kennedy, & Stevenson, 2002; Shields et al., 1995). It is intended to assist mothers and fathers to express their needs and concerns at the time of the initial drafting of a support plan (Bailey & Blasco, 1990). In our Manitoba survey of families with young children with developmental and intellectual disabilities, we found the FNS to have high internal reliability for both mothers and fathers (Trute

& Hiebert-Murphy, 2005). Our analysis suggested that the FNS comprised three main factors or subscales: Information Needs, Managing Resources Needs, and Facilitative Counselling Needs. The items that formed the Facilitative Counselling Needs subscale of the FNS reflect a parent's perceived need for professional assistance related to specific issues in interpersonal relations (e.g., explaining her/his child's disability to others, help to resolve emotional issues related to her/his child's disability in the family). In families with young children with disabilities, this subscale was found to be important in predicting, over a one year period, maternal and paternal perceptions of family maladjustment and maternal parenting stress. Empirical assessment tools such as the FNS may hold potential to serve a predictive function as well as supplementing the interview in the ongoing assessment of family service needs. They may help to identify families at risk for longer-term distress and deserving of a higher service priority for psychosocial support resources.

We are not suggesting that empirical tools such as the FNS be employed as a replacement for the interview. However, our experience has taught us that they can importantly serve to supplement and enhance the interview process. In our experience, most parents will respond positively when invited to complete needs inventories such as the FNS, as it serves as a way for them to quickly and systematically outline their needs for support. Some parents have reported to us that the FNS helped them identify needs that did not immediately come to mind when they were first asked to identify their service hopes and goals.

Measures such as the Family Needs Survey also assist families in identifying sensitive issues that are of concern that they wish to discuss with service providers. For example, a parent may indicate the following need listed as an item on the FNS: "My spouse needs help in understanding and accepting our child's condition." This acknowledgment of a need opens the door for the practitioner to gently explore the issue. In this way, a non-threatening measure may help a family member express a need that might be difficult to raise in an interview and gives the practitioner permission to explore issues in the emotional life of the family.

Intensity and complexity of service needs. We have suggested that in child health and developmental services many parents will only want assistance with practical family support resources that are immediately required for the well-being of their children and families. These needs can range from low-cost, short-term respite to more expensive needs such as a physical lift for a son or daughter with a serious mobility dis-ability, and who has grown to a size and weight that makes entry to a bath or a wheelchair a challenge for the parent (particularly the parent's arms and back). In such situations of practical or informational needs, the service assessment process can be brief, direct, and parsimonious in time required from the parent and professional. However, there will be families who will have need for more extensive psychosocial supports such as out-of-home respite or ongoing facilitative counselling. Much will depend on the service context (e.g., child health or child welfare) and whether services are voluntary or involuntary in their delivery. For example, child psychiatric services and child protection services will tend to have larger proportions of families in their caseloads with complex needs for psychosocial support resources. In these situations, the family-centred practitioner will be required to expand the scope of assessment and service planning to include a more in-depth consider-ation of family functioning and patterns of family resiliency.

The Ecological Perspective: A Key Conceptual Framework

The theoretical model that has been most useful in providing an over-arching conceptual model for assessment in family-centred practice is the ecological perspective, which has its roots in general systems the-ory (Freeman, 1981; Miller, 1978). The ecological perspective assists in the shift from a narrow focus on individual behaviour and functioning to an expanded scope of assessment that includes gathering informa-tion on relationships within the family, and further, on family-commu-nity interactions. A consideration of networks of social support, be they informal (e.g., family and friends) or formal (e.g., churches, hospital staff), is an important component of this assessment. The family is seen to be not only a supra-system to the individual but, simultaneously, a subsystem of the community. That is, the ecological perspective attends to human transactions within the family and also beyond the boundary of the family to include transactions between family members and their physical, social, spiritual, and cultural environments.

The ecological perspective as it is applied to child development was first explicated by Uri Bronfenbrenner (1979). He described a series of embedded and interrelated ecological niches that were salient to the understanding and study of child well-being and growth. When prac-ticing from an ecological perspective, one seeks to understand, activate, and enrich family support resources, while simultaneously strengthening the coping resources of individual family members, so that a better match can be achieved between family members' needs and priorities and the circumstances of their physical and social environments (Hartman & Laird, 1983). The ecological perspective influences family assessment and family-centred practice through the identification of five fundamental areas of concern (Rodway & Trute, 1993):

- personal and family adaptation and competency;
- interpersonal and inter-system transactions (particularly within the family);
- developmental themes which are salient at the levels of the person, family, and community;
- social network resources in promoting change and maintaining stability; and
- the cultural context which frames individual and family behaviours and beliefs.

(The assessment of social network support is more fully addressed in Chapter 7, and cultural implications of practice are considered in Chapter 12.)

Assessing Family Functioning and Resiliency

Exploring the family holons. Family systems theory has provided a succinct framework for the assessment of family functioning. In their explication of the implications of systems theory for family practice, Minuchin and Fishman (1981) identify the differentiation and function of the "holon" or subsystem as being a salient element of human systems. The holon is seen as corresponding to a subunit of a system, yet is also a system in its own right (e.g., the person is a holon of the family, the family is a holon of the community). Holons are independent yet part of each other in a "continuing, current, and ongoing process of communication and interrelationship" (Minuchin & Fishman, 1981, p. 13). Holons are created within families to accomplish basic tasks (e.g., parenting, regulating sibling relations). Human systems then are not simply a collection of individuals but are complex multilevel entities, entities in which one must look beyond the sum of the parts to see the interactional elements. These interactions in the family usually go beyond mechanistic linear relations (in which "a" causes or leads to "b"), to more often reflect recursive relations (in which "a" and "b" can be mutually linked in reciprocal and changing patterns of cause and effect). For example, in the parental holon (the subsystem that is the family executive authority or hub of family management), there may be permanent membership and roles (e.g., a mother and grandmother) or temporary membership and roles (e.g., the oldest sibling takes over in the parenting role when a single parent is not available).

The systems perspective represents a dramatic shift in assessment when compared to the paramount focus on the child in traditional children's services. The systems perspective expands the primary practice interest to include a wider emphasis on child and family relations and family functioning as a salient context for child development. The process of assessment of child and family well-being is dependent on many complex interrelated individual and family elements. For example, the systems principle of equifinality (e.g., there are many alternative routes to achieving a goal or "there are many roads to Mecca") replaces the idea of simple cause and effect, in which the "correct" diagnosis leads to the "correct" prescription for the "correct" treatment. Assessment of complex human systems, such as children within families, is recognized as an ongoing process that is responsive to new information about a changing entity. Family-centred practice therefore requires flexible strategies of assessment.

Assessing family holons. In their identification of major family holons (or subsystems) to serve as a guide to family assessment, Minuchin and Fishman (1981) differentiate between individual, spousal, parental, and sibling holons. In effect, this typology offers a basic framework for assessment of family membership and family organization which is consistent with family developmental theory (Walsh, 1993). When two people (i.e., individual holons) join each other in a committed, long-term relationship (i.e., spousal holon), the prototype of a family holon is created. This union becomes formalized through the development of mutual expectations (e.g., addressing emotional, instrumental, sexual, and financial needs) and requires reciprocal accommodations to establish mutually satisfying sexual, household, and lifestyle routines. The spousal holon as an entity goes through its own developmental stages as it evolves and matures over time. At first, infatuation and excitement is high in the spousal holon, which over time becomes tempered and expanded to include negotiation of mutually satisfactory sexual relations and partnership in household management. Development of the spousal subsystem sets the stage for future child-rearing. In the same way that it makes sense to collect adequate information to understand the needs and priorities of each member of the family, it also makes sense when working with families with young children to assess the organization and strengths of the spousal holon. Many parents of young children with serious developmental disabilities become so preoccupied with the needs of their child that they forget that their spousal relationship also needs attention and deserves nurturing. This is important to ensure that they will continue to remain together as partners, and it is important for their spousal relationship to mature and be stable over time. In the longer term, the investment of time and attention by conjugal partners to the spousal holon may be as essential to long-term child well-being as is ongoing parental attention to the child's developmental challenges. There are, of course, many families that do not fit the intact, two parent model. In these families there may not be a spousal relationship. In these instances, attention might be given to the ways in which the parent gets her/his needs for adult interaction met.

Assessing the parental holon. In the process of family assessment, an important distinction is made between the spousal and the parental holon. Spouses become parents with the entry of a child into the life of their family of procreation. The parental holon addresses child-rearing tasks such as childcare, discipline, and socialization. In some cases it might include different persons than does the spousal holon. For example, in a single parent family it may include a mother and the mother's mother (i.e., maternal grandmother). In families where there has been divorce, ex-spouses may continue to function as co-parents. Most family practitioners consider the parental holon the "hub" or "central authority" in typically functioning families. In families with young children, it is important to assess membership, organization, and functioning of each family's parental holon. I previously noted that in some heterosexual families with young children with severe developmental disabilities or health challenges, mothers and fathers are pulled into a traditional patriarchal pattern of parenting, even if they initially maintained their spousal relations on a highly egalitarian basis. The challenging family circumstances combine with structural factors (including cultural expectations about gender roles in families, the limitations of community services available to assist families in meeting children's needs, and the demands of workplaces) to create a context in which one parent must take primary responsibility for childcare. This responsibility more frequently falls on mothers, with fathers often focusing their energy and time on generating income for the family.

These situations call for a skilled balancing of spousal and parental responsibilities to ensure a distribution of family workload that is seen by family members to be fair, equitable, and efficient. Such a balance may require challenging the broader structural context that reinforces traditional family roles. This could include helping parents to allocate childcare duties in the family in a way that shifts away from traditional gender expectations. It might also involve advocating for change in the support services available to the family, for example, securing additional family support resources that would allow mothers to remain in the workplace if they wish to do so.

Assessing the sibling holon. The sibling holon is created as children enter the life of the family. Siblings can support and learn from each other, as well as seek to establish their own identity and place in the family. Larger families that are resilient or strong in their adaptation to serious childhood illness or disability often show a family pattern in which the child with the disability is viewed as "part of the family" rather than the "centre of the family." In this respect, each sibling is appreciated as a unique individual and has her/his individuality respected. There is a balance between sibling·"individuality" (i.e., being her/his own person) and "mutuality" (i.e., the responsibilities each sibling holds as a member of the family). This balance between individual autonomy and family allegiance is dependent on the capabilities, needs, and desires of each sibling. In assessment of the sibling holon in families with children with serious disabilities or health challenges, it is of interest to note when, how, and for what duration a sibling is drawn into the parental holon to provide care and direction to her/his brother or sister with special childcare needs.

Drafting a family genogram as a basic tool in family assessment. A tool that is often employed to graphically outline the membership and organization of a family is the family genogram (McGoldrick & Gerson, 1985). In its simplest application, the family diagram can offer a brief description of the membership of key family holons. For example, consider Figure 5.1.

This family diagram offers a graphic outline of the Smith family in which Michael and Sally Smith reside in the same community as do both of their mothers (with both maternal and paternal grandfathers being deceased, as is indicated by the "X" in their boxes). Each line of the genogram represents a generation of the family, with males represented by a square and females by a circle. The top line contains the maternal and paternal grandparents while the middle line contains the

Figure 5.1. The Smith Family Genogram

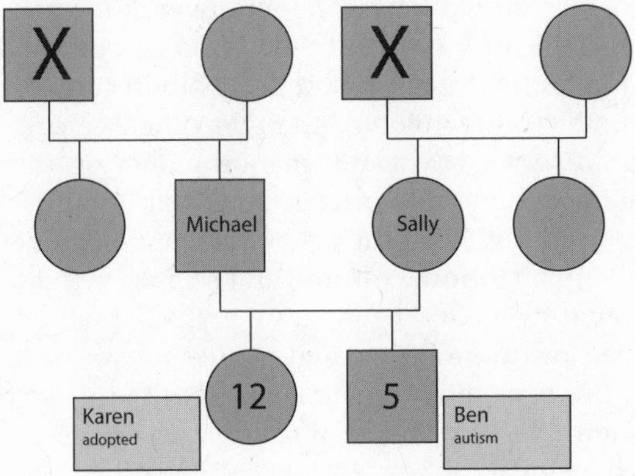

parents' generation (each is shown to have a sister). The bottom line contains the children in the family of procreation. There are two children. The youngest child, Ben, is a 5-year-old male that has been diagnosed with autism spectrum disorder (ASD). The oldest child, Karen, is a 12-year-old adopted daughter. If one wishes to practice from a family-centred perspective, then at a minimum one should know who is in the immediate family (with basic knowledge being three generations of the family: child, parents, and grandparents). It is beyond the scope of this chapter to offer a detailed instruction on the completion of the genogram. However, there are a number of sources available that provide more detailed directions (e.g., Hartman, & Laird, 1983).

As previously suggested, it is important when working with families of children with health or developmental disabilities to begin the process by assuming that these are ordinary families with special children (Seligman & Darling, 1997). The initial genogram therefore does not seek to delve deeply into the emotional life of the family, but serves as a tool to inform the practitioner about family membership and organization. The genogram should not be viewed as a static instrument which is completed at service intake, attached to the client's file, and then disregarded. It should be seen as a tool that is an ongoing guide and that can serve in the continuing process of information gathering. It can open the door to new and important information about the life of families. For example, in the genogram of the Smith family, the circumstances of there being an older sister and grandmothers living nearby may have implications for understanding who constitutes the parental holon. Is the older sister involved in helping with the parenting of her brother (since she is an adolescent who is seven years older)? Do the parents turn to their mothers for practical help in caring for their son? Is one grandmother more involved than the other?

The genogram serves as an information gathering framework that follows an interactive method of collecting and organizing important details about the family. It is a means of information gathering that can place the family in historical, cultural, and social context. Asking questions when preparing a family genogram is a skill that will evolve with practice and become more focused and efficient over time, as a service provider gains more experience and comfort with this approach to understanding family history and organization.

It is best to develop a capacity to ask simple questions that stimulate the sharing of important information about the family. For example, asking parents to describe the strengths or positive qualities they see in their child with a disability or developmental challenge, or asking parents about the positive influences their child with special needs has on a sibling, may lead to a greater understanding of family dynamics. Important events in the history of a family, and changes in the family circumstances over time as the child with special needs grows, can have saliency in the understanding of current family functioning.

It is important to think of the family in developmental terms, in that not only does a child grow older and go through developmental stages, but simultaneously, the siblings and parents of that child also age and develop. Furthermore, family structure, such as the place of the child with special needs in the span of sibling ages, can have important implications for family organization and functioning. Brothers and sisters can be influenced in different ways when a sibling with special needs is older versus younger. Other important contextual influences such as family culture and family religiosity can have profound implications for internal family organization, and for the patterns of relations that each family member has with friends and associates. These persons who are not family members, but who are an emotional or practical resource to a family member, can play an important role in how family members cope with and respond to situational crises or life challenges.

The McMaster Model of Family Functioning. Another conceptual model of the family that can be helpful in family assessment is the McMaster Model of Family Functioning (Epstein, Ryan, Bishop, Miller, & Keitner, 2003). This model leads to assessment of the family as a "working unit" and considers seven aspects or sub-dimensions of family functioning. These include

- *task accomplishment*, how well things get done in and by the family to maintain effective functioning;
- *role performance*, who does what tasks and carries what responsibilities in the family to complete family functions;
- *control*, how well rules are understood and how fair they are;
- *involvement*, the sense of belonging and mutuality in the family;
- *communication*, how well members communicate information to each other;
- *affective expression*, how openly and clearly emotions are expressed in the family; and
- *values and norms*, how closely beliefs and values are shared by family members.

Skinner, Steinhauer, and Santa-Barbara (1995) have developed the Family Assessment Measure which is in its third version (FAM-III). This empirical tool, which is based on the McMaster Model of Family Functioning, offers a comprehensive approach to assessing overall family functioning from the perspective of the adjustment of each individual in the family, key dyads in the family (e.g., father–eldest child), and the family as an overall entity. Norms are available for adults and adolescents, and the FAM-III is available in a number of languages including English, French, Spanish, and German. A short form of the FAM-III is available as a 14-item overall assessment of family well-being that can be employed, when it is appropriate in the flow of information that emerges in the family assessment process, as a supplement to the assessment interview. The total score allows the practitioner to consider if the family falls within the "normal range" of family functioning as perceived by a youth or parent. As well, the response to each individual item by family members opens the door to more dialogue about family issues and strengths.

Understanding family resiliency. Walsh (1998) provides guidance for family assessments that go beyond the study of family subsystems and family organization. She identifies three key assessment areas when considering patterns of family resiliency. These are

- *family belief systems*, which include the consideration of how a family makes meaning of threats or adversity, a family's propensity to

maintain a positive outlook, and the place and importance of spiri-
tuality in the life of the family;

- *organizational patterns*, which have to do with a family's flexibility in
  response to challenges, family members' ability to remain cohesive
  or connected to each other, and a family's social support and economic resources; and
- *communication processes*, which involve the openness and clarity of
  communication of information and of emotions as well as family
  members' abilities in collaborative problem solving. (p. 24)

Assessing family coping and adjustment. When parent or family distress becomes evident during the assessment process, then more careful
attention needs to be given to elements that underlie parenting stress or
family maladaptation and to the resources that are required to facilitate
positive adjustment or adaptation by the parent or family. This takes
the family-centred practitioner into a deeper level in the exploration of
parenting issues and family assessment in the completion of a support
plan. A theoretical model which is helpful in the assessment of family
response to life stresses and challenges is the classic ABCX Model of
family stress and coping (Hill, 1949). This model views the family as
responding to stress and managing resources, from both within and
outside the family, when coping with that stressor. Figure 5.2 offers a
graphic description of the components of this model.

In this model

- "A" represents the stressor or family challenge, such as the diagnosis of a developmental disability or chronic health challenge in a
  child or the emergence of significant behavioural issues.
- "B" represents coping resources that are mobilized in response to
  the perceived threat or stressor. These can be considered to be "internal" or psychological coping resources of the family members
  (such as self-esteem, morale, optimism, etc.) or "external" coping
  resources such as social network support. External coping resources
  are usually classified as "informal" (e.g., extended family, friends)
  or "formal" (e.g., paediatrician, child welfare agency, daycare
  centre).
- "C" is the meaning family members make of the threatening or
  challenging event. The challenging event may be seen as having
  negative, neutral, or positive influences on family life.

Figure 5.2. ABCX Model (Hill, 1949)

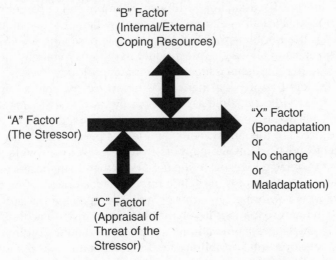

"B" Factor
(Internal/External
Coping Resources)

"A" Factor
(The Stressor)

"X" Factor
(Bonadaptation
or
No change
or
Maladaptation)

"C" Factor
(Appraisal of
Threat of the
Stressor)

- "X" is the level of family functioning that is achieved in response to the stressor or family challenge. Does the family deteriorate in its functioning as a result of the challenge, does it stay the same, or does it grow stronger?

The ABCX Model can serve as a template for the stress and coping aspects of family assessment. In particular, the B and C factors are important to explore in the development of a support plan. Consideration of the B factor leads to an exploration of the strength of internal and external coping resources of parents and family members. In terms of internal coping resources, family-centred practitioners should appreciate the importance of parenting self-esteem and sense of self-efficacy in the ability of parents to meet their ongoing childcare responsibilities. These issues can be gently explored during early assessment interviews, and there are brief empirical measures that can be employed as a supplement to the interview. For example, the Parenting Morale Index (PMI; Trute & Hiebert-Murphy, 2005) offers a 10-item questionnaire (see the appendix) that explores both positive and negative feelings in regard to parenting. Brief screening instruments such as the PMI can offer a non-threatening and minimally intrusive way of opening the door to a more extensive discussion of both positive and negative parenting experiences. The PMI allows parents to identify whether or not they wish to address the emotions they experience while parenting a child with special needs and allows the practitioner to follow the parent's lead in addressing the emotional issues the parent identifies.

The exploration of social network support, or external coping resources, should be a routine aspect of family-centred assessment. The scope of this assessment should be congruent with the support priorities and needs of the family. For example, if a parent simply seeks intermittent and brief respite support from the service provider, only information related to respite relief need be gathered. In the assessment of "external" coping resources, it is important for practitioners to appreciate what is "normal" in terms of family social networks and social support in family situations involving children with serious disabilities or health challenges. For example, families with young children with serious developmental disabilities tend to have sparse social networks composed of a few family members and friends (Trute & Hauch, 1988). Because of the importance of family support resources within family-centred practice theory, we devote a chapter of this book to this topic (Chapter 7). This chapter more fully considers the assessment of family social support resources and the building, mobilization, and/or coordination of social network resources as a fundamental aspect of family-centred practice in children's services.

The ABCX Model, in its C factor, emphasizes the importance of the construct of family meaning, or appraisal, of a stressor in understanding patterns of family coping and adaptation. The appraisal process is filtered through the family schema, which is a set of shared beliefs and values that serve as a basis in which family experiences are interpreted and understood (McCubbin, Thompson, Thompson, & McCubbin, 1993). When applying models of family stress and coping in children's services, it is important to view challenges or stressors as having an activating effect that can be positive or negative depending on the meaning that parents make of the challenge or stressor. Much depends on personal and social factors that mediate the impact of stressors, including the personal attributes or cognitive and emotional resources of the person under stress (Aldwin, 1994). For example, psychological coping resources that are often considered to be related to parenting stress are parent morale, self-esteem, and self-efficacy, and these can influence the meaning that is made of a stressor related to childcare. Thus, the C and B factors can be seen to be reciprocal and interrelated aspects in the process of coping. Further, coping can be viewed in terms of management rather than removal of a stressor, which is salient to the chronic nature of family demands associated with issues such as childhood disability (Beresford, 1994).

Impact of children's special needs on parents' well-being. Many professionals anticipate or assume that childhood disability or serious child health challenges will lead to parent chronic depression, high parenting stress, and frequent family distress. They do not understand that although parenting stress may be high at times, this does not directly or invariably lead to psychopathology in a parent or to family discord. Prior research has shown that although families with children with developmental challenges show relatively higher levels of parenting stress, they are within normal limits for family functioning (e.g., Mahoney, O'Sullivan, & Robinson, 1992; Seligman & Darling, 1997). There is evidence that positive transformation, where families develop a deeper appreciation of the meaning of family and a stronger sense of purpose, are potential outcomes of childhood disability (Abbott & Meredith, 1986; Mullins, 1987; Stainton & Besser, 1998; Seideman & Kleine, 1995). Aldwin (1994) summarizes the literature on stress and coping as showing that psychosocial stress can lead to positive effects such as the strengthening of social ties and "the development of mastery and self-esteem, enhanced perspectives on life, or a larger coping repertoire for use in future situations" (p. 274). Scorgie and Sobsey (2000) summarize positively perceived impacts in situations of childhood disability as "transformational" parenting experiences that include personal growth in family members, improved relations with others, and positive changes in philosophical or spiritual values.

Wolfensberger (1972), a pioneer in the development of "normalization" principles for people with intellectual disabilities, posited that parents go through a period of "novelty shock" when their child is diagnosed with a disability. He saw this as a temporary period that involved coming to terms with unanticipated losses that required both psychological adjustment and the development of confidence that the situation could be positively managed. Trute's (1995) survey of Manitoba families supported this assertion, in that levels of depression in mothers of young children with developmental disabilities was found to diminish over the preschool years, rather than increase. Parenting stress experienced by these mothers increased as their children grew older, but their psychological adjustment improved. This offers some important lessons for early parent and family assessment in childhood disability services. First of all, one must not take the early adjustment period as a time that reflects what will be "normal" functioning for a parent or for a family. Second, the cognitive appraisal, or the meaning that parents make of the impact of their child's challenges, may change over time as they live the experience, realize that they can competently handle the situation, and see that there are both positive and negative impacts that accrue as a consequence of the disability in the life of the family. Third, positive and negative appraisals may coexist, with parents recognizing that at times there are both negative and positive family impacts of childhood disability (Trute, Hiebert-Murphy, & Levine, 2007).

Negative cognitive appraisal has been found to be related to parenting stress associated with childhood disability (Saloviita, Itälinna, & Leinonen, 2003). However, Folkman and Moskowitz (2000) suggest that positive appraisal of the demands of family caregiving may be particularly important in helping people sustain coping efforts over long periods of time. This is consistent with research findings that positive perceptions and meaning attributed to aspects of child disability can assist coping in parents (Stainton & Besser, 1998; Tennen & Affleck, 1999). Therefore, it is important in the assessment of the C factor in the ABCX Model of family stress and adaptation that attention is given both to negative and positive appraisals of family impacts of childhood challenges and, further, that this is done with an understanding of, and a sensitivity to, the initial period of adjustment that many parents face when it is confirmed that their child has a disability or serious health challenge. When working within the context of childhood behavioural, health, or developmental challenges, The Family Impact of Childhood Disability Scale (FICD) can help in the assessment of the C factor, as it is a brief, 20-item scale (see the appendix) that gives a parent's appraisals of both the positive and negative family impacts of childhood disability (Benzies, Trute, Worthington, Reddon, Keown, & Moore, 2011; Trute & Hiebert-Murphy, 2005; Trute et al., 2007).

Assessing Needs for Psychosocial Supports, Facilitative Counselling, and Family Therapy

In family-centred practice, the meaning that parents make of their child's challenges and the perceived impacts that these challenges have on family life become salient in assessment. In families that do not appear to be coping adequately, this situation may lead to conversations with parents regarding their beliefs about the causes of their child's disability, and perhaps issues of parental attribution of blame. It may lead to conversations about "realistic" parent and family expectations, as well as perceived personal and family limitations that are consequent to their child's disability. These are examples of important issues that can be relevant in the assessment of family strengths and family needs for psychosocial supports. Earlier in this book (in Chapter 3) consideration was given to the differences between family-centred counselling and family therapy. It is important for family-centred practitioners to be able to make an assessment that would allow them to determine when a family would benefit from specialized therapeutic resources, such as those that are offered by family therapy and require a referral to professionals who have the expertise required to assist parents and families experiencing significant distress.

Issues in Information Gathering

Family assessment as an ongoing process. There will be times when families do not respond well or openly to assessments initiated by professionals. This may be a signal that all is not well with the process of information gathering, rather than an indication of "family pathology." That is, family members' reactions may have to do with their sense that the information being gathered is irrelevant to their understanding of what services should include or should have as their focus. As well, it may be based on feelings of intimidation or feelings of not being respected and understood. When this occurs, it is a signal that the process needs to be slowed, that more attention needs to be given to relationship building, and that working alliance is not sufficiently secured. There are often good reasons for families to be "resistant" or "non-compliant" when family assessment is initiated at the onset of services. First, the family may have had prior negative experiences with professionals. This is not unusual in child welfare services or when services are initiated with families living in poverty or in marginalized communities. Many of these families have had exposure to professionals who do not practice from a family-centred perspective. These families will have experienced service failures and believe that in the past they did not receive what was required by them and their family members, or that inadequate or inappropriate services were offered or delivered. If the assessment process is rushed or if too much information is sought too quickly, families may feel offended or not appreciate the relevance of the information gathering. If the procedures of assessment, or the forms that are employed to gather information, are not understood because of illiteracy or limited reading comprehension, this can be overwhelming or give rise to shame in family members. As well, some families will feel vulnerable because of the serious and extensive needs of their child and other family members. They may feel insecure about expressing their views and ideas, and feel pushed to proceed in ways that seem to them to be the priorities of the professional or agency, rather than in close concert with their priorities and needs.

When service providers are engaged in dialogues with family members for the purposes of gathering assessment information, the intent is to maintain "open awareness." That is, as practitioners, we must proceed with honest curiosity and respect for the views of the family. The primary intent is to clarify and understand the beliefs and perceptions of those we are assisting. Our intent should not be to implant or inject our opinions and interpretations (even when we are convinced that they are accurate). In this respect, our most powerful tools are our listening skills and relevant and well-timed questions (knowing that a crude and poorly timed question can be disrespectful or abusive). The intent is not primarily to make diagnoses and give people the "answers" to their challenges and dilemmas. The intent is to share understanding with those who seek our help, and to mutually explore and better understand the issues and hurdles that block progress towards more positive adjustment, meaningful problem resolution, and effective accommodation. When we engage in a family-centred assessment, it is done in the hope that it will serve to advance problem solving and capacity building; it is done with the understanding that the professional brings her/his own knowledge and perspective to the collaborative interpretation, as does the family, and that there is shared effort in this process. It does not identify the role of the professional as the expert who has the job of "fixing things," particularly when the professional enters the psychological realm or emotional life of the family. The first duty is to help family members grow stronger and take as much charge and self-agency as they can to advance their child's and their own well-being in their social, economic, and cultural world.

Understanding child with family: A strategy of information gathering. A sequential strategy of information gathering has been suggested in this chapter that starts with the assumption of parent and family "normality," that follows the lead of the parent(s) in terms of the identification and clarification of family support needs, and that includes the consideration of focused service goals that are of immediate relevance to the family. Attention has been given to the importance of two intertwined goals of the process of family assessment: building a working alliance between the professional and family members and gathering salient family information to guide support planning. As the family support plan becomes more complex or challenging, and as it addresses issues having to do with the emotional well-being of family members, there will be a greater need for the development of a deeper and more closely collaborative partnership. In this sense, assessment and working alliance are not mutually exclusive practice components but operate in tandem.

REFERENCES

Abbott, D.A., & Meredith, W.H. (1986). Strengths of parents with retarded children. *Family Relations, 35*(3), 371–5. http://dx.doi.org/10.2307/584363

Aldwin, C.M. (1994). *Stress, coping, and development: An integrative perspective.* New York, NY: Guilford Press.

Bailey, D.B., Jr, & Blasco, P.M. (1990). Parents' perspectives on a written survey of family needs. *Journal of Early Intervention, 14*(3), 196–203. http://dx.doi.org/10.1177/105381519001400302

Bailey, D.B., Jr, & Simeonsson, R.J. (1988). Assessing needs of families with handicapped infants. *Journal of Special Education, 22*(1), 117–27. http://dx.doi.org/10.1177/002246698802200113

Benzies, K.M., Trute, B., Worthington, C., Reddon, J., Keown, L.A., & Moore, M. (2011, June). Assessing psychological well-being in mothers of children with disability: Evaluation of the Parenting Morale Index and Family Impact of Childhood Disability Scale. *Journal of Pediatric Psychology, 36*(5), 506–16. http://dx.doi.org/10.1093/jpepsy/jsq081 Medline:20843877

Beresford, B.A. (1994, January). Resources and strategies: How parents cope with the care of a disabled child. *Journal of Child Psychology and Psychiatry, and Allied Disciplines, 35*(1), 171–209. http://dx.doi.org/10.1111/j.1469-7610.1994.tb01136.x Medline:8163627

Borrell-Carrió, F., Suchman, A.L., & Epstein, R.M. (2004, November-December). The biopsychosocial model 25 years later: Principles, practice, and scientific inquiry. *Annals of Family Medicine, 2*(6), 576–82. http://dx.doi.org/10.1370/afm.245 Medline:15576544

Bronfenbrenner, U. (1979). *The ecology of human development: Experiments by nature and design.* Cambridge, MA: Harvard University Press.

Davis, S.K., & Gettinger, M. (1995). Family-focused assessment for identifying family resources and concerns: Parent preferences, assessment information, and evaluation across three methods. *Journal of School Psychology, 33*(2), 99–121. http://dx.doi.org/10.1016/0022-4405(95)00001-3

Epstein, N.B., Ryan, C.E., Bishop, D.S., Miller, I.W., & Keitner, G.I. (2003). The McMaster model: A view of healthy family functioning. In F. Walsh (Ed.), *Normal family processes* (3rd ed., pp. 581–607). New York, NY: The Guilford Press.

Folkman, S., & Moskowitz, J.T. (2000, June). Positive affect and the other side of coping. *American Psychologist, 55*(6), 647–54. http://dx.doi.org/10.1037/0003-066X.55.6.647 Medline:10892207

Freeman, D. (1981). *Techniques of family therapy.* New York, NY: Jacob Aronson.

Hartman, A., & Laird, J. (1983). *Family-centered social work practice.* New York, NY: Free Press.

Hill, R. (1949). *Families under stress: Adjustment to the crisis of war, separation, and reunion.* New York, NY: Harper Row.

Krauss, M.W. (2000). Family assessment within early intervention programs. In J.P. Shonkoff & S.J. Meisels, (Eds.), *Handbook of early childhood intervention* (2nd ed., pp. 290–308). Cambridge, England: Cambridge University Press. http://dx.doi.org/10.1017/CBO9780511529320.015

Mahoney, G., O'Sullivan, P., & Robinson, C. (1992). The family environments of children with disabilities: Diverse but not so different. *Topics in Early Childhood Special Education, 12*(3), 386–402. http://dx.doi.org/10.1177/027112149201200309

McCubbin, H.I., Thompson, E.A., Thompson, A.I., & McCubbin, M.A. (1993). Family schema, paradigms, and paradigm shifts: Components and processes of appraisal in family adaptation to crises. In A. Turnbull, J. Patterson, S. Behr, D. Murphy, J. Marquis, & M. Blue-Banning (Eds.), *Cognitive coping, families, and disability* (pp. 239–55). Baltimore, MD: Paul H. Brookes.

McGoldrick, M., & Gerson, R. (1985). *Genograms in family assessment.* New York, NY: Norton.

Miller, J.M. (1978). *Living systems.* New York, NY: McGraw Hill.

Minuchin, S., & Fishman, H.C. (1981). *Family therapy techniques.* Cambridge, MA: Harvard University Press.

Mullins, J.B. (1987). Authentic voices from parents of exceptional children. *Family Relations, 36*(1), 30–3. http://dx.doi.org/10.2307/584643

Pit-ten Cate, I.M., Kennedy, C., & Stevenson, J. (2002, May). Disability and quality of life in spina bifida and hydrocephalus. *Developmental Medicine and Child Neurology, 44*(5), 317–22. http://dx.doi.org/10.1111/j.1469-8749.2002.tb00818.x Medline:12033717

Rodway, P., & Trute, B. (1993). Ecological family therapy. In P. Rodway & B. Trute (Eds.), *The ecological perspective in family-centered therapy* (pp. 3–19). Lewiston, NY: Edwin Mellon Press.

Saloviita, T., Itälinna, M., & Leinonen, E. (2003, May-June). Explaining the parental stress of fathers and mothers caring for a child with intellectual disability: A double ABCX Model. *Journal of Intellectual Disability Research, 47*(4-5), 300–12. http://dx.doi.org/10.1046/j.1365-2788.2003.00492.x Medline:12787162

Scorgie, K., & Sobsey, D. (2000, June). Transformational outcomes associated with parenting children who have disabilities. *Mental Retardation, 38*(3), 195–206. http://dx.doi.org/10.1352/0047-6765(2000)038<0195:TOAWPC>2.0.CO;2 Medline:10900927

Seideman, R.Y., & Kleine, P.F. (1995, January-February). A theory of transformed parenting: Parenting a child with developmental delay/mental retardation. *Nursing Research, 44*(1), 38–44. Medline:7532298

Seligman, M., & Darling, R.B. (1997). *Ordinary families, special children: A systems approach to childhood disability* (2nd ed.). New York, NY: Guilford Press.

Shields, G., Schondel, C., Barnhart, L., Fitzpatrick, V., Sidell, N., Adams, P., ..., & Gomez, S. (1995). Social work in pediatric oncology: A family needs assessment. *Social Work in Health Care, 21*(1), 39–54. http://dx.doi.org/10.1300/J010v21n01_04 Medline:8553190

Skinner, H.A., Steinhauer, P.D., & Santa-Barbara, J. (1995). *FAM III – Family Assessment Measure version III. Technical manual*. Toronto, ON: Multi-Health Systems.

Slentz, K.L., & Bricker, D. (1992). Family guided assessment for IFSP development: Jumping off the family assessment bandwagon. *Journal of Early Intervention, 16*(1), 11–19. http://dx.doi.org/10.1177/105381519201600102

Stainton, T., & Besser, H. (1998). The positive impact of children with intellectual disability on the family. *Journal of Intellectual & Developmental Disability, 23*(1), 57–70. http://dx.doi.org/10.1080/13668259800033581

Tennen, H., & Affleck, G. (1999). Finding benefits in adversity. In C.R. Snyder (Ed.), *Coping: The psychology of what works* (pp. 279–304). New York, NY: Oxford University Press.

Trute, B. (1995, October). Gender differences in the psychological adjustment of parents of young, developmentally disabled children. *Journal of Child Psychology and Psychiatry, and Allied Disciplines, 36*(7), 1225–42. http://dx.doi.org/10.1111/j.1469-7610.1995.tb01367.x Medline:8847382

Trute, B., & Hauch, C. (1988). Building on family strength: A study of families with positive adjustment to the birth of a developmentally disabled

child. *Journal of Marital and Family Therapy, 14*(2), 185–93. http://dx.doi.
    org/10.1111/j.1752-0606.1988.tb00734.x

Trute, B., & Hiebert-Murphy, D. (2005). Predicting family adjustment and par-
    enting stress in childhood disability services using brief assessment tools.
    Journal of Intellectual & Developmental Disability, 30(4), 217–25. http://dx.doi.
    org/10.1080/13668250500349441

Trute, B., Hiebert-Murphy, D., & Levine, K. (2007, March). Parental appraisal
    of the family impact of childhood developmental disability: Times of sad-
    ness and times of joy. *Journal of Intellectual & Developmental Disability, 32*(1),
    1–9. http://dx.doi.org/10.1080/13668250601146753 Medline:17365362

Walsh, F. (1993). *Normal family processes* (2nd ed.). New York, NY: Guilford
    Press.

Walsh, F. (1998). *Strengthening family resilience*. New York, NY: Guilford Press.

Weston, W.W. (2005). Patient-centered medicine: A guide to the biopsy-
    chosocial model. *Families, Systems & Health, 23*(4), 387–92. http://dx.doi.
    org/10.1037/1091-7527.23.4.387

Wolfensberger, W. (1972). *Normalization: The principle of normalization in human
    services*. Toronto, ON: National Institute on Mental Retardation.

6 Capacity Building and Empowerment Practice

KATHRYN LEVINE

The Concept of Empowerment

The concept of empowerment is widely embraced in the human services and there is an extensive literature on empowerment initiatives within the theory and practice of social science disciplines (Gutierrez, 1990, 1995; McWhirter, 1991; Suarez-Balcazar, Harper, & Lewis, 2005). Empowerment is also at the forefront of the majority of policy directives that guide human services, and it would be difficult to discover a program that does not seek to "empower" its clients in some way. However, the use of the term empowerment has become a cliché to the extent that the rhetoric significantly outweighs practitioners' comprehensive knowledge of the components and procedures of empowerment. That is, people talk about it but do not necessarily know how to incorporate its methods and goals into their practice routines.

Empowerment has been conceptualized as both a process (i.e., an element of professional practice) and as an outcome (i.e., change in the client as a consequence of professional practice), and there continue to be debates as to which perspective should prevail (Carr, 2003). Although process definitions remain the dominant focus in the social sciences, in practice, empowerment is most often evaluated as an outcome through assessment of the attainment of specific short-range goals and objectives or outcomes. In this context, successful empowerment generally means that individuals act on issues that they define as important, with the intent of securing desired personal control, needed resources, or both. From this perspective, empowerment can be achieved when parents of a child with special needs obtain needed resources, such as mobility devices or respite services, or obtain access to a desired educational program.

In contrast, process definitions of empowerment imply long-term achievements with services directed to enhance psychological empowerment in their clients, which is consequently often less able to be achieved within the short term. Process definitions suggest that empowerment can refer to developmental or lifespan perspectives in which one achieves a sense of personal power (Zimmerman, 1995), the interactions between persons and their environments that encourage them to take action (Herrenkohl, Judson, & Heffner, 1999), experiences that break a negative chain of events (King, Willoughby, Specht, & Brown, 2006), or simply, participating in shared decision-making (Turnbull & Stowe, 2001). Therefore, within family-centred practice, empowerment may be understood as a lifelong and intergenerational process for families, in which the professional or service provider acts only as an instigator or catalyst of heightened self-agency or self-efficacy. For families of children with special needs, empowerment is defined as having a real say in decisions that affect their family and the lives of their children. It is not something that suddenly appears one day, but is a process that develops over time and involves full participation, decision-making, and responsibility.

Empowerment may be evidenced when families with children with special needs

- move from positions of passive recipients of service to ones in which they take an active role in managing the full range of issues related to their child;
- identify multiple choices and courses of action for themselves and their child;
- engage with the service system in meaningful roles at various stages of their child's life;
- express confidence in their abilities to manage difficult situations;
- accept their own personal perspectives on their families as authoritative; and, for some,
- take on advocacy and social action challenges.

Zimmerman (1995) conceptualized empowerment as a developmental process and proposed three domains of psychological or individual empowerment that occur as outcomes of an empowering process: intrapersonal, interactional, and behavioural. The intrapersonal domain consists of a positive self-concept, an internal locus of control, competence, and motivation. The interactional domain refers to the attainment of knowledge and a critical awareness and understanding of the sociopolitical environment. The behavioural domain is manifest in taking on more responsibility oneself for decision-making and participation in collective action. Empowerment therefore occurs in the context of "a series of experiences in which individuals learn to see a closer correspondence to their goals and how to achieve them" (p. 583). This perspective may be most valuable, as it suggests that individuals begin from a particular position and, through critical self-analysis, determine that their current situation may be a function of powerlessness, rather than their perceived inherent deficiencies. Within children's services, this may be evidenced as the recognition by parents that the purpose and content of existing programs are not congruent with their families' needs, are imposed from above with little opportunity for parental input or feedback, and are delivered by professionals who do not respond to family-identified needs.

Conceptualizations of capacity building are subject to similar criticisms in that there is "a striking lack of shared definitions of capacity building, its features and essential elements" (Philbin, 1998, p. 4). As with empowerment, capacity building can refer to initiatives undertaken at the level of the individual, family, group, or community. Capacity building at a parent or family level suggests themes of

- generating knowledge in order to build capacity for change and development,
- facilitating choices and control,
- unfettered access to concrete and material resources,
- recognition of the value of mutual aid and self-help strategies,
- recognition that families have the capacity to address their own issues at a community level, and
- the development of family-accountable policies and service provision.

Through capacity building, people are made aware of new possibilities and are empowered by gaining new skills, upgrading existing skills, and having clear and continuous access to information resources. Although principles of capacity building have their roots in organizational theory and planning, there are significant implications for services delivered within family-centred programs. For example, participatory help-giving models emphasize family responsibility for finding solutions to their identified problems through the acquisition of skills and knowledge and are rated more family-centred by parents than traditional models of help-giving (Dunst, Boyd, Trivette, & Hamby, 2002). What this means is that capacity building within children's services needs to go beyond abstract theoretical conceptualizations and move towards actual implementation through service provider action. The role of the service provider subsequently becomes one of assisting parents to access the knowledge and skills to think critically about their problems and to develop strategies to act on and change these problems.

The translation of family-centred principles into practice remains a challenge, as it requires commitment from both families and professionals to examine existing service delivery policy and practice issues. Dunst et al. (1991, p. 123) have referred to the discrepancy between policies of family-centredness and actual "street level" practices as "implementation lag." Given that the current state of knowledge regarding family-centred practice suggests that it is simply best practice, the continuing discrepancy between principles of family-centredness and the implementation of actual practice requires additional attention from service providers.

Using an integrated framework of capacity building, within an empowerment model, provides practice directives that are applicable in the implementation of family-centred services. First, both concepts are intrinsically linked to ideas about power and control. The concept of power is relational, and both empowerment and capacity-building models refer to processes in which families gain the ability to access and control economic, social, physical, and political resources. However, in order for parents of children with special needs to understand that some of their challenges stem from a lack of power, they must first acknowledge how parents of children with special needs were historically understood. As a result of the "charity" and "medical" models that have been dominant in the delivery of the human services, parent-professional relations have historically limited families' roles to being passive recipients of service. This translated into professional attitudes towards families in which family members were often characterized as "change resistant," considered a part of the problem rather than the solution, and viewed as targets for service rather than partners in collaboration. In contrast, empowerment within family-centred service describes a practice context that recognizes the power differential that typically exists between parents and service providers. From this position, the balance of power is shifted by removing professional barriers to family participation in planning services and recognizes family-based power wherein families have the power to choose to accept or receive service in a manner that reflects their unique family needs and preferences. For example, an empowerment perspective would acknowledge that parental "resistance" is more likely a reflection of values and beliefs in which family problems are best resolved by the family rather than by professionals. For some professionals, empowerment within family-centred service is as much about facilitating a process whereby families define their needs and make their concerns known as it is about providing service. Through the parent-professional relationship, the practitioner shifts the balance of power by projecting a new way of doing business, which involves high and purposeful engagement and involvement of family members, and recognizes them as mutual experts in the process.

Second, capacity-building and empowerment models emphasize the importance of information and knowledge exchange in order for families to participate in decision-making processes. At an individual level, parents can become empowered by assuming responsibility for their own learning about the needs of their family and how the service system may best assist them. However, their learning is dependent upon the service provider making certain that parents have comprehensive information about their child's diagnosis, the range of existing remedial, therapeutic, and adjunct support services, and the choices available to them, as well as offering other referrals/services that can include connections with other parents. Parents are only able to make appropriate decisions for their children when they are in possession of all of the necessary information. Ensuring straightforward access to information is therefore a tangible approach to power-sharing.

Within conventional service models, when families are viewed solely as recipients of service rather than as interconnected members of the service system, service delivery models neglect to avail themselves of the power and expertise of parents. Empowerment within a capacity-building framework therefore requires professionals to recognize the importance of family-based knowledge as legitimate and essential to service provision. With respect to service provision, acknowledging that parents are the experts on their families is an important first step. The critical second step is for the service provider to facilitate an organized approach to translating this knowledge into action.

Third, both empowerment and capacity-building models stress the importance of using support networks, linking with necessary resources, skill development, and collective action. An important component of empowerment-based service provision is to advise parents about the potential positive impact of social networks. Creating linkages between diverse groups of parents of children with special needs who possess expertise, information, connections, and resources can provide parents with important support and information that may assist them in finding solutions to their particular challenges.

Components of Empowerment Practice

McWhirter (1994) defined empowerment as

> the process by which people, organizations, or groups who are powerless or marginalized (a) become aware of the power dynamics at work in their life context, (b) develop the skills and capacity for gaining some reasonable control over their lives, (c) which they exercise, (d) without infringing on the rights of others, and (e) which coincides with actively supporting the empowerment of others in their community. (p. 422)

From this position, she identified the five interdependent components of capacity building within an empowerment framework as context, collaboration, competence, critical consciousness, and community.

The remainder of this chapter will describe how these principles of capacity building within an empowerment framework may be translated into practice and program delivery within children's services.

Contextual Domains of Family-Centred Practice

Understanding and helping people in the context of their environment is the defining orientation of the ecological perspective, in that human behaviour is inseparable from the context in which it occurs (Bronfenbrenner, 1979). There are multiple contextual domains that need to be considered in terms of providing family-centred services which employ a capacity-building framework. The fundamental assumption of the importance of context acknowledges that there are important historical, sociopolitical, and institutional forces that impact parent and family experiences. The multiple environmental contexts of family life are significantly more diverse, embedded, and interactive than professionals may have initially understood. According to Chronister and McWhirter (2003), important elements of family context include culture and cultural value systems, family structure (e.g., single parent or blended families), religious or spiritual beliefs, adaptive coping strategies, economic situation, quality and depth of social support, and characteristics of the surrounding community, including available services and programs for children with disabilities. In addition, the history of families' relationships with previous service providers will have a profound influence on the nature of current parent-professional relationships. Families may enter the service relationship having been criticized, blamed, or simply not listened to with respect to service planning, and there is often a need to acknowledge the legacy of family struggle with past professional services.

Collaboration in Family-Centred Practice

The concept of parent-professional collaboration is no longer viewed as innovative; rather, it has become an expected component of service provision. In addition, the health and social service literature that focuses on parent-professional relationships unequivocally concludes that parent satisfaction with service delivery is overwhelmingly related to parent-professional collaboration (Dechill, Koren, & Schultze, 1994; MacKean, Thurston, & Scott, 2005; Summers et al., 2005; Hiebert-Murphy, Trute, & Wright, 2011). There are, however, multiple definitions of collaboration, and there is minimal research describing how collaboration may be measured. While there is agreement that collaboration is desirable, there is often a difference in definition and how it is translated into practice (Franck & Callery, 2004). Definitions are constructed along a continuum – ranging from the occasional "courtesy communication" to transdisciplinary teamwork. As previously stated, the ecological systems perspective provides the strongest rationale for working in collaborative relationships. This framework highlights the transactional nature of relationships between children, families, and communities and emphasizes the significance of interdependence among individuals, families, and society. Building capacity within families therefore necessitates paying attention to how collaborative processes between families and service providers are fostered and developed and, by extension, paying attention to understanding how the policy and legislative context in which service is provided will influence the parent-professional dynamic.

Although collaboration as an outcome is valued, there is a need to improve professionals' and families' capacities for collaboration (Leiter, 2007; Pinkus, 2005). The key to successful collaborative relationships appears to be professionals' attitudes towards collaboration, their professional preparation in terms of skills for collaboration, and institutional or agency support for collaboration (Dinnebeil, Hale, & Rule, 1999; Pinkus, 2003). Attitudes of service providers that are necessary preconditions for collaborative relationships include a belief in the sharing of power, as evidenced by an absence of criticism, judgment, need for control (authoritarianism), and possessiveness. Moreover, it is important for service providers to value the parent-professional connection by being supportive, accessible, honest, respectful, and appreciative of parents' contributions. Although seemingly obvious, it is further important for the professional to genuinely enjoy her/his work, and enjoy working with people.

Generally, service providers receive very little training on how to collaborate, and empowerment skills are assumed to be embedded within knowledge of the "helping relationship." However, when professionals are provided with an orientation to what collaborative practice is, how they think about the process of collaboration, and strategies to promote collaboration, their development of collaborative relationships can also alter parents' perspectives about service delivery. This shift in parental perspectives and expectations can then result in changed professional practices.

The development of a collaborative relationship also includes changing family members' perceptions so that they see themselves as an integral part of the service delivery team and as persons who have an important contribution to make. From a family-centred perspective, collaboration becomes an opportunity for families to envision what might be possible, rather than limiting service provision to simply responding to identified problems. The development of new norms regarding involvement is only possible when families are involved in all stages of service delivery. That includes articulating their preferred vision of their family, having a voice in the development of plans for how their service goals may be accomplished, facilitating the implementation of a service plan, evaluating the effectiveness of action plans, and determining what new actions are needed.

To utilize concepts from family therapy, this describes the shift from "first-order" change to "second-order" change (Watzlawick, Weakland, & Fisch, 1974). Applied to strategies of service delivery, first-order change involves making minor alterations in how children's services are provided (e.g., simplifying service access, making services more "friendly" to parents); no fundamental alteration is made to the traditional role of the professional as the expert and the family as unskilled, uninformed, and therefore in need of clear direction. Although service may on the surface look more "sensitive to consumers," the underlying values, basic structure, and mandate of the program or organization are maintained. In contrast, second-order change invites a meaningful transformation of the service system and its capacities, including a shift in roles, relationships, and rules. This shift may be evidenced through the professional encouraging parents to develop their own strategies for managing their children's special needs, to take risks when necessary, to provide access to diverse ways of managing challenging circumstances, and to maintain the position that the parents' knowledge is valued.

Collaborative relationships are committed to sharing ideas, resources, expertise, responsibility, and decision-making. They are rooted in ideas about partnerships, working alliances, and equality of power. It is important that collaboration is not translated into the service provider maintaining a rigid position of uncritical acceptance of all ideas expressed by the family or other significant persons. Both parents and professionals possess comparable, albeit different, information, and the heart of a collaborative relationship is the desire for each partner to learn and acquire knowledge and skills from each other. The professional takes an egalitarian stance without minimizing the expertise that she or he brings to the relationship and, at the same time, respects and values the family's contributions. Capacity building stresses the importance of "local knowledge" (i.e., the intimate knowledge that parents have about their families and other key family members) that forms the foundation for determining what type of services they feel will best benefit their children and families. Parents are understood to have knowledge that is rooted in family experience, to be capable or hold the potential of negotiating with the range of professionals, to understand the impact of the disability on the family and siblings, and to be capable of rearranging roles and responsibilities to suit the needs of their child and family.

Collaboration is fundamentally about doing the work together, and it is important that the partnership be mutually beneficial; service providers need to experience their work as valued, and families need to experience a sense of personal power within helping relationships.

Developing collaborative relationships with mutual respect requires a commitment from both the parent and the professional. It requires flexible communication styles based on individualized family needs and attention to things that may seem like small details such as language (e.g., the use of jargon or acronyms) and styles of interaction, which might include how people are referred to and addressed. Specific skills include

- recognizing that families' voices have frequently been silenced within many service systems,
- working with people to overcome feelings of distance and isolation that are often part of families' experiences,
- building on families' strengths and resources,
- refraining from interpreting families' experiences through one's own perceptions and experiences,
- assisting families to increase their access to power in the service system,
- acknowledging that problem definition is owned by the family, and
- encouraging families to seek social change.

Indicators of Good Collaboration

Trust. True parent-professional partnerships share a common philosophy and a demonstrated commitment towards the mutual goal of wanting children and families to succeed. A key goal in collaboration is the early establishment of a relationship based on trust that is evidenced by a mutual belief in the honesty, integrity, and reliability of each partner. It has been noted that "the cost of repairing trust is much higher than preventing its loss" (Stoner & Angell, 2006, p. 186). The process of building trust, as a foundation for parent-professional partnerships, involves an appreciation of one another's strengths and abilities and leads to a more integrated model of service delivery. We have referred to this as "working alliance" (see Chapter 4). Trust develops in many ways: through acknowledging each partner's life experiences, unique knowledge, and skills; expressing confidence in each other's abilities; promoting emotional cohesion and a sense of belonging; listening to and learning from each other; and sharing both personal and professional issues. Furthermore, once trust is established, it is important for service providers to continue to care about and work on the relationship. Strengthening and maintaining trust is a process that requires consistency, sustained involvement, and ongoing confidence that each partner will share her/his knowledge and resources.

Although partners in collaborative relationships generally share common values, the development of trust also comes from acknowledging differences and communicating respect for these differences. Common goals do not preclude the divergence of opinions, nor is collaboration inconsistent with providing specific information, stating overt values, or being directive. It means that differences in experiences, resources, perspectives, and goals are acknowledged in the parent-professional relationship, rather than being denied. Moreover, although honesty is critical, it does not preclude tact. The essential skill for the family-centred practitioner is to create a service atmosphere that fosters the effective and respectful exchange of ideas.

Clear and open communication. Communication and the use of language can shift the power balance between parents and service providers, and open and respectful communication has been identified as a crucial element to the success of collaborative relationships (Watson, Kieckhefer, & Olshansky, 2006). Asking questions is of central importance to fostering the exchange of unshared information and to collaborative problem solving and decision-making. Asking appropriate questions is not a simple task – and the way in which people navigate regular turn-taking affects collaboration. In addition, collaboration requires the repeated negotiation of shared goals that is best accomplished through active and regular communication and face-to-face meetings. A major consideration is the time needed to authentically integrate the capacity-building process within service provision. For example, although service providers may believe that they are always "available," regular and direct connections (whether family members prefer it to be face-to-face, by telephone, or by email) create opportunities for help-seeking that may not necessarily be taken up in the absence of regular, personal contact. In addition, parents have frequently identified how important it is to them that service providers spend time with them and their children (Nelson, Summers, & Turnbull, 2004). Although service providers may often perceive face-to-face time with their clients as a luxury, there is evidence that spending time with families will foster greater independence and capacity (Pinkus, 2005).

Partnership accountability. Family-centred service has at times been erroneously misinterpreted as offloading the majority of responsibility onto families, in the absence of the availability of resources in the community network of services. The key to successful collaborative relationships is mutual accountability. This is a helpful concept as it invites a transactional relationship that openly acknowledges the power dynamics that form the basis of an empowerment model. In order to be mutually accountable, each partner needs to participate in all aspects of the service delivery process. Professional accountability is dependent upon the commitment to actively engage with families, to be clear and explicit about the professional's agenda, and to actively encourage and explore parent/family contributions prior to enacting service plans. Although service planning may be based on best professional practices, it is critical for families to have a voice in defining/redefining the service agenda. Families are accountable for their actions and values and must accept responsibility for informed and autonomous decision-making.

Developing collaborative relationships has required a paradigm shift in children's services – moving away from the traditional "professional as expert" model towards one in which both families and professionals value the contribution that each of them brings to the relationship. Professionals can no longer see themselves as the experts or the "gatekeepers" of services but more as the facilitators and bridge builders, as those who do not come with a prescribed service plan based on diagnosis, but develop the plan based on what the family and children say they need and want. Families must be seen as bringing intimate knowledge and understanding of their child and family, their strengths, and their needs. In turn, professionals are viewed as a resource to the family by bringing skills, knowledge, and program linkages to service planning.

Joint skill in implementation. The history of parent education initiatives parallels the hierarchal and paternalistic models of service provision for children with special needs in that these initiatives were frequently perceived as insulting or threatening to parents (Winton, Sloop, & Rodriguez, 1999). With the advent of family-centred service, these traditional models of parent education, as a key component of early intervention services, have been greatly de-emphasized as a result of perceived inconsistencies in philosophies (Kaiser et al., 1999). Examples of traditional parent education include training parents on how to facilitate speech and language development, or how to conduct regular physiotherapy sessions with their children. In essence, traditional models frequently focused on training parents to act as pseudo-professionals as substitutes for service provision. Current perspectives recognize that families want to help their children develop and learn, and that this may be accomplished within a context of family-centred practice (Bailey et al., 2006). Rather than acting as pseudo-professionals, parents are encouraged to facilitate their children's development within the context of typical, day-to-day parenting activities such as family swim days, library "read-along" programs, or spending time with their children on the community park's play structure.

One means of facilitating parents' development of expertise in managing their children's special needs is to provide joint professional-family information/training opportunities. Although preparation for collaborative practice may be provided to novice service providers through a university-based program, it is only the first step towards implementation. Parents and professionals need opportunities to work and learn together. Although these opportunities rarely exist in programs of professional education, research indicates that parents and professionals who participate in joint training initiatives have more positive perceptions of each other (Gallagher, Rhodes, & Darling, 2004).

In order for joint training to be successful, it is important for professionals to respond to parent-identified preferences for service and family outcomes. Although parent participation in and of itself is a positive outcome, parents are primarily concerned with the well-being of their children. Professionals need to expand their roles, from those that focus on the provision of individualized specialized services, to being members of a team that places families' needs first. Families also would benefit from the opportunity to learn about how professionals are oriented towards practice and the current research findings of individual disciplines. By learning the language and issues of the organizations they work with, parent and service providers will develop shared language and ways of communicating. This will also enhance more seamless service delivery and, most importantly, facilitate the development of family-identified goals and hopes for the future.

Competence

A key element of building capacity within an empowerment framework is competence, or the acquisition of skills through continuous learning and a progression of skill development. Service providers need to acknowledge that families are fully capable of demonstrating a complexity of abilities such as critical thinking, analytical skills, and communication skills. For many families who may have experienced a sense of disempowerment in their prior interactions with professional services, capacity building includes the reclaiming of competence.

Within a family-centred model, competence refers to recognizing the skills, resources, and experiences that parents/family members possess that contribute to achieving their family-identified needs. In addition, a key component of competence is the recognition of which skills may not be present, and the implementation of plans to address these gaps. It is important that the skills that parents need to navigate the service system are identified and learned. In these situations, the practitioner will need to take the time to assist the family to learn about the service system in ways that the family can understand. Further, they will need to provide emotional and informational support as parents begin to manage some of the tasks of brokering therapeutic or remedial services.

Families may lack confidence in expressing themselves and may not be able to articulate their needs, opinions, and experiences. There are a myriad of reasons for this that can range from prior experience with service systems in which their perspectives were minimized, judged, or pathologized to having a limited personal repertoire of coping responses. The acquisition of skills can allow individuals to understand the resources and competencies needed for empowerment. Although practitioners may feel that skill building is not part of their service mandate, building capacity may involve professionals assisting parents through modelling, practicing alternatives, role play, assertiveness training, the use of "I" statements, and other communication strategies. With the acquisition of greater knowledge and confidence in themselves, parents can develop strategies that better meet their needs and the needs of their children.

Critics may note that the building of competence takes a good deal of time, and family goals may best be accomplished with a practitioner skilled in the knowledge of brokering systems. This highlights the dichotomy of empowerment: long-term achievement versus short-term gains. Although it may be easier for the service provider to obtain a particular resource, the recognition of empowerment as a process emphasizes the importance of supporting parents as they negotiate with resource providers to build lasting skills in parents.

Parental competence is intrinsically related to their morale and self-confidence. Although no longer the sole focus of professional intervention, the themes of loss, fear, and feeling out of control remain a part of the experience for many parents when they have a child with special needs. We know that there continues to be stigma and blame experienced by families of children with emotional or behavioural disturbances, and it is important for service providers to acknowledge how this may influence family members' functioning and attitudes. One outcome of experiencing their situation as unmanageable is the perpetuation of the belief within a family that they are not capable of handling difficult or problematic situations. This can be seen when the parent/family member defers to the professional in the role of "expert" or when the professional assumes the role of an authority figure in a family meeting, maintains control of the agenda at team meetings, or makes decisions on behalf of the family or their fellow professionals. For example, recipients of social services are often assumed by professionals to lack the ability to make decisions or, more specifically, the ability to make the "correct" decision. Consequently, contrary to the goals of empowerment, professionals may adopt the paternalistic stance of limiting the number or quality of decisions that parents are allowed. For example, parents may be able to decide on whether they wish to receive day-care services, but not on which daycare they may send their child to or who will be hired as the care provider. Parents are unlikely to feel confident in their decision-making unless they have the opportunity to make important decisions about their lives, which includes having a range of options from which to make choices and not simply "yes/no" or "either/or" dichotomies.

Empowerment within family-centred services is directed towards fostering parent-professional dynamics that generate greater self-efficacy within parents. Self-efficacy refers to the belief that one is confident and capable of undertaking and succeeding at a particular task (Bandura, 2001). In order to encourage greater parental self-efficacy, practitioners need to be aware of the conditions that foster an increased sense of control. Past performance is generally the strongest indicator of an individual's confidence. Some families enter children's services with an extensive history of interactions with formal service agencies, and for others, the first contact with the professionals who have entered the life of their child and their family may be their first contact with a service agency. If parents have been successful at a particular skill in the past, they are more likely to believe that they will be successful in the future (Bandura, 2001). It is therefore important for service providers to link prior successes with potential future success. However, many families may express a high degree of unfamiliarity with the service system, and learning how to navigate the myriad of services can be fraught with fear, frustration, and failure.

Service providers need to use these parameters to guide their interactions with service recipients with a view towards increasing their self-efficacy. Service providers need to create a service context and a working alliance that encourages families to transform beliefs that they lack ability into beliefs that they have the ability. A key practice principle is that effective support from outside the family is necessary to build internal family capacity and is a prerequisite to family empowerment. An important strategy is to provide parents with positive feedback as they interact with the service system. Providing feedback, however, is not a simple task and practitioners need to assess how and when to provide meaningful and constructive feedback. First, it is important that the service provider communicate with the parent that they are receptive to feedback. Providing feedback in the absence of requests for assistance may contribute towards parents feeling inadequate or incapable of undertaking the tasks related to their children. Second, effective feedback requires mindfulness on the part of the service provider that recognizes and emphasizes parental abilities, rather than to resorting to professional action as the more expedient way to achieve a goal. Third, part of the skill of the service provider is to ensure that positive feedback is genuine. Part of what service providers can do is to clearly communicate specific information to families that invites them to manage issues independently. However, not all families may be at this stage, and families who appear frustrated with their perceived inabilities to navigate service systems need to be given greater guidance and more carefully structured information.

A second means by which practitioners can contribute towards improved self-efficacy is through collaborating in the establishment of service goals with the family. Parents/family members who set specific goals for themselves and their family are more likely to feel confident in their abilities to achieve these goals. Service providers may facilitate the process of goal setting by assisting families to compartmentalize large goals into smaller, achievable pieces. It is also important to "check in" with families to ensure that their service goals are specific and clear, so that success is unambiguous.

A third way to increase self-efficacy is through observing others in similar situations. In this respect, professionals can sometimes be most effective by facilitating linkages between and among parents. Parents who are struggling with a particular issue may best be helped by learning from other parents in similar situations. Parent-to-parent modelling can provide families with tangible knowledge of how to manage particular situations experienced by other families. It is important for service providers, however, to facilitate linkages between parents who have some degree of commonality – either in their children's diagnoses, ages, or setting.

Critical Consciousness

Paulo Freire (1970) first introduced the term *conscientização* that describes the construct of "critical consciousness" or the process of developing knowledge and "personal concern" for social justice leading to action. McWhirter (1998) has defined critical consciousness as involving the dual processes of power analysis and critical self-reflection. The processes of developing critical consciousness and empowerment are closely related. They each require an examination of the social, political, and economic environments that, over time, have impacted children's services. The concept of self-awareness is an important beginning point of strengths-based practice and a crucial element in professional education of future service providers. This has included education modules directed towards the development of self-awareness through the consideration of family practitioners' "early learning" through analysis of their own family autobiographies, with a focus on the study of their own family-of-origin history, to better appreciate their assumptions and beliefs relating to "normal" family life and to advance their capabilities as mindful practitioners. Students are encouraged to examine their own socialization processes to understand how their ideas about family, disability, and society were developed and perpetuated. This can become a painful process for professionals as this may make evident previously held beliefs that are uncovered to reveal unconscious racism, ableism, or sexism. It is clearly important that professionals engage in a self-reflective process to identify their feelings regarding disability, or the types of family systems that may trigger some negative feelings (such as families living in poverty, with a history of family violence, etc.). It is only when the worker has developed her/his own awareness that s/he is able to facilitate the development of a critical consciousness in parents and family members. We believe that you cannot help to take others any further than you have gone yourself in strengthening social and cultural consciousness. Unfortunately, the increasing pace of work and reduced personnel resources do not often provide opportunities for service professionals to focus upon reflective practice. Instead, workload demands and professional training tend to advance traditional practice and ideology about the "helping process," leaving insufficient time and attention to critical reflection as an integral aspect of positive professional action.

The process of developing a critical consciousness is equally important for parents. The historical legacy of "disability as shame" is a powerful influence that shapes relationships among parents and their families and friends, as well as their relationships with professionals. We are not that far removed from the historical trauma of institutionalizing children that continues to reverberate in the consciousness of some families of children with disabilities.

The development of a critical consciousness also emphasizes the role of current sociopolitical dynamics. The shift towards family-centred practice in early intervention and childhood disability services was initiated by parents who demanded a change in service culture by enacting their abilities to analyse their experiences as participants and not as targets. In applying these principles to childhood disability services, critically conscious parents become aware of (a) the historical, political, and social implications of the service context; (b) their own social locations in the service context; (c) the intersectionality of multiple identities (e.g., race, class, gender); and (d) the discrepancies that exist between a vision of social justice and current societal conditions. For example, the development of a critical consciousness within families involves the acknowledgment and recognition that ableism remains an overt barrier for families with children with disabilities. By introducing and facilitating a discussion on the concept of ableism, the service provider may assist families to deconstruct messages that disability is synonymous with deficiency and to gain a clearer understanding of how these powerful social beliefs become internalized within individual family systems.

What this suggests is that in order for children's services to become truly family-centred, professionals need to facilitate the development of a critical consciousness within themselves, as well as facilitate the process within family systems. At the family systems level, this may take the form of engaging in discussions that explicitly discuss the meaning that disability holds for the family and the level of congruence with societal views, and how they may be perceived differently by friends, extended family members, and/or service systems as a result of their child's special needs. There may be salient family issues such as how being a single parent family, immigrant family, or family living in poverty may differentially influence a family's experiences with service providers. Finally, parents need to grapple with systems issues such as how "inclusive" environments can take on many different meanings for their children. For example, parents are frequently given the "choice" of having their child with special needs placed in a segregated school setting with learning supports or an integrated school setting with an absence of adequate special learning support. Although these may represent "inclusivity" at a systems level, this may not conform to the parents' definitions.

Community Connections

Becoming a parent of a child with special needs is often a catalyst to move towards engaging in a community advocacy role and can greatly facilitate the growth of critical consciousness. A fundamental element of capacity building is the recognition of the importance of "social capital" and community connections that are an integral component of parental well-being.

Participating in mutual self-help groups brings benefit not only to the participants, but also to the communities in which the activities occur. Families of children with special needs have expressed feelings of isolation and often withdraw from contact with friends and family members as a consequence of feeling ashamed, angry, or hopeless. Mutual self-help can assist in reducing feelings of isolation, as well as act as an important source of social and emotional support. An important practice principle is the group dimension. It is necessary for professionals to recognize that although individual parents may experience a feeling of empowerment, it often comes from experiencing a sense of connectedness with other people. With respect to service provision, it is important that parents have the opportunity to be linked with other parents in similar circumstances to facilitate mutual support and sharing of experiences. Facilitating parent-to-parent connections through participation in support groups or other activities can be a source of important information, provide emotional and social support and opportunities for belonging and contribution, and ultimately, be empowering for parents. Unfortunately, as there continue to be decreases in resources available to meet the needs of families, there is correspondingly less emphasis on efforts directed towards community building.

However, in recognition of contemporary circumstances, parents of children with health challenges and developmental disabilities are routinely using the Internet as a resource to access information and support. The benefits of using the Internet as a means to connect with community include the ability to access a wide range of information resources, social networking as a means of assisting with decision-making, an accessible way to connect with other parents, and sharing of affirmative and supportive messages with other parents. Although personal empowerment may not be the identified goal, participation in online support groups, including writing, expressing emotions, collecting information that is not filtered through an "authority," developing social relationships, and enhancing decision-making skills, serves as a possible generator of a sense of personal empowerment for people in distress (Barak, Boniel-Nissim, & Suler, 2008).

Community may also act as a catalyst for parents to cultivate their sense of personal empowerment by engaging with the broader community at a volunteer level. Engagement in community-based work is both a process and outcome of individual empowerment (Pinderhughes, 1995; Zimmerman, 1995, 2000). Community advocacy involves mobilizing other parents of children with special needs to address common concerns and increase their presence in the systems (and decisions) that affect their children. Creating opportunities for parents to participate in community can provide an alternative context, one in which parents see themselves as contributing to the collective good, rather than being only recipients of services.

Conclusion

It is clear that the parent-professional relationship is dynamic in children's services and has undergone a significant transformation over the past several decades. We have moved from past prevalence of professional-centred services, to the present where family-centred principles provide the context to build and maintain new relational ways of working, into the future where parents may hold the balance of power whenever it is possible. In order to accomplish this, those who are in positions of decision-making will need to be open to relinquishing their authority, and parents who were previously disempowered will gain greater control over their families' lives. True empowerment may translate into a pattern of parent-professional relations wherein parents who have become more self-defined and self-directed may begin to challenge, negotiate, and at times alter the decisions of those previously in control of services they receive.

REFERENCES

Bailey, D.B., Bruder, M.B., Hebbeler, K., Carta, J., Defosset, M., Greenwood, C., ..., & Barton, L. (2006). Recommended outcomes for families with young

children with disabilities. *Journal of Early Intervention, 28*(4), 227–51. http://
dx.doi.org/10.1177/105381510602800401

Bandura, A. (2001). Social cognitive theory: An agentic perspective. *Annual Review of Psychology, 52*(1), 1–26. http://dx.doi.org/10.1146/annurev.
psych.52.1.1 Medline:11148297 .

Barak, A., Boniel-Nissim, M., & Suler, J. (2008). Fostering empowerment in
online support groups. *Computers in Human Behavior, 24*(5), 1867–83. http://
dx.doi.org/10.1016/j.chb.2008.02.004

Bronfenbrenner, U. (1979). *The ecology of human development.* Cambridge, MA:
Harvard University Press.

Carr, E. (2003). Rethinking empowerment theory through a feminist lens: The importance of process. *Affilia, 18,* 8–20. http://dx.doi.
org/10.1177/0886109902239092

Chronister, K., & McWhirter, E. (2003). Applying social-cognitive career
theory to the empowerment of battered women. *Journal of Counseling and
Development, 81*(4), 418–25. http://dx.doi.org/10.1002/j.1556-6678.2003.
tb00268.x

DeChillo, N., Koren, P.E., & Schultze, K.H. (1994, October). From paternalism
to partnership: Family and professional collaboration in children's mental health. *American Journal of Orthopsychiatry, 64*(4), 564–76. http://dx.doi.
org/10.1037/h0079572 Medline:7847572

Dinnebeil, L., Hale, L., & Rule, S. (1999). Early intervention program practices
that support collaboration. *Topics in Early Childhood Special Education, 19*(4),
225–35. http://dx.doi.org/10.1177/027112149901900403

Dunst, C.J., Boyd, K., Trivette, C.M., & Hamby, D.W. (2002). Family-oriented
program models and professional helpgiving practices. *Family Relations,
51*(3), 221–9. http://dx.doi.org/10.1111/j.1741-3729.2002.00221.x

Dunst, C.J., Johanson, C., Trivette, C.M., & Hamby, D. (1991, October-November). Family-oriented early intervention policies and practices: Family-centered or not? *Exceptional Children, 58*(2), 115–26. Medline:1836180

Franck, L.S., & Callery, P. (2004, May). Re-thinking family-centred care
across the continuum of children's healthcare. *Child: Care, Health and Development, 30*(3), 265–77. http://dx.doi.org/10.1111/j.1365-2214.2004.00412.x
Medline:15104587

Freire, P. (1970). *Pedagogy of the oppressed.* New York, NY: Herder and Herder.

Gallagher, P., Rhodes, C., & Darling, S. (2004). Parents as professionals in
early intervention: A parent educator model. *Topics in Early Childhood Special Education, 24*(1), 5–13. http://dx.doi.org/10.1177/02711214040240010101

Gutierrez, L. (1990). Working with women of color: An empowerment perspective. *Social Work, 35,* 149–54.

Gutierrez, L. (1995). Understanding the empowerment process: Does consciousness make a difference? *Social Work Research, 19*, 229–37.

Herrenkohl, G., Judson, T., & Heffner, J.A. (1999). Defining and measuring employee empowerment. *Journal of Applied Behavioral Science, 35*(3), 373–89. http://dx.doi.org/10.1177/0021886399353008

Hiebert-Murphy, D., Trute, B., & Wright, A. (2011). Parents' definition of effective child disability support services: Implications for implementing family-centered practice. *Journal of Family Social Work, 14*(2), 144–58. http://dx.doi.org/10.1080/10522158.2011.552404

Kaiser, A., Mahoney, G., Girolametto, L., MacDonald, J., Robinson, C., & Spiker, D. (1999). Rejoinder: Toward a contemporary vision of parent education. *Topics in Early Childhood Special Education, 19*(3), 173–176.

King, G., Willoughby, C., Specht, J.A., & Brown, E. (2006, September). Social support processes and the adaptation of individuals with chronic disabilities. *Qualitative Health Research, 16*(7), 902–25. http://dx.doi.org/10.1177/1049732306289920 Medline:16894223

Leiter, V. (2007). Families and childhood disabilities. *Blackwell Encyclopedia of Sociology*. Blackwell Reference Online. Retrieved 8 April 2008.

MacKean, G.L., Thurston, W.E., & Scott, C.M. (2005, March). Bridging the divide between families and health professionals' perspectives on family-centred care. *Health Expectations, 8*(1), 74–85. http://dx.doi.org/10.1111/j.1369-7625.2005.00319.x Medline:15713173

McWhirter, E. (1991). Empowerment in counseling. *Journal of Counseling and Development, 69*(3), 222–7. http://dx.doi.org/10.1002/j.1556-6676.1991.tb01491.x

McWhirter, E. (1994). *Counseling for empowerment*. Alexandria, VA: American Counseling Association.

McWhirter, E. (1998). Emancipatory communitarian psychology. *American Psychologist, 53*(3), 322–3. http://dx.doi.org/10.1037/0003-066X.53.3.322

Nelson, L., Summers, J., & Turnbull, A. (2004). Boundaries in family-professional relationships. *Remedial and Special Education, 25*(3), 153–65. http://dx.doi.org/10.1177/07419325040250030301

Philbin, A. (1998). Capacity building work with social justice organizations: Views from the field. Submitted to Anthony Romero, Director, Human Rights and International Cooperation, The Ford Foundation.

Pinderhughes, E. (1995). Empowering diverse populations: Family practice in the 21st century. *Families in Society, 76*, 131–40.

Pinkus, S. (2003). All talk and no action: Transforming the rhetoric of parent-professional partnership into practice. *Journal of Research in Special Educational Needs, 3*(2), 115–21. http://dx.doi.org/10.1111/1471-3802.00004

Pinkus, S. (2005). Bridging the gap between policy and practice: Adopting a strategic vision for partnership working in special education. *British Journal of Special Education, 32*(4), 184–7. http://dx.doi.org/10.1111/j.1467-8578.2005.00395.x

Stoner, J., & Angell, M. (2006). Parent perspectives on role engagement: An investigation of parents of children with ASD and their self-reported roles with education professionals. *Focus on Autism and Other Developmental Disabilities, 21*(3), 177–89. http://dx.doi.org/10.1177/10883576060210030601

Suarez-Balcazar, Y., Harper, G.W., & Lewis, R. (2005, February). An interactive and contextual model of community-university collaborations for research and action. *Health Education & Behavior, 32*(1), 84–101. http://dx.doi.org/10.1177/1090198104269512 Medline:15642756

Summers, J., Hoffman, L., Marquis, J., Turnball, A., & Poston, D. (2005). Relationship between parent satisfaction regarding partnerships with professionals and age of child. *Topics in Early Childhood Special Education, 25*(1), 48–58. http://dx.doi.org/10.1177/02711214050250010501

Turnbull, H., & Stowe, M. (2001). Five models for thinking about disability: Implications for policy development. *Journal of Disability Policy Studies, 12*(3), 198–205. http://dx.doi.org/10.1177/104420730101200305

Watson, K.C., Kieckhefer, G.M., & Olshansky, E. (2006, May). Striving for therapeutic relationships: Parent-provider communication in the developmental treatment setting. *Qualitative Health Research, 16*(5), 647–63. http://dx.doi.org/10.1177/1049732305285959 Medline:16611970

Watzlawick, P., Weakland, J.H., & Fisch, R. (1974). *Change: Principles of problem formation and problem solution*. New York, NY: W.W. Norton & Co.

Winton, P.J., Sloop, S., & Rodriguez, P. (1999). Parent education: A term whose time is past. *Topics in Early Childhood Special Education, 19*(3), 157–61. http://dx.doi.org/10.1177/027112149901900306

Zimmerman, M.A. (1995, October). Psychological empowerment: Issues and illustrations. *American Journal of Community Psychology, 23*(5), 581–99. http://dx.doi.org/10.1007/BF02506983 Medline:8851341

Zimmerman, M.A. (2000). Empowerment theory: Psychological, organizational and community levels of analysis. In J. Rappaport & E. Seidman (Eds.), *Handbook of community psychology* (pp. 43–63). New York, NY: Plenum Press. http://dx.doi.org/10.1007/978-1-4615-4193-6_2

7   Social Network Analysis and Practice

DIANE HIEBERT-MURPHY

Introduction

The view that individuals are part of multiple environments (both physical and social) that influence growth and development is core to Bronfenbrenner's (1979) concept of social ecology. Consistent with social systems theory, social ecology emphasizes that individuals both influence and are influenced by the interactions that occur in these environments. As applied to children with special needs, these concepts suggest that the multitude of relationships that exist between the child and his/her social and physical environments must be examined to understand the child's development. While the family is central, providing the most immediate and enduring environment within which the child lives and develops, other social relationships are also important. Thus, attention must be given to the broader environment which includes friends, extended family, neighbourhoods, schools, and community organizations and groups. Given the demands of raising a child with special needs, professional services and helpers often become prominent in the lives of children and families and play an influential role in helping parents respond to the unique needs of the child. Social ecology and systems theory have proven to be useful as conceptual frameworks for making sense of the interactions between families with children with special needs and the multitude of systems that provide assistance to them and their children (Kazak, 1987).

Family stress theory also provides a framework for understanding the experiences of families raising children with special needs (Xu, 2007). This model views families as responding to various stressors that arise during their day-to-day functioning (Malia, 2006; McCubbin &

McCubbin, 1987). Some of these stressors are expected or "normative" and are experienced by many families as they progress through the life cycle. Other stressors are less common and emerge out of a unique set of life circumstances. Families respond to these stressors in an effort to adapt or adjust. These responses constitute the family's coping. Within this model, coping resources and the use of coping strategies moderate the effects of stress on families. This process model suggests that both personal resources (e.g., physical health, problem-solving skills) and socioecological factors are important to family coping and adaptation (Beresford, 1994). Social support is a one of the socioecological factors that plays a central role in a stress and coping model of family functioning (McCubbin & McCubbin, 1987). An extensive literature documents the importance of social support in parental functioning and in mitigating the effects of a wide range of family stressors including both normative stressors (e.g., birth of a child, transition of children to adolescence) and non-normative stressors (e.g., raising a child with special needs, chronic illness of a family member; Belsky, 1984; Carnes & Quinn, 2005; Dunst, Trivette, & Cross, 1986).

Building on these theoretical concepts, the goal of family-centred practice is to empower families by building on their capabilities. The family's social network is a primary source of support and resources for helping families meet their needs (Dunst & Trivette, 2009). Support may come from the family's "natural" or "informal" support network (e.g., friends, family, neighbours) and/or the "formal" support network (e.g., professionals, community organizations, self-help groups). Given the important role that social support plays in outcomes for families as well as the changing nature of family needs, the fit between a family's needs and the support available is a central focus of assessment in family-centred practice (Dunst, Trivette, & Deal, 1994). Enhancing the capacity of the natural and professional network to provide support is a key activity of family-centred practitioners. Practice moves beyond a focus on linking families with established services to considering how support within the family's informal and formal social network can be mobilized and/or expanded to meet family-identified needs.

Social Support: Definitions and Core Concepts

Social support is generally used to describe resources that are provided by individuals or groups that promote competence in dealing with short-term crises and life transitions as well as longer-term stress

(Caplan & Killilea, 1976). The form that support can take is broad, including, for example, material aid, behavioural assistance, intimate interaction, feedback, and positive social interaction (Barrera & Ainlay, 1983). There is a vast literature that documents the important role that social support plays in mediating between a host of life stressors and both physical and mental health and well-being (e.g., Kawachi & Berkman, 2001; Uchino, 2006).

While there are variations in how social support has been defined, there appears to be agreement that it is composed of two dimensions: structure and function (Pillay & Rao, 2002). The structure of social support is often assessed by the analysis of social networks. Such analysis identifies persons and groups who provide support, the interrelationships between these persons, and the types of support that is provided. Social network analysis permits the examination of structural characteristics of social support including, for example, network size (the number of individuals with whom the focal person has direct contact), network density (the extent to which members of the network know and interact with one another), network reciprocity (the degree to which various types of support are both given and received), and network dimensionality (the number of functions served by a particular relationship; Kazak & Wilcox, 1984). Thus, the structure of social support addresses the following questions:

- Who provides support to the family?
- What types of support are provided?
- How well do members of a family's support network know each other?
- To whom does the family provide support?

The functional aspect of social support refers to what is expected in terms of social support and what is received (Pillay & Rao, 2002). The function of support addresses the following issues:

- What types of support does the family expect?
- What support does the family think is available?
- How satisfied are family members with the support they receive?

It is important to note that the needs of families are not static; families' needs change in response to their life cycle as do their unique circumstances and the needs of their children. As a family's needs change,

so do the demands on the social network. The support network also un-
dergoes changes as members and groups providing support enter and
exit. The types and amounts of support the network is able to provide
may shift over time. Hence, this is a dynamic process with changing
needs and resources, requiring ongoing assessment of the adequacy of
the fit between the two.

While at first glance the concept of social support may appear quite
simple, research has demonstrated the construct to be multifaceted and
complex (Haber, Cohen, Lucas, & Baltes, 2007). For example, there has
been much discussion about the differences between perceived social
support (the support an individual perceives is available and/or general satisfaction with the support available) and received support (the
types and amount of support that is actually received), with research
demonstrating limited agreement between the two (Haber et al., 2007).
These findings suggest that how much support is provided is only one
among many factors that affect the level of social support that an individual perceives to be available. Other factors, including culture, influence how social support is perceived and used (Pillay & Rao, 2002). It
is essential in practice to consider not only the supports that are provided to a family but also how this support is experienced by the family
within its unique social context.

Social Support and Families with Children with Special Needs

Families with children with special needs deal not only with the
changes experienced by all families as they progress through the developmental life cycle, but also face a myriad of transitions related to the
specific needs of their children (Hanline, 1991). For example, a child's
entry into public school marks a transition for all families; children and
their families must adapt to a different routine and a change in childcare arrangements as well as to the demands associated with the start
of formal education. Families with children with special needs often experience this transition as much more disruptive. For many, this developmental shift means transitioning from early intervention programs
and supports to a completely new service delivery system with different policies, services, and providers. It is during such transitions that
families are especially vulnerable to experiencing stress and are called
on to cope with the demands and adjust to changing circumstances.
During such times, families are likely to seek support from their informal and formal network (e.g., friends, extended family, professionals).

The adaptation of families with children with special needs is best understood as a lifelong process that occurs within the context of the family's developmental life cycle (Hanline, 1991).

A body of literature has examined social support among families with children with special needs (e.g., Armstrong, Birnie-Lefcovitch, & Ungar, 2005; Barakat & Linney, 1992; Bristol, 1987; Jones, Rowe, & Becker, 2009; Trivette & Dunst, 1992). A positive relationship has been found between social support in times of crisis and life satisfaction among families with children with disabilities (Sloper & Turner, 1993). Social networks can provide support in various ways to families with children with special needs. For example, Lindblad, Holritz-Rasmussen, and Sandman (2007) found that parents reported that various types of support were helpful, such as practical assistance (e.g., transportation, help with the daily care of the child and siblings) and emotional support (which they called "being provided a room for sorrow and joy" [p. 243]). Informal supports can also be important in helping families develop formal supports. In their study of families with children with disruptive behaviours, Arcia, Fernández, Jáquez, Castillo, and Ruiz (2004) found that network members were important in the entry of families into professional services. Members of the network encouraged help-seeking in a variety of ways, including providing instructions for accessing services, providing personal testimonies, suggesting medication, identifying a service provider, reframing help-seeking in an acceptable manner, making the initial appointment, and in some cases, coercing the mother to seek help.

Researchers have examined the structure of the networks of families of children with special needs. Some studies have found the networks of families of children with special needs to be smaller than comparison families (e.g., Kazak & Marvin, 1984; Kazak & Wilcox, 1984), although other research has not found this to be the case (e.g., Kazak, 1988). A number of studies have found that the networks have a higher density, meaning that more people within the network are known to each other (Kazak, 1987; Kazak & Marvin, 1984). Not surprisingly, the networks of families with children with special needs have been found to include more professional helpers compared to other families (Kazak, Reber, & Carter, 1988). It has been suggested that positive adaptation is linked to small, intense networks in which extended family and friends provide different types of support (Trute & Hauch, 1988a).

The families' perceptions regarding the support that is available appears to be particularly important to understanding the link between social support and family outcome. For example, in one study comparing families with children with disabilities living in a kibbutz with families in the city, Margalit, Leyser, Ankonina, and Avraham (1991), contrary to what they expected, did not find evidence that additional resources available to families living in the kibbutz were related to more positive family outcomes. They interpreted this finding as evidence of the importance of parents' subjective experiences of support rather than the actual support that is provided in predicting outcome.

A frequently asked question refers to who in the network is most helpful in providing support to families with children with special needs. Marital partners (Trute & Hauch, 1988b), siblings of the child with disabilities, friends, and professionals (Levy, Rimmerman, Botuck, Ardito, Freeman, & Levy, 1996) have all been identified as major sources of support for families with children with special needs. Extended family members have also been identified as key members of the support network. Grandparents in particular have been identified as an important source of support for parents (Lindblad et al., 2007; Seligman, 1991; Trute, 2003; Trute, Worthington, & Hiebert-Murphy, 2008).

Although members of the social network are possible resources for families, they can also be sources of stress. Jones and Passey (2005), for example, found that the majority of the parents (66.7%) in their study of families with children with developmental disabilities and behaviour problems reported that dealing with friends and family on a daily basis was extremely stressful. Dealing with doctors and other professionals was also rated as extremely stressful by many parents (82.4%). It must also be recognized that asking for and accepting help may be a difficult process. Brett (2004) found that some parents view receiving support as a measure of failure and experience a sense of vulnerability when asking for help. Furthermore, it should not be assumed that having members in a network ensures that support is forthcoming. In their study of mothers of children with cognitive disabilities, Levy et al. (1996) found that mothers received little support from family and frequently found the support offered unhelpful. Many mothers in their study reported that they did not receive support from their parents, their relatives, their partner's parents, or their partner's relatives.

Conclusions based on theory and research. Based on existing literature regarding support for families with special needs, a number of conclusions can be drawn:

- Social support is an important resource for families and can mitigate the effects of stress, including the demands placed on families that result from having a child with special needs.

- Social support is multifaceted and can involve instrumental help as well as emotional support.
- Support can be received from informal sources (e.g., friends, family) as well as formal sources (e.g., professionals, social service programs).
- It should not be assumed that the existence of a social network necessarily translates into the provision of support. Interactions within a social network have the potential to be sources of stress as well as resources for support.
- A family's perception of the availability and adequacy of support may be as important as the actual amount of support provided.
- The experience and utilization of social support can be influenced by many factors within the individual, family, and sociocultural environment.

Social Support and Family-Centred Practice

Knowledge of the importance of social support to family functioning, and more specifically, the evidence that social support plays an important role in understanding the experience of families with children with special needs, provides a foundation for a family-centred approach to practice with these families. It has long been recognized that families with children with special needs have many relationships with professional helpers and that social network analysis can be a useful conceptual tool in understanding the complex relationships between formal helpers and families (Kazak, 1987). Recognition of the needs of children and their families has led to the development of services to address these needs. The uniqueness of family needs combined with the complexity of the service delivery system has further resulted in professionals assuming the role of "case manager" or "service coordinator." One of the primary functions of this role is to facilitate links between the children and families and services and supports in the community and within the informal helping network (Levy et al., 1996).

Family-identified unmet needs might be best interpreted as gaps in support. Research on families with children with special needs provides evidence of the link between needs and supports. In their study of families with children with chronic health conditions, Farmer, Marien, Clark, Sherman, and Selva (2004) found that the perceived level of social support predicted the number of unmet family needs even after controlling for demographic factors and child functioning. Mothers who felt more supported identified fewer needs for information about how to promote their child's health and well-being as well as fewer needs for strategies to promote effective family interactions. Farmer et al. (2004) conclude that with adequate support, families may be able to access more resources and function more effectively, thereby promoting child health and reducing overall family needs. It is this relationship between unmet needs and supports that is key to a family-centred practice model. Within this model, assessment must include not only an identification of family-defined needs but also an evaluation of the family's resources (which includes the social network) and, most importantly, the fit between the needs and resources. The adequacy of the support network and the ability of the family to mobilize and utilize available resources is a major focus of assessment. Family-centred intervention seeks to increase the ability of the family to meet its needs by enhancing the family's skills in recognizing and defining its needs and in securing the resources necessary to address those needs. Thus, intervention should result in family empowerment (Dunst & Trivette, 1996; Dunst, Trivette, & Deal, 1988).

Assessment of Social Network Resources

The assessment of social network resources within a family-centred practice model includes the following: (a) identifying existing sources of support in the family's social environment; (b) determining the family's perceptions of the support that is available and the family's satisfaction with that support; (c) understanding the family's beliefs, values, expectations, and preferences about asking for and receiving help; and (d) engaging the family in the assessment so that family strengths are identified and family members are encouraged to see themselves as problem-solvers who have competence to identify the needs that they have and secure the resources necessary to ensure that those needs are met. Thus, assessment must be concerned not only with information gathering (the content) but also with the process (the how).

The "what" of social support assessment. A number of issues must be addressed in understanding a family's social support resources:

Who is relevant in the life of the child and the family? The beginning point to understanding the support network of the family is to identify the individuals, groups, and organizations that are important in the life of the family. Social support assessment must begin with knowledge of the persons outside of the immediate family who play important roles in family life. Key assessment questions include: With whom do family members interact? Who do family members consider to be important in their daily life?

Who currently provides support to family members, and what types of support are given? The next step in assessment is to clarify who among the people in the family's life provide family members with support. There are many different aspects to support (Barrera & Ainlay, 1983); it is important to consider all types of support that are given, including tangible help, emotional support, guidance, social feedback, and positive social interaction. These broad areas guide the practitioner in developing specific questions that are relevant to the family's context.

Knowledge of the demands faced by all families as they progress through the life cycle as well as the challenges that families may face given their unique circumstances should be incorporated into specific questions that explore the demands that exist in the many areas of family life. For example, if a family has just experienced the birth of a child, it would be relevant to explore the types of support that might be needed by first-time parents (e.g., babysitting so that the parents are able to get a short reprieve from parenting, emotional support to deal with the stress associated with caring for an infant, information about accessing daycare, the provision of feedback to the parents that they are doing a good job). In addition to these normative demands, unique circumstances of the family will create a context in which additional demands emerge. For example, following the birth of a child with complex medical needs, many of the normative issues identified above may be relevant to the family. Furthermore, the family may have the need for additional types of support to address specific demands associated with this circumstance (e.g., who is available to help with transportation to medical appointments, who can provide emotional support for the parents as they come to terms with the implications of the diagnosis, who can provide information about the medical condition and how to access professional support services).

The family's particular sociocultural environment must also be considered as specific stressors (and supports) will emerge within this context. For example, a family that has recently immigrated will have needs related to integrating into Canadian culture. Such integration will pose additional demands if family members are in the process of learning English. Families living in poverty have fewer financial resources to address demands and may experience needs that are different from families who have substantial financial resources. The complex inter-play of life cycle stages, critical events, and social context means that practitioners must carefully consider the unique circumstances of each family and tailor the assessment of social support accordingly.

How satisfied are family members with the support that is available? In addition to identifying sources of support in the family, practitioners must listen carefully to the family's assessment regarding its satisfaction with the support that is provided. While it might appear that minimal sources of external support exist for a family, it may be that the family prefers to be self-reliant and feels little need to "burden" friends and family with requests for help. The family may also prefer to have limited contact with professional services. In other families, although it may appear that there are abundant sources of support available to the family, the family may experience the level of support as inadequate. Exploring a family's satisfaction with support will begin to illuminate the family's beliefs and expectations about social support and will also provide information about a family's preferred coping style. This information is critical, as intervention will only be effective if there is a fit between a family's coping style and the plan developed to address the family's needs.

What is the fit between the support that is available and the needs that are identified? The purpose of any assessment is to guide intervention. What is critical within a family-centred model is to understand the unmet needs of the family and work with the family to develop a family support plan to address those needs (Bennett, Lingerfelt, & Nelson, 1990). The assessment of social support addresses the question of the adequacy of the support network as a resource to families as they manage the demands they face. Such an assessment must ask: (a) Are there sufficient resources in the network to meet the needs of the family? (b) Is there an adequate fit between the types of support that is available and the needs that the family has identified? (c) If resources are available, do barriers exist that interfere with the family accessing those supports? Answers to these questions give direction to the planning process. For example, consider the family that recently relocated from another province. It is possible that the family is competent in terms of the family members' skills at accessing support. Given their recent move, however, the family's network has been disrupted. Sources of support have diminished and the family finds itself quite isolated. Intervention may need to attend to helping the family re-establish a social support system. In another family, there may be a relatively large network of friends and family who are available to provide emotional support to the family and advice on childcare matters. The family may also have interactions with other families of children with special needs; these connections provide them with emotional support and information and advice that helps them navigate the professional service delivery system. Given the limited financial resources of this family, however, they may have unmet needs that relate more to the provision of concrete help. Accessing help with transportation to medical appointments and babysitting for other children may be pressing needs. Although emotional support is forthcoming, concrete help is largely unavailable. In yet another family, it may appear that there are many potential sources of social support but the family is unable to access the support. In some cases, the family's beliefs about asking for help may be a barrier to accessing support. It is also possible that the ways in which professional services are organized and delivered create barriers to families accessing the support they provide (e.g., supportive therapies for the child may be available but only during daytime hours which interfere with the parent's work schedule). These examples illustrate the twofold nature of the assessment of support; the assessment should uncover sources of support and gaps in support as well as result in a better understanding of the nature of the mismatch between needs and resources.

What potential resources exist that are untapped? In order to be useful for intervention planning, the assessment of social network resources must not only identify gaps but also explore potential sources of support. There may be supports that exist in the network that are currently untapped. There may also be individuals/groups/organizations that can be added to the network to help the family address a need. This type of assessment requires a shift from a focus solely on "what is" to a consideration of "what could be." Uncovering potential resources can be a more difficult task than identifying current sources of support. It may be helpful to talk with the family about who has provided support in the past and what changes have occurred in the network that have affected the resources that are currently available. Considering with the family who they could imagine helping them with particular needs might open up possibilities that can be further explored.

What interactions with the social network are sources of stress? Given the potential for members of a network to be sources of stress as well as support, a thorough assessment is required to identify how members of the network contribute to family stress. Effective intervention can sometimes involve decreasing reliance on a network member that increases the family's stress rather than strengthening a network connection. It is also possible that a particular connection in the network can be both a source of support as well as a source of stress. For example, a parent may identify a grandparent as useful in providing concrete help (e.g., loaning money, providing babysitting) but also note that the grandparent is a source of stress because of her/his criticism of the parenting style or denial of the disability. Network connections can be complicated. The issue is not simply who can provide what types of support but, rather, who is able to provide what types of support under what circumstances and at what cost to the family. In the example given above, it may be reasonable for the parent to ask the grandparent to help care for siblings while the parent attends medical appointments with the child with special needs, but not to discuss specific parenting concerns with the grandparent or ask for advice about accessing disability services.

The process of assessment. In addition to providing information which should inform planning, assessment should begin a process of creative problem solving. To be effective, the family and practitioner must work in partnership. Encouraging the use of support in a way that is incongruent with the family's values or preferences will not be effective in addressing an unmet need. It will lead to a plan that will either not be implemented or not be sustained.

Working in partnership with families is a defining feature of family-centred practice (Dunst, 2002; Roberts, Rule, & Innocenti, 1998). Collaborative transactions between professionals and families strengthen the family's existing competencies and promote the acquisition of new competencies. To promote family empowerment, the assessment of social resources must involve families in the exploration of supports and remain attentive to the values and beliefs that families hold regarding the use of network resources. This can be accomplished through a variety of practitioner behaviours. To begin, the practitioner must have a genuine interest in understanding the life experience of the family and be curious about the ways that the family has dealt with the myriad of demands it has faced in the past. Some of these demands may be directly related to the reason for the practitioner's current involvement in the family (e.g., the demands of caring for a child with complex medical needs) although much can also be learned from understanding how the family has adjusted to other stressors related to normative family life cycle events as well as extraordinary circumstances. The practitioner must begin with an assumption that the family has strengths and that the assessment should further an understanding of these strengths and how they have served the family as it has set about to accomplish its tasks. The practitioner must also assume that the family will have preferences about how family needs are to be met and will have beliefs or family rules that govern who is looked to for support, what types of support are sought and accepted, how the family accesses supports, and under what conditions the family seeks help from external sources. It is through investigating the nature of exchanges between the family and external supports that the practitioner develops an understanding of the family's relationships with its social network and has the opportunity to explore potential sources of support. The family must be invited to participate not only by providing information but also by being engaged in a problem-solving and decision-making process. The assessment of social support should begin by working with the family to identify possible resources that could be incorporated into the intervention plan.

The expertise of the family-centred practitioner does not exist in the ability to make the "best" decisions for the family but in the skills required to facilitate a process whereby needs can be identified and articulated, resources can be identified, and a plan can be developed to address unmet needs. The practitioner brings to the relationship specific information and knowledge that may be of assistance to families. It is frequently reported that families have the need for relevant and accessible information related to their child's special needs and the formal support services available (e.g., Mitchell & Sloper, 2002; Sloper & Turner, 1992). This information can be shared with families as part of the process of identifying new resources that might be accessed to address needs.

The process of social support assessment, therefore, becomes one in which existing supports within the family's network of informal and formal supports are described and potential sources of support within both the informal network and the formal service delivery system are explored in order to generate possible resources to address unmet family needs. These external supports are considered in conjunction with internal family resources (e.g., family coping style) during the development of a support plan.

In order to accomplish the goals of social support assessment, a number of practice approaches can be used. One approach focuses on identifying members of the social network and the types of support that are provided. The other approach focuses on assessing satisfaction with support received from the network. Frequently, these two approaches are combined within an assessment.

A range of tools, varying in complexity and sophistication, have been developed to assist practitioners in the assessment of social networks and social support (Bailey & Simeonsson, 1988). The use of an eco-map (Hartman, 1978), for example, is a simple tool commonly used in practice that provides a visual representation of the nature of the interactions between the family and friends, extended family, and social institutions, including the flow of resources between the different systems. Interviews with the family provide a basis for the information contained on the eco-map. Other approaches that have been developed for research purposes have more involved procedures. For example, Hirsch (1980) developed a procedure that includes a simple self-report questionnaire that asks respondents to list up to 20 people with whom they have had contact during a 4- to 6-week period. Further assessment is completed by a self-report log of daily interaction, a support system map, and interviewer ratings of the support. In their research with families of children with disabilities, Kazak, Reber, and Carter (1988) assessed networks using a social network listing (adapted from Hirsch, 1980), a social network density grid, and a questionnaire to assess qualitative aspects of the network. Tracy and Whittaker (1990) developed a procedure for assessing support in clinical practice. Their approach takes into account both the structure and function of a person's social network. Dunst and his colleagues have also developed a number of measures that can be useful in practice (Dunst et al., 1988; Dunst, Trivette, & Hamby, 1994). These measures include (a) the Family Support Scale (which lists individuals and groups that are often helpful to members of families raising a young child and asks respondents to rate how helpful each source is for her/his family), (b) the Inventory of Social Support (which lists people and groups and asks respondents to indicate how often they have contact with those people and then asks respondents to indicate which of these people/groups provides them with various types of help that people sometimes need), and (c) a Personal Network Matrix (which involves an assessment of contacts that the respondent has, 10 needs or aspirations important to the respondent and who has offered assistance with those needs, and the respondent's perceptions of the extent to which s/he can depend on different network members for various kinds of support). Other questionnaires have been developed which focus exclusively on the satisfaction of respondents with the support that they receive rather than who actually exists in the network (e.g., Procidano & Heller, 1983).

Social Network Intervention

Whatever the method of assessing social network resources, the purpose of the assessment is to provide a foundation upon which a plan can be developed that addresses the unmet needs and aspirations of the family. The role of service coordination for professionals working with families is often emphasized. A service coordinator engages in a variety of activities, including coordinating evaluations and assessments, facilitating and participating in service plan development, helping families identify prospective service providers, coordinating and monitoring the delivery of services, informing families of the availability of advocacy services, coordinating early intervention services with medical services, and facilitating the development of a transition plan (Stepanek, Newcomb, & Kettler, 1996). While coordinating the delivery of formal services addresses an important family need (Sloper, 1999), a family-centred practitioner is not limited to looking to the relationships between the family and existing services. While formal services may play an important role in meeting family needs, there may be family needs that extend beyond the resources of the professional service delivery system and/or may be more effectively met through the family's informal support system. The assessment of resources contained in the entire social support network (including both informal and formal resources) identifies a broader range of options for addressing the family's unmet needs.

Fostering the linkage between the family and both formal and informal resources expands the role of the practitioner beyond service coordination. Rather than merely informing the family of the services that are available and determining which services might be helpful to the family, intervention focuses on helping the family articulate its needs and priorities and then working collaboratively with the family to identify resources (from potentially the formal or informal network or both) that can be accessed to meet the identified needs. This requires a shift in focus from what is available to a focus on what is needed. This can be a difficult shift for professionals to make – exploring what is needed may uncover needs for which the service delivery system is not well equipped to respond. Once identified, families may look to the professional for assistance in meeting those needs (a potentially uncomfortable position for the professional who does not have services to offer). The practitioner might need to acknowledge the limitations of the service delivery system and either work with the family to advocate for the development of services and/or engage the family in a process of identifying ways in which the informal network may be accessed to assist in meeting the needs. When resources are not readily available in either the informal or formal network, the family-centred practitioner may need to engage with the family in a more active process of developing needed resources. In this situation, the role of the practitioner moves beyond service coordination to resource development.

The Importance of Resource Development in Family-Centred Practice

While in some situations the practitioner may focus on coordinating professional services that are being provided to the family, there are other situations in which the practitioner may be called upon to fill the role of resource developer, seeking to work with the family to expand its resource base. This is distinct from linking the family to existing sources of support – it requires the development of new support resources in either the informal or the formal network.

Expanding the resource base for families can occur in a variety of ways. In the informal network, resource development can involve efforts to expand the social network by introducing new people into the network. It can also involve using people in the existing network to provide support in new ways. Within the network of formal supports, resource development can link casework and policy development; practitioners can provide input about gaps in service provision and can serve an advocacy role.

Network building. Intervention with families may involve working towards the goal of expanding and strengthening the parenting support network. Fuchs (1993) has identified five strategies that can be used to accomplish this goal: consulting, coaching, connecting, convening, and constructing. Using these constructs, practitioners can work with families to make changes to the network that increase support and reduce stress. For example, practitioners can work with parents to identify and map support networks, provide information on resources that might help them make connections with other people, teach parents the skills needed to initiate new connections, restore or repair links, or sever links that are unhelpful and facilitate the bringing together of people to provide opportunities for the formation of new network ties.

One of the approaches to network building that has received attention in the literature is developing strategies to connect parents with other parents who are dealing with similar situations. The opportunity to exchange experiences with other parents who have a child with similar challenges has been reported by parents to be very helpful (Taanila, Syrjälä, Kokkonen, & Järvelin, 2002). Some research has found that while few mothers with children with disabilities received support from parent groups, those who had access to this type of support found it helpful (Levy et al., 1996). Belonging to a mutual support group has been found to benefit parents on sociopolitical, interpersonal, and intraindividual levels by helping parents develop a sense of control in the outside world, develop a sense of belonging to a community, and engage in self-change (Solomon, Pistrang, & Barker, 2001). It is important to note that the extent to which parents may want and need this type of support will vary. For example, Perrin, Lewkowicz, and Young (2000), in a study of parents of children with chronic health conditions, found that mothers reported a higher need for contact with other families of children with chronic conditions than did fathers.

Family-group conferencing. One type of intervention that has been used with various types of families experiencing difficulty is family-group conferencing (e.g., Baffour, 2006; Connolly, 2006a, 2006b). This intervention involves bringing together extended family and other key members of a family's support network to work towards meeting specific needs. This approach could be applied to work with families with children with special needs as a way to identify new sources of support and mobilize members of a network to help the family meet its needs. Given the important role that extended family can play in providing support (especially grandparents; Lindblad et al., 2007; Trute, 2003; Trute et al., 2008), this may be an intervention that could be adapted for use with families with children with special needs, particularly in times of crisis or when unmet needs are high.

Supports for network members. Individuals in a family's network who provide support may themselves need to be provided with assistance in order to know how best to be a resource to the family. In some families, there may be a role for practitioners to play in providing support to those providing support. In their study of families with children with disabilities, Lindblad et al. (2007) found that parents valued interventions for those members providing informal supports such as providing them with information and education about the child's disability and treatment. Intervention with members of a network may indirectly serve to enhance the well-being of families by strengthening sources of support.

Advocacy. Focusing on social resources in intervention may create opportunities for practitioners to assume the role of advocate. Advocacy can occur at the level of the family by working to ensure that the rights of the family and the child are protected and that the family is able to access services to which it is entitled (Bennett et al., 1990). Practitioners may also have the opportunity to serve as advocates at a policy level (Bennett et al., 1990). Because of their direct involvement with families, practitioners are in a position to provide valuable insights regarding gaps in resources for families and/or policies that create barriers for families accessing the supports that they need (Zipper, Weil, & Rounds, 1993). As an advocate, practitioners can create opportunities to influence policymakers as well as support families in developing the skills and knowledge that they need to be stronger advocates for themselves and their children.

Social Support and Family-Centred Practice: Summary

One important component of a family-centred practice model is acknowledgment of the importance that social support plays in the lives of families. Engaging the family in an assessment of social resources that exist in the family's network and are provided by friends, extended family, professionals, and organizations is central to family-centred practice. The knowledge gained from such an assessment is used in the development of a plan aimed at addressing the unmet needs that the family identifies. Interventions that seek to strengthen sources of support available to the family can serve not only to meet the immediate needs of the family but can enhance the family's ability to meet the needs that emerge in the future.

REFERENCES

Arcia, E., Fernández, M.C., Jáquez, M., Castillo, H., & Ruiz, M. (2004, November). Modes of entry into services for young children with disruptive behaviors. *Qualitative Health Research, 14*(9), 1211–26. http://dx.doi.org/10.1177/1049732304268784 Medline:15448296

Armstrong, M.I., Birnie-Lefcovitch, S., & Ungar, M.T. (2005). Pathways between social support, family well being, quality of parenting, and child resilience: What we know. *Journal of Child and Family Studies, 14*(2), 269–81. http://dx.doi.org/10.1007/s10826-005-5054-4

Baffour, T.D. (2006). Ethnic and gender differences in offending: Examining family group conferencing interventions among at-risk adolescents. *Child & Adolescent Social Work Journal, 23*(5-6), 557–78. http://dx.doi.org/10.1007/s10560-006-0075-4

Bailey, D.B., & Simeonsson, R.J. (1988). *Family assessment in early intervention.* Englewood Cliffs, NJ: Macmillan Publishing Company.

Barakat, L.P., & Linney, J.A. (1992, December). Children with physical handicaps and their mothers: The interrelation of social support, maternal adjustment, and child adjustment. *Journal of Pediatric Psychology, 17*(6), 725–39. http://dx.doi.org/10.1093/jpepsy/17.6.725 Medline:1484335

Barrera, M., Jr, & Ainlay, S.L. (1983, April). The structure of social support: A conceptual and empirical analysis. *Journal of Community Psychology, 11*(2), 133–43. http://dx.doi.org/10.1002/1520-6629(198304)11:2<133::AID-JCOP2290110207>3.0.CO;2-L Medline:10299305

Belsky, J. (1984, February). The determinants of parenting: A process model. *Child Development, 55*(1), 83–96. http://dx.doi.org/10.2307/1129836 Medline:6705636

Bennett, T., Lingerfelt, B.V., & Nelson, D.E. (1990). *Developing individualized family support plans: A training manual.* Cambridge, MA: Brookline Books.

Beresford, B.A. (1994, January). Resources and strategies: How parents cope with the care of a disabled child. *Journal of Child Psychology and Psychiatry, and Allied Disciplines, 35*(1), 171–209. http://dx.doi.org/10.1111/j.1469-7610.1994.tb01136.x Medline:8163627

Brett, J. (2004, October). The journey to accepting support: How parents of profoundly disabled children experience support in their lives. *Paediatric Nursing, 16*(8), 14–18. Medline:15537108

Bristol, M.M. (1987, December). Mothers of children with autism or communication disorders: Successful adaptation and the double ABCX Model. *Journal of Autism and Developmental Disorders, 17*(4), 469–86. http://dx.doi.org/10.1007/BF01486964 Medline:3680150

Bronfenbrenner, U. (1979). *The ecology of human development.* Cambridge, MA: Harvard University Press.

Caplan, G., & Killilea, M. (1976). *Support systems and mutual help.* New York, NY: Grune & Stratton.

Carnes, S.L., & Quinn, W.H. (2005). Family adaptation to brain injury: Coping and psychological distress. *Families, Systems & Health, 23*(2), 186–203. http://dx.doi.org/10.1037/1091-7527.23.2.186

Connolly, M. (2006a). Fifteen years of family group conferencing: Coordinators talk about their experiences in Aotearoa New Zealand. *British Journal of Social Work*, *36*(4), 523–40. http://dx.doi.org/10.1093/bjsw/bch273

Connolly, M. (2006b, September). Up front and personal: Confronting dynamics in the Family Group Conference. *Family Process*, *45*(3), 345–57. http://dx.doi.org/10.1111/j.1545-5300.2006.00175.x Medline:16984075

Dunst, C.J. (2002). Family-centered practices: Birth through high school. *Journal of Special Education*, *36*(3), 139–47. http://dx.doi.org/10.1177/00224669020 360030401

Dunst, C.J., & Trivette, C.M. (1996, July-August). Empowerment, effective helpgiving practices and family-centered care. *Pediatric Nursing*, *22*(4), 334–7, 343. Medline:8852113

Dunst, C.J., & Trivette, C.M. (2009). Capacity-building family-systems intervention practices. *Journal of Family Social Work*, *12*(2), 119–43. http://dx.doi.org/10.1080/10522150802713322

Dunst, C.J., Trivette, C.M., & Cross, A.H. (1986, January). Mediating influences of social support: Personal, family, and child outcomes. *American Journal of Mental Deficiency*, *90*(4), 403–17. Medline:2418680

Dunst, C.J., Trivette, C.M., & Deal, A.G. (1988). *Enabling and empowering families: Principles & guidelines for practice*. Cambridge, MA: Brookline Books.

Dunst, C.J., Trivette, C.M., & Deal, A.G. (Eds.). (1994). *Supporting & strengthening families: Methods, strategies and practices*. Cambridge, MA: Brookline Books.

Dunst, C.J., Trivette, C.M., & Hamby, D.W. (1994). Measuring social support in families with young children with disabilities. In C.J. Dunst, C.M. Trivette, & A.J. Deal (Eds.), *Supporting & strengthening families: Methods, strategies and practices* (pp. 152–60). Cambridge, MA: Brookline Books.

Farmer, J.E., Marien, W.E., Clark, M.J., Sherman, A., & Selva, T.J. (2004, July-August). Primary care supports for children with chronic health conditions: Identifying and predicting unmet family needs. *Journal of Pediatric Psychology*, *29*(5), 355–67. http://dx.doi.org/10.1093/jpepsy/jsh039 Medline:15187174

Fuchs, D. (1993). Building on the strengths of family and neighbourhood social network ties for the prevention of child maltreatment: An ecological approach. In M.R. Rodway & B. Trute (Eds.), *The ecological perspective in family-centered therapy* (pp. 69–97). Lewiston, NY: The Edwin Mellen Press.

Haber, M.G., Cohen, J.L., Lucas, T., & Baltes, B.B. (2007, March). The relationship between self-reported received and perceived social support: A meta-analytic review. *American Journal of Community Psychology*, *39*(1-2), 133–44. http://dx.doi.org/10.1007/s10464-007-9100-9 Medline:17308966

Hanline, M.F. (1991). Transitions and critical events in the family life cycle: Implications for providing support to families of children with disabilities. *Psychology in the Schools, 28*(1), 53–9. http://dx.doi. org/10.1002/1520-6807(199101)28:1<53::AID-PITS2310280109>3.0.CO;2-E

Hartman, A. (1978). Diagramming assessment of family relationships. *Social Casework, 59,* 465–76.

Hirsch, B.J. (1980). Natural support systems and coping with major life changes. *American Journal of Community Psychology, 8*(2), 159–72. http:// dx.doi.org/10.1007/BF00912658

Jones, J., & Passey, J. (2005). Family adaptation, coping and resources: Parents of children with developmental disabilities and behaviour problems. *Journal on Developmental Disabilities, 11,* 31–46.

Jones, L., Rowe, J., & Becker, T. (2009). Appraisal, coping, and social support as predictors of psychological distress and parenting efficacy in parents of premature infants. *Children's Health Care, 38*(4), 245–62. http://dx.doi. org/10.1080/02739610903235976

Kawachi, I., & Berkman, L.F. (2001, September). Social ties and mental health. *Journal of Urban Health: Bulletin of the New York Academy of Medicine, 78*(3), 458–67. http://dx.doi.org/10.1093/jurban/78.3.458 Medline:11564849

Kazak, A.E. (1987, March). Families with disabled children: Stress and social networks in three samples. *Journal of Abnormal Child Psychology, 15*(1), 137–46. http://dx.doi.org/10.1007/BF00916471 Medline:3553273

Kazak, A.E. (1988). Stress and social networks in families with older institutionalized retarded children. *Journal of Social and Clinical Psychology, 6*(3-4), 448–61. http://dx.doi.org/10.1521/jscp.1988.6.3-4.448

Kazak, A.E., & Marvin, R.S. (1984). Differences, difficulties and adaptation: Stress and social networks in families with a handicapped child. *Family Relations, 33*(1), 67–77. http://dx.doi.org/10.2307/584591

Kazak, A.E., Reber, M., & Carter, A. (1988, June). Structural and qualitative aspects of social networks in families with young chronically ill children. *Journal of Pediatric Psychology, 13*(2), 171–82. http://dx.doi.org/10.1093/jpepsy/13.2.171 Medline:3171811

Kazak, A.E., & Wilcox, B.L. (1984, December). The structure and function of social support networks in families with handicapped children. *American Journal of Community Psychology, 12*(6), 645–61. http://dx.doi.org/10.1007/BF00922617 Medline:6395691

Levy, J.M., Rimmerman, A., Botuck, S., Ardito, M., Freeman, S.E., & Levy, P.H. (1996). The support network of mothers of younger and adult children with mental retardation and developmental disabilities receiving case management. *British Journal of Developmental Disabilities, 42,* 24–31.

Lindblad, B.M., Holritz-Rasmussen, B., & Sandman, P.O. (2007, June). A life enriching togetherness – meanings of informal support when being a parent of a child with disability. *Scandinavian Journal of Caring Sciences, 21*(2), 238–46. http://dx.doi.org/10.1111/j.1471-6712.2007.00462.x Medline:17559443

Malia, J.A. (2006). Basic concepts and models of family stress. *Stress, Trauma and Crisis, 9*(3-4), 141–60. http://dx.doi.org/10.1080/15434610600853717

Margalit, M., Leyser, Y., Ankonina, D.B., & Avraham, Y. (1991). Community support in Israeli kibbutz and city families of children with disabilities: Family climate and parental coherence. *Journal of Special Education, 24*(4), 427–40. http://dx.doi.org/10.1177/002246699102400404

McCubbin, M.A., & McCubbin, H.I. (1987). Family stress theory and assessment: The T-Double ABCX Model of family adjustment and adaptation. In H.I. McCubbin & A.I. Thompson (Eds.), *Family assessment inventories for research and practice* (pp. 3–32). Madison, WI: University of Wisconsin.

Mitchell, W., & Sloper, P. (2002, March). Information that informs rather than alienates families with disabled children: Developing a model of good practice. *Health & Social Care in the Community, 10*(2), 74–81. http://dx.doi.org/10.1046/j.1365-2524.2002.00344.x Medline:12121265

Perrin, E.C., Lewkowicz, C., & Young, M.H. (2000, January). Shared vision: Concordance among fathers, mothers, and pediatricians about unmet needs of children with chronic health conditions. *Pediatrics, 105*(1 Pt 3), 277–85. Medline:10617736

Pillay, U., & Rao, K. (2002). The structure and function of social support in relation to help-seeking behavior. *Family Therapy, 29,* 153–67.

Procidano, M.E., & Heller, K. (1983, February). Measures of perceived social support from friends and from family: Three validation studies. *American Journal of Community Psychology, 11*(1), 1–24. http://dx.doi.org/10.1007/BF00898416 Medline:6837532

Roberts, R.N., Rule, S., & Innocenti, M.S. (1998). *Strengthening the family-professional partnership in services for young children.* Baltimore, MD: Paul H. Brookes Publishing Co.

Seligman, M. (1991). Grandparents of disabled grandchildren: Hopes, fears, and adaptation. *Families in Society, 72,* 147–52.

Sloper, P. (1999, March). Models of service support for parents of disabled children. What do we know? What do we need to know? *Child: Care, Health and Development, 25*(2), 85–99. http://dx.doi.org/10.1046/j.1365-2214.1999.25220120.x Medline:10188064

Sloper, P., & Turner, S. (1992, September-October). Service needs of families of children with severe physical disability. *Child: Care, Health and Development, 18*(5), 259–82. http://dx.doi.org/10.1111/j.1365-2214.1992.tb00359.x Medline:1394855

Sloper, P., & Turner, S. (1993, February). Risk and resistance factors in the adaptation of parents of children with severe physical disability. *Journal of Child Psychology and Psychiatry, and Allied Disciplines, 34*(2), 167–88. http://dx.doi.org/10.1111/j.1469-7610.1993.tb00978.x Medline:8444991

Solomon, M., Pistrang, N., & Barker, C. (2001, February). The benefits of mutual support groups for parents of children with disabilities. *American Journal of Community Psychology, 29*(1), 113–32. http://dx.doi.org/10.1023/A:1005253514140 Medline:11439824

Stepanek, J.S., Newcomb, S., & Kettler, K. (1996). Coordinating services and identifying family priorities, resources, and concerns. In P.J. Beckman (Ed.), *Strategies for working with families with young children with disabilities* (pp. 69–89). Baltimore, MD: Paul H. Brookes Publishing Co.

Taanila, A., Syrjälä, L., Kokkonen, J., & Järvelin, M.R. (2002, January). Coping of parents with physically and/or intellectually disabled children. *Child: Care, Health and Development, 28*(1), 73–86. http://dx.doi.org/10.1046/j.1365-2214.2002.00244.x Medline:11856190

Tracy, E.M., & Whittaker, J.K. (1990). The social network map: Assessing social support in clinical practice. *Families in Society, 71*, 461–70.

Trivette, C., & Dunst, C. (1992). Characteristics and influences of role division and social support among mothers of preschool children with disabilities. *Topics in Early Childhood Special Education, 12*(3), 367–85. http://dx.doi.org/10.1177/027112149201200308

Trute, B. (2003). Grandparents of children with developmental disabilities: Intergenerational support and family well-being. *Families in Society, 84*, 119–26.

Trute, B., & Hauch, C. (1988a). Social network attributes of families with positive adaptation to the birth of a developmentally disabled child. *Canadian Journal of Community Mental Health, 7*(1), 5–16.

Trute, B., & Hauch, C. (1988b). Building on family strengths: A study of families with positive adjustment to the birth of a developmentally disabled child. *Journal of Marital and Family Therapy, 14*(2), 185–93. http://dx.doi.org/10.1111/j.1752-0606.1988.tb00734.x

Trute, B., Worthington, C., & Hiebert-Murphy, D. (2008). Grandmother support for parents of children with disabilities: Gender differences in parenting stress. *Families, Systems & Health, 26*(2), 135–46. http://dx.doi.org/10.1037/1091-7527.26.2.135

Uchino, B.N. (2006, August). Social support and health: A review of physiological processes potentially underlying links to disease outcomes. *Journal of Behavioral Medicine, 29*(4), 377–87. http://dx.doi.org/10.1007/s10865-006-9056-5 Medline:16758315

Xu, Y. (2007). Empowering culturally diverse families of young children with disabilities: The double ABCX Model. *Early Childhood Education Journal,* *34*(6), 431–7. http://dx.doi.org/10.1007/s10643-006-0149-0

Zipper, I.N., Weil, M., & Rounds, K. (1993). *Service coordination for early intervention: Parents & professionals.* Cambridge, MA: Brookline Books.

PART THREE

Partnership in Planning and Action

8 Parent Preparation for Family-Centred Services

DIANE HIEBERT-MURPHY

Introduction

There is widespread acknowledgment of the importance of parent involvement in services directed towards enhancing child well-being (e.g., Mahoney & Wiggers, 2007; Saint-Jacques, Drapeau, Lessard, & Beaudoin, 2006). Parents play both a direct and an indirect role in child outcomes, and thus the involvement of parents in children's services is essential to achieve intervention goals. While professionals may initiate intervention to enhance child development, parents are key to ensuring that the changes are supported and reinforced in the home environment. Intervention with parents that assists them in learning how to promote their children's development through daily activities directly influences the child's functioning. Providing more general support to parents can also improve outcomes for children, albeit in an indirect way. By providing parents with the supports they require, the family environment is enhanced, creating a context that facilitates positive child development.

Parent involvement in intervention is encouraged by a range of approaches to service delivery (Dunst, Boyd, Trivette, & Hamby, 2002). In family-focused models, parents support professionals who maintain the primary responsibility for identifying goals for intervention and developing the intervention plan. Parents may be involved in service delivery, but the relationship with service providers is not one of meaningful partnership. Within family-centred practice, a qualitative shift occurs in parental roles; parents are expected not only to be involved in intervention but to act as partners in intervention (Dunst et al., 2002; Epley, Summers, & Turnbull, 2010; Law et al., 2003).

Within family-centred practice, relationships between professionals and parents are based on parents having an equal voice in decision-making about the desired goals of intervention, the priorities for intervention, and the particular services received. Parents are not seen primarily as pathological requiring treatment (although therapeutic interventions may be part of the support plan) nor are they seen as only important in supporting their child's treatment. Rather, parents are seen as having strengths and as capable of engaging in partnership with professionals in the intervention process. Parents play this central role by identifying needs that exist within the family and working collaboratively with professionals to develop and implement a plan to address those needs. In order for children's services to be family-centred, parents must have opportunities to be actively engaged in the definition of family needs, the development of a support plan, and the ongoing evaluation of the effectiveness of the plan in addressing their needs and priorities.

A challenge for family-centred services is to identify ways in which to promote the participation of parents in service delivery. Facilitating the development of parent-professional collaboration and partnership often requires shifts in service delivery policies and practices. The changes in organizational structures needed to support the implementation of the principles of family-centred practice have been identified (Lotze, Bellin, & Oswald, 2010; Wright, Hiebert-Murphy, & Trute, 2010). It has been recognized that training and ongoing support for service providers is essential to successful implementation (Beatson, 2008; Tomasello, Manning, & Dulmus, 2010). Less attention has been given to developing specific strategies for helping parents prepare for engaging as partners in service planning and delivery. This chapter explores the issue of parent participation in family-centred practice with a focus on discussing specific interventions that can prepare parents for involvement with family-centred services and enhance their participation in parent-professional collaborations.

Assessment for Enhancing Parent Participation

McCurdy and Daro (2001) provide a useful theory for conceptualizing parent involvement in family support programs. They emphasize that factors impacting parent involvement exist at the levels of the individual, service provider, program, and neighbourhood. This theory speaks to the complex interplay of factors that must be considered in understanding parent participation and implies that a range of inter-ventions might be needed to enhance parental participation in ser-vices. Increasing the participation of any particular parent may require change in the community, the service delivery system, the family, and/or the parent. It is important to note that focusing intervention at the level of the family or parent will likely be of limited success in increas-ing parent participation if barriers at other levels remain unchanged. Developing strategies that enhance parent participation in family-centred services requires an analysis of factors at multiple levels that promote or hinder parent involvement so that relevant goals for inter-vention can be identified.

Key components of assessment for parent participation include

- evaluating the service delivery context,
- assessing parents' preferences for participation,
- assessing parents' need for information regarding their role in family-centred practice, and
- assessing parents' skills for participation.

Evaluating the service delivery context. Family-centred practice is based on the belief that it is the responsibility of the service system to provide services, to the greatest extent possible, in a manner which is consistent with family values and traditions (Dunst, Trivette, & Deal, 1988). Service providers must be motivated to change service delivery practices in order to better meet the needs of parents and children and not focus on how parents need to change in order to adapt to the ser-vice delivery system. Families should not be expected to radically alter their beliefs and practices in order to fit with existing service models; service providers should constantly be working towards adapting the service delivery system to make the services that are offered acceptable and accessible to families.

Assessment for parent participation, then, must strive to understand parents' experiences of the service delivery system and be responsive to parent feedback. Parent input is central to identifying changes in policy and practice that will be meaningful to parents. Research sug-gests that even when parents have positive experiences with services, they can identify ways in which services can be improved. For example, Siebes et al. (2007), in their evaluation of parent participation in paedi-atric rehabilitation, found that despite being generally satisfied, par-ents had suggestions for how their involvement could be enhanced by improvements in the communication between professionals and parents, parents' involvement in goal setting, and parents' involvement in treatment. Obtaining this type of feedback is a critical step in working towards the goal of increased participation of a specific family or for program planning for broader system change. The key point is that the focus of intervention for enhanced parent participation may be changes in policies, programs, and practice rather than, or in addition to, direct interventions with parents.

In exploring parents' experiences of the service delivery system that may impact on their participation, a number of issues might be considered. For example, are services offered at locations that are accessible to parents so that parents are able to engage with professionals? Are services provided in the family's home when transportation is a challenge and a barrier to participation? Can professionals arrange to accommodate parents' work schedules so that parents can participate in meetings regarding their child? Do program policies allow flexibility so that parents are able to have input into how program resources can be tailored to best meet the unique needs of their families? Is there collaboration and coordination between various service sectors (e.g., mental health and child welfare) and/or service providers (e.g., different community organizations and government programs) so that service providers are consistent in the value placed on partnership with parents? Is information about family-centred practice and service delivery available to parents so that they can become familiar with the philosophy of family-centred practice and parent-professional partnerships? Are supports available to parents to help them develop the skills and knowledge needed to participate in partnership? These questions will help to evaluate the context in which parent participation occurs and may be useful in identifying shifts in the service delivery system that could support greater engagement with parents.

In addition to considering the organization of services, it is also important to examine the ability and willingness of professionals within the system to engage in partnerships with parents. The shift from engaging parents in intervention to working in meaningful partnership with parents is not easy for professionals. As illustrated by Campbell and Halbert's (2002) research, professionals may voice support for engaging parents in intervention, but are often more familiar with, and comfortable with, parent involvement and not true partnership. In their study, practitioners expressed the desire for increased parent participation; however, they placed the responsibility for increased involvement on parents. These practitioners did not see parents as partners and did not identify the need for professionals to improve their practices to encourage the involvement of families. It appears that while professionals wanted increased parent involvement, they wanted this involvement within a context of traditional professional-directed service delivery. Interventions that help professionals embrace family-centred practice principles and train them in the skills required to facilitate parent empowerment are needed to prepare professionals for engaging in partnership with parents. Assessing the extent to which professionals in a service delivery system have these supports may identify changes that need to occur on an organizational level to enhance parent participation.

Assessing parents' preferences for participation. Assessing interest and capacity for parent participation is a component of the broader assessment of family needs and includes both content and process considerations. In addition to the assessment of the goals, aspirations, and priorities parents have for their child and family, family-centred assessment must also examine parents' assumptions and expectations of service delivery and their preferred role for involvement in services.

There will be differences between families regarding expectations for service delivery, desired level of involvement, and perceived barriers to achieving their preferred level of participation. Exploring each family's perceptions and experiences provides a nuanced picture of each family's needs and preferences for participation. Examining the unique circumstances and preferences of each family assists in understanding the strengths and challenges in developing a partnership with a particular family and provides insights into the types of interventions that might be helpful in enhancing parents' participation in family-centred services. While assisting in direct practice with families, this type of assessment can also result in the identification of common themes across families and can contribute to the evaluation of the family-centredness of services, including the care that families deem important (Nijhuis et al., 2007). These themes can identify and give direction to needed changes at an organizational or system level.

Service providers must remain aware that the overall goal of parent engagement and involvement in family-centred practice is the empowerment of families, that is, the increased capacity of families to be effective in meeting their needs. As Boehm and Staples's (2002) research demonstrates, there are differences in how consumers of services define empowerment. They found the need for different sets of assumptions and predictions regarding empowerment for different populations. Put simply, different families will define empowerment differently and will require different approaches to assist them in increasing their ability to meet their own needs. To add to the complexity, there is variability in the extent to which parents present for service ready and willing to engage in a collaborative relationship with professionals. Given this variability between families, flexibility, creativity, and openness to new ways of engaging and involving parents remain a challenge for service providers committed to family-centred practice. This may be particularly challenging when working with families who, for various reasons, present as reluctant or resistant to engage in the process. Practitioners may need to be trained in specific techniques that equip them to work towards engagement. For example, motivational interviewing has been discussed as one technique that might be useful for engaging parents in family-centred services (Gance-Cleveland, 2007).

One of the factors that should be emphasized in the assessment of parent participation is the ways in which culture affects a family's expectations and preferences for participation. Understanding the ways in which a family's cultural values and experiences influence how parents perceive professionals and service delivery and the expectations they have for participation must be integrated into any planning that occurs with the family around support for participation. Many barriers to the participation of culturally and linguistically diverse families have been identified, including, for example, insensitivity to cultural diversity, use of jargon, inflexible scheduling of conferences, lack of language-appropriate information materials, and a shortage of bilingual/bicultural personnel (Zhang & Bennett, 2003). Consideration should also be given to the influence that individuals in the families' social networks have on parents' beliefs about involvement with professionals and the appropriateness of accessing formal supports. Attention must be given to the extent to which the families' communities support parental involvement. For some families, practitioners may need to expand the role of the extended family in family-centred services in order to engage the families and identify ways in which parents and other caregivers important in the family can be supported in working collaboratively with professionals (Ochieng, 2003). Hamilton, Roach, and Riley (2003) also emphasize the importance of paying attention to cultural traditions and values and note that there is not a single successful approach to involving parents in family-centred practice but rather, multiple alternative approaches are needed depending on the context.

This speaks to the need for an individualized assessment of each family's desire for involvement and preparation for participation.

While parent participation is a goal within family-centred services, it is important that practitioners not be judgmental about a family's preference for involvement. While practitioners continuously work towards enhancing participation, there will be families who, for a variety of reasons, are limited in their ability or willingness to engage as partners. These families may look to professionals to take responsibility and may opt for a limited role in decision-making. The family's preference for involvement should be accepted and efforts should be made to engage the family to the greatest extent possible. It should also be recognized that the preference for involvement may change as the demands on the family and the resources available to them change. Thus, practitioners should consider ways to enhance a family's sense of empowerment given their current situation while being sensitive to shifts in circumstances that may allow for an expanded role for parents.

Assessing parents' need for information about their role in family-centred practice. Much has been written about how providing information is an important (and often unmet) need in family-centred services (Dyke, Buttigieg, Blackmore, & Ghose, 2006; Raghavendra, Murchland, Bentley, Wake-Dyster, & Lyons, 2007). Stewart et al. (2006) review the literature on the importance of information for parents of children with special needs and make the point that studies of family-centred practice consistently find that the provision of information is rated lower than other aspects of family-centred practice. Information relevant for parents can be specific to their child (e.g., information about a diagnosis, recommendations for therapeutic services, parenting strategies for enhancing the child's development) or can be more general (e.g., information about the organization of the service delivery system, available services, eligibility for services). Although family-centred services should address the needs of parents for both types of information, information about the service delivery system and the roles, rights, and responsibilities of parents and service providers within family-centred services is the type of information that is critical to enhancing parent participation in service delivery.

Within family-centred practice, parents are considered the experts on their child (Tomasello et al., 2010). By virtue of their central role in the child's life, parents have a unique perspective on their child's functioning, including areas of difficulty as well as strengths. In contrast, parents typically enter the world of formal support services without prior knowledge or experience with formal services and are faced with the daunting task of navigating a complex service delivery system. Parents must acquire knowledge about the roles of various service providers, the policies and procedures that govern the delivery of services, and the philosophy of service delivery systems while simultaneously managing the ongoing challenges associated with parenting a child with special needs in addition to other home and work responsibilities. Given these demands, it is not surprising that some parents do not participate in services to the extent deemed optimal by practitioners.

Providing parents with information about family-centred practice is one step that can help to prepare parents to participate as partners with professionals. The information that might be helpful to parents includes the philosophy of family-centred practice, the role of parents in defining the needs of their child and family, what individualized family support plans are and how they are developed, the importance of ongoing evaluation of needs and the effectiveness of the plan, reasonable expectations of service providers, the range of services that are available, eligibility requirements for services, and procedures for obtaining formal supports. Knowledge of the rights of parents as consumers of service and how to access advocacy services can also help parents to feel empowered in their role as collaborators in service delivery.

Assessing parents' skills for participation. According to Dunst and Trivette (1996), participatory experiences are a major component of empowerment and consist of a wide range of collaborative transactions that bring together people who share common interests or concerns and who bring knowledge and wisdom together to solve problems and attain desired goals. A meta-analysis of the relationships between family-centred help-giving practices and child, parent, and family outcomes provides strong evidence of the importance of both relational and participatory elements of practice (Dunst, Trivette, & Hamby, 2007).

While it is the responsibility of practitioners to facilitate interactions that work towards empowerment, parents bring skills and experiences to the interactions with professionals that can influence the extent to which those interactions are participatory. Identifying and strengthening the skills of parents that facilitate partnership can be important in moving towards greater empowerment and participation. For example, some parents may benefit from opportunities that help them develop their communication skills so that they are better able to articulate their perceived needs and priorities for service to professionals. Assertiveness training may support parents in expressing their needs and providing input on the support plan, especially if they hold an opinion that differs from the professional. These skills may also help parents hold professionals accountable in their delivery of services. Problem-solving skills may equip parents to participate in the development of an individualized family support plan while advocacy skills may help parents be better able to obtain the supports that they need.

Summary. Assessment of the barriers that interfere with parent participation as well as the challenges and strengths that parents bring to the parent-professional relationship is the foundation for planning how to most effectively engage parents in family-centred services. This assessment is broad and must consider factors in the service delivery system and the family (see the appendix at the end of this chapter for a summary of assessment questions). The assessment is both situated in the present (where the family is at this point in time) as well as oriented to the future (in what ways might the capacity of the family be enhanced). Thus, the nature and extent of participation is not static; a family-centred service provider is constantly working towards facilitating increased parental capacity not only to engage in service provision but also to be active in ensuring that the needs of the family are met. As with all elements of family-centred practice, practitioners must develop skills in completing this assessment in a way which sets the stage for ongoing participation. The assessment of interest, preference, and capacity for parent participation should itself invite parents to participate in exploring their assumptions about their role in service delivery, respect their desired level of involvement, and attempt to better understand the family culture and values that influence their participation. It is through the process of engaging with practitioners that parents experience first-hand the benefits of parent-professional partnership and increase their motivation and skill for participating in the relationship, which in turn promotes parent empowerment.

Practical Strategies for Enhancing Parent Participation in Family-Centred Practice

Notwithstanding that the particular interventions used to enhance parental participation in family-centred practice must be based on an individualized assessment of each family's unique situation and may involve interventions beyond the parent and family, there are a number of general strategies that can be developed within family-centred services that can further the goal of parent participation.

Developing resources for parents. One of the challenges for family-centred services is to respond to parents' needs for information. Resources that assist service providers in responding to this need can be beneficial in enhancing parents' knowledge. Providing parents with written materials that contain information about formal services that are available as well as educating parents about family-centred practice can enhance parents' ability to engage in a partnership with service providers. Any written material must be provided in a way that is accessible to parents; attention must be given to the literacy level of information as well as the language (Lehna & McNeil, 2008). A variety of formats should also be considered. Based on their study of providing health information about their children to parents, Lehna and McNeil (2008) suggest that information be provided to caregivers in a variety of formats (e.g., booklets, pictures, audio, and video). Increasingly, information about family-centred services is available through a variety of websites. Some parents will be familiar with using the Internet to meet a range of information needs. Directing these parents to web-based resources that provide information about family-centred services will be a convenient way to make this type of information accessible to them.

In addition to providing information, resources can also be provided that help parents organize the vast amount of information that they obtain when dealing with the service delivery system. Stewart et al. (2006), for example, have developed a tool to help parents manage the information relevant to their child. Their tool assists parents to get, give, and use information effectively. Their research provides evidence that the use of the tool improved parents' perceptions of their ability, confidence, and satisfaction using information and increased their perceptions of the family-centredness of services. Expanding such tools to help parents integrate and organize the information that they acquire about family-centred practice and services may further assist parents in engaging in family-centred services.

Developing educational opportunities for parents. In addition to developing resources that can be given to parents, there has been some interest in exploring the benefits of providing educational opportunities for parents whereby they can learn about the family-centred practice service delivery model as well as obtain information about the services that are available to assist them in meeting their needs (Camara, 2003). This type of training focuses on preparing parents to engage as partners in relationships with professionals and is distinct from educational interventions aimed at increasing parents' knowledge of their child's needs and/or helping them develop skills to address developmental or behavioural concerns. The focus is on providing parents with the knowledge and skills that they need to be fully involved as partners in the identification of family needs and the development of a support plan. Families develop skills and knowledge for engagement through both informal and formal training (Beverly & Thomas, 1999). In terms of preparation for participation in family-centred practice, informal training can occur through a variety of experiences including, for example, involvement in the decision-making process and observing how professionals work from a family-centred model. Formal training involves more structured intervention aimed at providing parents with information about the philosophy of family-centred practice, what to expect from service coordinators, how the service delivery system is organized, what services are available, and what is involved in being a partner with professionals. This training can also involve helping parents develop skills for identifying and articulating their needs, exploring supports that are available in their social networks, participating in the development of the individualized family support plan, and advocating within the service system.

Developing parent-to-parent support. There has been a great deal of interest in the benefits of parents of children with special needs connecting with other parents who have similar experiences. This interest has been driven by evidence that parent-to-parent support is beneficial (e.g., Ireys, Chernoff, Stein, DeVet, & Silver, 2001; Solomon, Pistrang, & Barker, 2001) as well as by parents' requests for this type of support. For example, Mitchell and Sloper (2003), in their study of parents of children with disabilities and/or chronic illness, found that parents welcomed opportunities to network with other parents. Sax (2007) suggests that family members need to form alliances with people who have "been there" and need to feel connected to the community. Peer support provides parents with a variety of forms of support including concrete help as well as advocacy and self-determination (Sax, 2007). Ireys et al. (2001) identify three forms of support provided by parent-to-parent support programs: informational, emotional, and affirmational (messages that enhance a parent's confidence). These various forms of support assist parents in dealing with the myriad of challenges that they face when working to meet the needs of their child and family.

In addition to providing emotional support, parent-to-parent support can be a way of preparing parents for participation in family-centred service delivery and enhancing parents' involvement in services. Winch and Christoph (1988), in their work within a paediatric hospital, found that parent groups not only provided opportunities for sharing and listening, problem solving, and sharing of information, but also provided education and the development of skills (e.g., advocacy and communication). Furthermore, they found that participation in such groups promoted parental participation in the care of the child. It would appear, then, that parent-to-parent support can be a mechanism for providing parents with both information and skills to enhance their engagement in family-centred services.

There are various models of how to facilitate the development of parent-to-parent support, including structured parent groups that provide the opportunity for parents to meet other parents, less structured mutual aid groups that are parent-run, and programs that link parents with other parents (Parent to Parent USA, 2010; Stuntzner-Gibson, Koroloff, & Friesen, 1990). Each of these ways of connecting parents could be used to facilitate parents learning from other parents about family-centred services and how to engage with professionals. In developing these types of supports, consideration must be given to what types of linkages are likely to be most useful to the parents. Decisions need to be made about whether the connections will be categorical (made on the basis of children having the same diagnosis or needs) or non-categorical (made not on the basis of children having identical needs, but on parents being involved in similar service delivery systems). If attempting to form a group, attention must be given to the homogeneity of the members in order to increase the chances that parents will develop the desired connections. In this respect, factors such as the families' needs, values, and culture must be assessed. If a group is the chosen method of promoting parent connections, decisions must be made about other factors relevant to establishing successful connections such as accessibility, format, and purpose.

Practitioners should not be limited to thinking that helping parents learn about family-centred practice from other parents requires the development of a new program requiring extensive resources. Intervention can occur as simply as developing a protocol that permits introducing parents who are new to the service delivery system with parents who have experience with family-centred services. Parent-to-parent support as a means of learning about family-centred practice can be a component of other interventions for preparing parents for family-centred practice (e.g., parent training opportunities) and/or can be integrated into existing interventions that encourage parent-to-parent connections (e.g., mutual support groups, parent mentorship programs). What must remain central is the belief that parents with experience with family-centred services can be a tremendous resource to other parents; the challenge is to develop ways to promote the linkages between parents so that this resource can be used.

Expanding the involvement of parents in family-centred services. Parent participation in family-centred services should not be limited to collaborations between parents and professionals involved in addressing the particular needs of their families. To be truly family-centred, service systems need to look for ways in which to expand parent participation beyond the individual case level to include meaningful involvement in policy development, service planning, and training of professionals for family-centred practice. Parent participation should be encouraged at all levels of decision-making and planning. Engaging parents in processes that shape the service system sends the clear message that parent participation is central to family-centred practice.

While the principle of involving parents in policy development and decision-making for services may be appealing, it can be challenging to implement. Inviting consumers of service to participate in decisions about the allocation of resources and the organization of service delivery requires a radical shift in thinking about health and social service administration. Making planning processes transparent and open to evaluation creates a level of vulnerability that is not comfortable for many policymakers and administrators. It is also challenging to identify practical ways in which to involve parents. Not all parents will be interested or able to commit to this level of participation. How then should parents' perspectives be included? How can parent feedback be gathered and used? What processes need to be put in place to ensure that there is not simply token parent input? It is not usually feasible to invite all parents involved in services to be active in all decision-making. What is the best way to ensure that parents have representation on decision-making bodies? By what means should parent representatives be chosen? Full involvement in decision-making processes requires a substantial commitment of time and energy. In what ways should parents be compensated? These and other questions must be addressed in order to develop structures that create opportunities for full parent participation.

While there are many challenges to involving parents in service planning, development, and delivery, there are ways in which these challenges can be addressed. For example, Gallagher, Rhodes, and Darling (2004) describe how parents were hired into a role of "parent educators" in one early intervention program. These parents linked families with resources and with other families, represented the parent perspective on local and state committees, and paid attention to the special issues of parents (e.g., cultural diversity, single-parenting). The overall goal for these parent educators was to make services more parent-friendly. This model benefited other parents who saw the parent educators as useful in disseminating information, encouraging family involvement, and helping families feel like an important part of the service delivery team. The model also had personal benefits for the parent educators; it assisted them financially and helped them develop a range of skills.

Parents can also play a valuable role in training professionals to engage with parents and support parental participation in services. There is a continuum of roles for parents ranging from inviting parents to share their experiences to including parents as co-instructors responsible for course planning and delivery of core content (Iowa Department of Education, 2003). Parent involvement has been found to benefit the students (Whitehead, Jesien, & Ulanski, 1998) as well as the parent and professional instructors (McBride, Sharp, Hains, & Whitehead, 1995). Curran and Murray (2008) have documented the benefits of a nontraditional approach to teaching skills for parent-professional partnerships in which family members team-teach with university faculty and parents of children with disabilities participate in the course with undergraduate students.

Summary

The engagement of parents and their involvement as partners with professionals in all aspects of the intervention process is a central goal of family-centred practice. Understanding parents' preferences for involvement and their ability to engage in partnership is the starting point for intervention aimed at enhancing the family's capacity for participation. Notwithstanding that parents will vary in their ability and desire for participation, the responsibility of the practitioner and the service delivery system is to create a context where parents can participate as fully as they desire. Ongoing encouragement for parent involvement, the provision of supports for acquiring the knowledge and skills that enhance participation, and the creation of opportunities to participate as partners at all levels of service delivery are required to create such an environment.

APPENDIX. ASSESSMENT QUESTIONS FOR ENHANCING PARENT PARTICIPATION

- In what ways does the current system deliver services in a manner that fits/does not fit with the family's style and preferences?
- How do the ways services are delivered make it difficult for parents to participate in the process?
- How do existing services engage parents in service delivery? In what ways could programs and policies be changed to encourage greater parent participation?
- To what extent do professionals embrace family-centred principles and what training and support is needed for professionals to facilitate greater parent participation?
- What opportunities exist for parent participation beyond the case level? What changes are needed to engage parents in policy development, program planning, and training of professionals?
- What are parents' expectations about their role in service delivery and what do they expect from professionals?
- What previous experiences have parents had with the service system and are these prior experiences congruent with a family-centred approach to service delivery? What, if any, shifts are needed in their expectations of professionals?
- What roles do parents want to play in the services that their child and family receive?
- What factors (e.g., numerous children, language barriers, poverty, lack of experience with the service delivery system) in the family's environment may impact on their ability to engage in partnership?
- What resources does the family have that make it more likely that the parent may be able to engage in partnership with the service providers (e.g., time, experience, social support, assertiveness, confidence, transportation to attend meetings)? What supports might be needed to increase participation?
- What knowledge do parents have about family-centred practice? What information might be helpful to the parents to increase their awareness of family-centred practice and clarify their role as parents

in service delivery? What might be the best way to share this information with the family?

- What skills do the parents have that will facilitate their engagement in the parent-professional partnership?
- Are the parents able to articulate their needs and priorities for service? What might help the parents assert their needs?
- What experiences and/or training might enhance the parents' skills for partnership in service planning?
- Given the family's values, culture, and preferences, what interventions might be most effective in enhancing their preparation for participation?

REFERENCES

Beatson, J.E. (2008). Walk a mile in their shoes: Implementing family-centered care in serving children and families affected by autism spectrum disorder. *Topics in Language Disorders, 28*(4), 309–22. http://dx.doi.org/10.1097/01.TLD.0000341126.16405.e9

Beverly, C.L., & Thomas, S.B. (1999). Family assessment and collaboration building: Conjoined processes. *International Journal of Disability Development and Education, 46*(2), 179–97. http://dx.doi.org/10.1080/103491299100623

Boehm, A., & Staples, L.H. (2002, October). The functions of the social worker in empowering: The voices of consumers and professionals. *Social Work, 47*(4), 449–60. http://dx.doi.org/10.1093/sw/47.4.449 Medline:12450015

Camara, D.M.C. (2003). *Parent education in family-centered practice with families of children with special needs: A partnership towards family empowerment.* Unpublished master's practicum report, University of Manitoba, Winnipeg, MB.

Campbell, P.H., & Halbert, J. (2002). Between research and practice: Provider perspectives on early intervention. *Topics in Early Childhood Special Education, 22*(4), 213–26. http://dx.doi.org/10.1177/027112140202200403

Curran, E., & Murray, M. (2008). Transformative learning in teacher education: Building competencies and changing dispositions. *Journal of the Scholarship of Teaching and Learning, 8*, 103–18.

Dunst, C.J., Boyd, K., Trivette, C.M., & Hamby, D.W. (2002). Family-oriented program models and professional helpgiving practices. *Family Relations, 51*(3), 221–9. http://dx.doi.org/10.1111/j.1741-3729.2002.00221.x

Dunst, C.J., & Trivette, C.M. (1996, July-August). Empowerment, effective helpgiving practices and family-centered care. *Pediatric Nursing, 22*(4), 334–7, 343. Medline:8852113

Dunst, C.J., Trivette, C.M., & Deal, A.G. (1988). *Enabling and empowering families: Principles & guidelines for practice.* Cambridge, MA: Brookline Books.

Dunst, C.J., Trivette, C.M., & Hamby, D.W. (2007). Meta-analysis of family-centered helpgiving practices research. *Mental Retardation and Developmental Disabilities Research Reviews, 13*(4), 370–8. http://dx.doi.org/10.1002/mrdd.20176 Medline:17979208

Dyke, P., Buttigieg, P., Blackmore, A.M., & Ghose, A. (2006, March). Use of the measure of process of care for families (MPOC-56) and service providers (MPOC-SP) to evaluate family-centred services in a paediatric disability setting. *Child: Care, Health and Development, 32*(2), 167–76. http://dx.doi.org/10.1111/j.1365-2214.2006.00604.x Medline:16441851

Epley, P., Summers, J.A., & Turnbull, A. (2010). Characteristics and trends in family-centered conceptualizations. *Journal of Family Social Work, 13*(3), 269–85. http://dx.doi.org/10.1080/10522150903514017

Gallagher, P.A., Rhodes, C.A., & Darling, S.M. (2004). Parents as professionals in early intervention: A parent educator model. *Topics in Early Childhood Special Education, 24*(1), 5–13. http://dx.doi.org/10.1177/02711214040240010101

Gance-Cleveland, B. (2007, March-April). Motivational interviewing: Improving patient education. *Journal of Pediatric Health Care, 21*(2), 81–8. http://dx.doi.org/10.1016/j.pedhc.2006.05.002 Medline:17321907

Hamilton, M.E., Roach, M.A., & Riley, D.A. (2003). Moving toward family-centered early care and education: The past, the present, and a glimpse of the future. *Early Childhood Education Journal, 30*(4), 225–32. http://dx.doi.org/10.1023/A:1023335523871

Iowa Department of Education. (2003). *Families as presenters: A manual and directory.* Des Moines, IA: Department of Education.

Ireys, H.T., Chernoff, R., Stein, R.E.K., DeVet, K.A., & Silver, E.J. (2001). Outcomes of community-based family-to-family support: Lessons learned from a decade of randomized trials. *Children's Services, 4*(4), 203–16. http://dx.doi.org/10.1207/S15326918CS0404_04

Law, M., Hanna, S., King, G., Hurley, P., King, S., Kertoy, M., & Rosenbaum, P. (2003, September). Factors affecting family-centred service delivery for children with disabilities. *Child: Care, Health and Development, 29*(5), 357–66. http://dx.doi.org/10.1046/j.1365-2214.2003.00351.x Medline:12904243

Lehna, C., & McNeil, J. (2008, May). Mixed-methods exploration of parents' health information understanding. *Clinical Nursing Research, 17*(2), 133–44. http://dx.doi.org/10.1177/1054773808316730 Medline:18387884

Lotze, G.M., Bellin, M.H., & Oswald, D.P. (2010). Family-centered care for children with special health care needs: Are we moving

forward? *Journal of Family Social Work, 13*(2), 100–13. http://dx.doi.
org/10.1080/10522150903487099

Mahoney, G., & Wiggers, B. (2007). The role of parents in early intervention: Implications for social work. *Children & Schools, 29*(1), 7–15. http://dx.doi.
org/10.1093/cs/29.1.7

McBride, S.L., Sharp, L., Hains, A.H., & Whitehead, A. (1995). Parents as co-instructors in preservice training: A pathway to family-centered practice. *Journal of Early Intervention, 19*(4), 343–55. http://dx.doi.
org/10.1177/105381519501900408

McCurdy, K., & Daro, D. (2001). Parent involvement in family support programs: An integrated theory. *Family Relations, 50*(2), 113–21. http://dx.doi.
org/10.1111/j.1741-3729.2001.00113.x

Mitchell, W., & Sloper, P. (2003). Quality indicators: Disabled children's and parents' prioritizations and experiences of quality criteria when using different types of support services. *British Journal of Social Work, 33*(8), 1063–80. http://dx.doi.org/10.1093/bjsw/33.8.1063

Nijhuis, B.J.G., Reinders-Messelink, H.A., de Blécourt, A.C.E., Hitters, W.M.G.C., Groothoff, J.W., Nakken, H., & Postema, K. (2007, July). Family-centred care in family-specific teams. *Clinical Rehabilitation, 21*(7), 660–71. http://dx.doi.org/10.1177/0269215507077304 Medline:17702708

Ochieng, B.M.N. (2003, June). Minority ethnic families and family-centred care. *Journal of Child Health Care, 7*(2), 123–32. http://dx.doi.
org/10.1177/1367493503007002006 Medline:12841530

Parent to Parent USA. (2010). Endorsed practices for parent to parent support. Retrieved from http://www.p2pusa.org/

Raghavendra, P., Murchland, S., Bentley, M., Wake-Dyster, W., & Lyons, T. (2007, September). Parents' and service providers' perceptions of family-centred practice in a community-based, paediatric disability service in Australia. *Child: Care, Health and Development, 33*(5), 586–92. http://dx.doi.
org/10.1111/j.1365-2214.2007.00763.x Medline:17725781

Saint-Jacques, M., Drapeau, S., Lessard, G., & Beaudoin, A. (2006). Parent involvement practices in child protection: A matter of know-how and attitude. *Child & Adolescent Social Work Journal, 23*(2), 196–215. http://dx.doi.
org/10.1007/s10560-005-0042-5

Sax, P. (2007). Finding common ground: Parents speak out about family-centered practices. *Journal of Systemic Therapies, 26*(3), 72–90. http://dx.doi.
org/10.1521/jsyt.2007.26.3.72

Siebes, R.C., Wijnroks, L., Ketelaar, M., van Schie, P.E.M., Gorter, J.W., & Vermeer, A. (2007, March). Parent participation in paediatric rehabilitation treatment centres in the Netherlands: A parents' viewpoint. *Child: Care,*

Health and Development, 33(2), 196–205. http://dx.doi.org/10.1111/j.1365-2214.2006.00636.x Medline:17291324

Solomon, M., Pistrang, N., & Barker, C. (2001, February). The benefits of mutual support groups for parents of children with disabilities. *American Journal of Community Psychology, 29*(1), 113–32. http://dx.doi.org/10.1023/A:1005253514140 Medline:11439824

Stewart, D., Law, M., Burke-Gaffney, J., Missiuna, C., Rosenbaum, P., King, G., Moning, T., & King, S. (2006, July). Keeping It Together™: An information KIT for parents of children and youth with special needs. *Child: Care, Health and Development, 32*(4), 493–500. http://dx.doi.org/10.1111/j.1365-2214.2006.00619.x Medline:16784504

Stuntzner-Gibson, D., Koroloff, N.M., & Friesen, B.J. (1990). *Developing and maintaining mutual aid groups for parents and other family members: An annotated bibliography.* Portland, OR: Portland State University, Research and Training Center on Family Support and Children's Mental Health.

Tomasello, N.M., Manning, A.R., & Dulmus, C.N. (2010). Family-centered early intervention for infants and toddlers with disabilities. *Journal of Family Social Work, 13*(2), 163–72. http://dx.doi.org/10.1080/10522150903503010

Whitehead, A., Jesien, G., & Ulanski, B.K. (1998). Weaving parents into the fabric of early intervention interdisciplinary training: How to integrate and support family involvement in training. *Infants and Young Children, 10,* 44–53.

Winch, A.E., & Christoph, J.M. (1988, Fall). Parent-to-parent links: Building networks for parents of hospitalized children. *Children's Health Care, 17*(2), 93–7. http://dx.doi.org/10.1207/s15326888chc1702_6 Medline:10290558

Wright, A., Hiebert-Murphy, D., & Trute, B. (2010). Professionals' perspectives on organizational factors that support or hinder the successful implementation of family-centered practice. *Journal of Family Social Work, 13*(2), 114–30. http://dx.doi.org/10.1080/10522150903503036

Zhang, C., & Bennett, T. (2003). Facilitating the meaningful participation of culturally and linguistically diverse families in the IFSP and IEP process. *Focus on Autism and Other Developmental Disabilities, 18*(1), 51–9. http://dx.doi.org/10.1177/108835760301800107

9 The Family-Centred Support Plan: An Action Strategy for Parent and Professional Partners

TRICIA KLASSEN, BARRY TRUTE, AND
DIANE HIEBERT-MURPHY

A cornerstone in the planning and delivery of family-centred services is the implementation and ongoing use of a Family-Centred Support Plan (FCSP). The early development of this service planning process was profoundly influenced in Canada by federal legislation in the United States. The legislation in the United States required the implementation of the Individualized Family Service Plan (IFSP) to qualify for federal funding. Public Law 99-457 of the United States Congress detailed the specific components of the IFSP. Within that law, part H, section 677, requires that the plan be developed by a team that includes participation by parents or guardians.

This legislative initiative in the United States was aimed at encouraging states to advance their early intervention services for infants and toddlers with disabilities. However, as children's services have a mandate that extends beyond early intervention with infants and toddlers, there has been a need for family support planning protocols that are relevant to a wide age range, from infancy to young adult. Parent-professional joint service planning for services to children and youth needs to be an ongoing process that begins when a child enters children's services and continues on until that child reaches adulthood and enters the adult service delivery system.

The IFSP, as initiated in the United States, is created through a formal, systematic assessment and planning process that incorporates parent concerns and priorities, that explores a child's and family's strengths and needs, that establishes service goals for the child and the family, and that designates the resources needed to reach those goals (Boone, Moore, & Coutler, 1995; Joanning, Demmitt, Brotherson, & Whiddon,

1994). The IFSP ties together all assessment information into a comprehensive understanding of the child and family needs, serves to establish service priorities, and employs these priorities as a fundamental guide to intervention (Moroz & Allen-Meares, 1991). It is important to recognize that although an IFSP can be viewed as a concrete product or formal service agreement that directs immediate action to meet child and family needs, the collaborative process whereby the plan is created is of critical importance. The process followed in designing each IFSP sets the stage for all subsequent IFSPs that will emerge as the needs of the "child with family" evolve and change over time.

We believe that it is more consistent with family-centred practice principles, and more congruent with a partnership approach to the care of children, to refer to the planning process as one involving "family support" rather than "family service"; thus, we prefer to use the term "Family-Centred Support Plan" in place of "Individualized Family Service Plan." Bennett, Lingerfelt, and Nelson (1990) suggest that the use of the word support instead of service denotes an emphasis on enabling the family through encouragement and support, rather than putting the emphasis on an intervention to solve the family's problems. Further, a family-centred approach recognizes the importance of both formal (e.g., professional services and programs) and informal (e.g., support from friends and family) resources in responding to family needs. Within this framework, planning should include a consideration of all supports available to a family, and not be limited to resources available through the formal service system. Finally, the IFSP is often associated with the field of child disability; there is a need to expand the planning process to other areas including services for children with complex medical needs, children in need of protection, and children with mental health challenges. While we will use the term FCSP, it should be noted that there is important wisdom that has guided the evolution of the IFSP as well as a substantial literature explicating its design and completion. The FCSP can be seen to be directly derived from the IFSP.

This chapter highlights the key elements in the development of the FCSP. The specific components of the FSCP are described along with strategies for how to enhance the planning process. The importance of a partnership between service providers and parents is emphasized with a consideration of how to enhance parent participation in the process.

Components of the FCSP

The FCSP mirrors the IFSP in that it contains seven basic elements. These elements include

1 A statement of the child's present level of development
2 A statement of the family's needs and strengths related to enhancing the child's development
3 A statement of the major outcomes expected to be achieved through parent and professional action for the child and family
4 A statement of services/supports required to meet the needs of the child and family
5 The projected dates for initiation of services and anticipated duration of these services
6 The identification of a "case manager," either parent or professional, who will oversee the activities delineated in the support plan (McGonigel & Garland, 1988) (We prefer the use of the term service coordinator instead of case manager, as the term case manager implies a hierarchy of decision-making in what should be a collaborative venture between the parent and professional [Turbinville, Lee, Turnbull, & Murphy, 1993])
7 Procedures of transition (e.g., preschool to elementary school program).

Statement of the child's current level of development. The FCSP begins with a statement about the child's current functioning. An assessment that follows family-centred principles will involve the full participation of parents as "experts on their child and family" (Joanning et al., 1994). Such parent involvement in the assessment process may take different forms, depending upon a particular family's preferences and needs. Although mothers are typically more involved in the assessment process, a family-centred approach seeks to involve both parents in two parent families (Joanning et al., 1994). Any key parenting figures for a child should also participate, such as grandmothers or siblings of the child's parents, if they share childcare responsibilities.

An assessment of the child's abilities is generally based on a variety of assessment procedures and methods, which are usually compiled by the service coordinator or primary service provider prior to the first FCSP meeting. The goal of the child assessment in preparing a support plan is to identify child needs and strengths that are immediately relevant, and to recognize and to support the parents' competencies to meet child development and social adjustment goals (Bailey, McWilliam, Winton, & Simeonsson, 1992). It is important to note that assessment is an ongoing process; young children's needs and abilities may change rapidly, and thus assessment information requires ongoing review and verification (Campbell, 1991).

Woods and Lindeman (2008) recommend that assessment and intervention occur in a family's natural environment so that the routines, activities, and events that occur regularly for children are identified and allow for outcomes that are authentic, relevant, and have greater likelihood of making a difference. Meeting with families in their homes often facilitates a reciprocal approach to assessment and planning, in which there is a dynamic exchange between parent and professional, that can increase efficiency and accuracy in information gathering. A great deal of developmental information can be identified by family members and, in a reciprocal manner, can be provided to parents by service providers throughout their mutual information exchanges. As well, much can be learned through the observation of children and their parents in daily interactions and routines. Woods and Lindeman (2008) note that a developmental assessment that is truly family-centred will underscore the relevance of the family members' perspectives of their child.

The assessment should be done in a manner that includes a review of a child's strengths, interests, and favourite activities. Most parents readily identify a variety of qualities about their children that can be seen as strengths. For example, instead of asking parents to describe their "child's strengths" in general terms, professionals may ask more focused questions like "What about your child shows her/his abilities or pleasing features?" Positive child qualities that are often reported by parents include the children being highly sociable, sensitive to others, of happy disposition, determined, well-mannered, independent, and thoughtful. Most parents are also able to see positive aspects in child attributes that many others would see as challenging. For example, a family may describe their child as dramatic, charismatic, and full of energy (rather than hyperactive and stubborn). Although these child characteristics can contribute to stress in the home, many parents can recognize the potential for their child to use these qualities in a positive way. Parents are usually able to identify positive impacts that their child has had on family members and on family life. For example, they may assert that their child has contributed to personal growth, taught them what is important in life, and made life more meaningful for family members.

Family assessment and the FCSP. While the special needs of a child may trigger initial involvement with the service delivery system, within family-centred practice the focus is on the child in the family. Thus, attention must be given to the needs of both the child and the family, as the family context is integral to the developmental functioning and well-being of the child. The purpose of family assessment activities, in support of the preparation of the FCSP, is to determine ongoing ways that supports may be used to address family concerns and enhance the strengths of the family (Campbell, 1991). Brown, Thurman, and Pearl (1993) assert that any family assessment must be congruent with the parents' priorities and service agenda, rather than being solely focused on securing a clinical assessment of overall family adjustment and well-being from a pathology or deficiency frame of reference. That is, the emphasis should be on strengthening and mobilizing family resources and supports for the child, rather than searching for, and then analysing, inadequacies or pathology that need to be "fixed" by professionals (Dunst, Trivette, & Deal, 1994).

Beckman and Bristol (1991) suggest that having a child with a disability or special needs does not give the service provider the right to subject families to time consuming and intrusive assessments when these are not appropriate to the service needs and priorities of the family. Parents will often indicate their preferences for what order and scope of assessment information makes sense in their family situation, and will want a voice in terms of what family information is shared between service providers. Parents will often interweave information about their family routines, activities, settings, resources, and needs into the discussion of child development issues, both obviously and incidentally (Woods & Lindeman, 2008). Through their response to the use of multiple information-gathering strategies (conversations, questionnaires, eco-mapping, problem solving, environmental scan, etc.), families will often provide clear indications of the types of information they want to share. In general, when service issues to be explored are simple and direct, the scope of the assessment should begin as simple and direct. Complex matters such as the psychosocial adjustment of the child or the psychological well-being of that child's family members may be addressed when and if the need arises, and (as discussed in Chapter 3) requires skilful and more comprehensive assessment methods.

Service providers sometimes struggle with a clear way to sequence information collection during the assessment process. As part of this, they weigh the costs and benefits of using standardized (or empirical) assessment measures and question the appropriateness of gathering information that the professional knows is important but that might be seen as personally intrusive by family members. The literature on service planning processes and procedures supports the use of both structured and non-structured interview and information collection formats (Beckman & Bristol, 1991; Fewell, Snyder, Sexton, Bertrand, & Hockless, 1991; Sexton, Snyder, Rheams, Barron-Sharp, & Perez, 1991). Some parents initiate service contacts due to a particular need (e.g., respite, child developmental services). These parents are usually clear about the services they desire and require little prompting to discuss the relevant child and family needs. Some parents who have been receiving services over many years, and who are not accustomed to completing standardized information-gathering or assessment forms, will often respond more positively to an interview approach in which they can share information verbally. These parents may be encouraged to begin the assessment process by identifying the strengths and abilities of their child and be invited to express what is important to them and their family (Campbell, Strickland, & Forme, 1992). When parents clearly verbalize their needs, gathering information through the use of an informal interview will typically be the most appropriate. However, the introduction of standardized assessment measures early in the FCSP process may be appropriate when parents are unsure of how to articulate their needs, are unsure of the services available to them, and would evidently benefit from a range of different support resources (examples of brief, empirical assessment tools are offered in Chapter 5). The best strategy in times of professional indecision is to move slowly in gathering information and to give more central attention to strengthening the working alliance with the parent and family. Many of these professional concerns about how to conduct an assessment dissipate as a strong working alliance evolves with family members.

Regardless of the method used to collect information, attention to parental and family strengths is an important component of the family assessment. Parents will demonstrate a variety of ways in which they cope with stresses of caregiving related to their child's developmental, behavioural, or health challenges. Coping mechanisms often include adaptive appraisals of one's situation, active problem solving, and reliance on social supports. Examples of adaptive coping might include emphasizing child and family strengths, recognizing small accomplishments, appreciating the unique qualities of family members, having optimism about the future, relying on religious beliefs, and perceiving all families as unique. Parents will identify a variety of methods in which they actively cope with what they see as their personal stressors (e.g., taking time for their own individual needs, developing regular family routines, planning ahead, developing assertiveness and advocacy skills, relying on humour as a way of handling disappointment, and engaging in activities and careers that are enjoyable and meaningful).

Many parents will identify more strengths in their family life than they identify needs and concerns, if asked about both. Although families with children with special service needs may experience additional stressors due to frequent appointments with professionals and involvement with a large number of service providers, most parents typically do not perceive these stressors as impacting upon their family's ability to function well. Some parents will report that their child's qualities facilitate positive family functioning in some areas. For example, a family may indicate that the child's gregarious and high-energy personality provides family members with more social opportunities than they may have had otherwise. Families also tend to view their daily routines as just a natural part of their lives, rather than viewing child needs as impacting negatively upon their schedules and everyday functioning.

When positive attributes of their children are identified by parents, an opportunity is provided to professionals to acknowledge parental strengths. Child qualities such as good manners and assistance with household chores can be attributed to effective parenting skills. There usually are a variety of positive parental qualities that can be recognized and acknowledged, including creative teaching and stimulation, skill in the recognition of child cues, flexibility and ability to match the pace of the child, consistency in discipline and applying consequences, provision of a safe and structured home, the ability to organize and plan ahead, and the ability to ensure their child's needs are met.

Identification of priority needs. As part of the FCSP process, parents identify important concerns in the life of their family and in regard to the well-being of their child with a disability or complex health, mental health, or behavioural challenges. These identified concerns are then translated into support needs (Dunst et al., 1994). The term "needs" is a broad concept that is used to define a variety of activities, events, or goals. Some families will define needs in general terms (e.g., indicating that they desire to be better parents or that they wish for their child to be more independent). Other families will define needs concretely (e.g., they would like an adapted bike for their child or transportation for their child to daycare). Needs can also be framed in terms of the kinds of services and resources families wish to access. It is helpful to discuss what the actual desired outcome is for parents (e.g., for the child to eat more independently) and then to determine what is required in order for that outcome to be achieved (e.g., referral to an occupational therapist for adapted utensils). The role of the service provider is often to assist families to break down broad needs into more focused, workable goals. The more specific and simply stated the outcome statements, the more adaptable the plan will be to family change. Furthermore, it is more effective to address a small number of immediate needs at a time rather than devising several long-term plans, unless parents identify a need such as planning for the future care of their child as their first priority.

Concerns are commonly identified that relate to child development and social needs, or to the child's access to medical, educational, and community services. Parents can often provide detailed information related to specific physical, cognitive, communicational, social, and personal care needs of their child. The most common concern expressed by parents at the time of diagnosis of a health challenge or developmental disability is the need for information about the child's diagnosis and services specifically responding to this diagnosis. Parents will want as much information as they can get about the service system and their role in accessing services. For example, families will often express confusion as to whether they need a referral to an agency or whether they can make contact directly. Parents are often unsure about their options for gaining child-related supports, how different services are connected with each other, and whether funding or subsidies are available for particular services.

Parents may identify a variety of their own personal needs such as relief from the stress of caregiving, a desire to meet other parents facing similar challenges, more personal time for themselves or with their spouse, assistance in gaining more support from family members and friends, and knowing how to explain their child's needs to others. Some will feel somewhat "trapped" in their role as a parent of a child with special needs and will be interested in pursuing other "outside family" relationships, activities, and employment opportunities. Some parents will show low levels of self-esteem and express emotional issues that they feel need to be resolved. Parent needs will vary widely depending on their present child concerns. Gowen, Christy, and Sparling (1993) summarize basic parent support needs as including help to access information on how to promote the positive development of their child, support in dealing with the emotional and time demands of parenting, the identification of community resources, planning for the child's future, and understanding the child's legal rights.

Some parents will also speak about needs of their entire family, which may not be directly related to their child's disability or behavioural or health challenges. For example, they may face barriers to achieving basic employment for themselves, financial support for the family, household management resources, or recreational opportunities (all of which are often exacerbated by child concerns and challenges). Ridgley and Hallam (2006) examined the concerns of rural, low-income families and the content of their service plan documents and found that the formal service plans primarily addressed issues related to parenting the child, even when family-related concerns were emphasized by families. Given that family-related concerns such as access to health care, food and nutrition, and financial limitations can profoundly impact the functioning of the family and affect how well the parent is able to address the needs of their child, these needs should be acknowledged by the service provider and addressed in the FCSP.

It is important for service providers to be aware that families' broader context (including their class, cultural background, and/or family form) will influence their definition of needs. For example, a family's socioeconomic status will influence the types of needs that are expressed (DeGangi, Wietlisbach, Poisson, Stein, & Royeen, 1994; Johnson et al., 1994). Families with lower socio-economic status tend to focus more on global family and parental needs, rather than defining specific needs for their children (Kalyanpur & Rao, 1991). Needs such as assistance with parenting, a daycare subsidy, assistance in gaining employment, transportation assistance, neighbourhood safety, and recreational opportunities are common priorities for families with financial challenges. When basic family needs are not being met, it is difficult to focus solely on the needs of the child. Service providers must be aware of, and sensitive to, the diversity between families and the ways in which contextual factors influence their life experiences and their definition of child and family needs.

A family-centred approach emphasizes that families should identify what they perceive as needs and not be pressured to address areas that are not of immediate concern to them (but that the professional may feel is important). One example that families have given us is the push by professionals for them to send their child to summer camp when they have good reasons not to want to use this resource. Families will usually respond openly to being asked what they want for their child and family and what kinds of supports would be most helpful to them. It appears that too often service providers tend to make observations and recommendations without asking what the parents feel is a priority need for their child and family. Questions such as "What would you like to see for your child in the next 6 to 12 months?" and "What are your immediate needs as a family?" are simple ways of determining what the top service goals are for families. Such specific questions assist parents and professionals in jointly developing goals that are based on parent-identified needs. Furthermore, as the assessment proceeds, parents may share information that provides an opportunity for further discussion of needs that might not be easily articulated by the parents. For example, asking parents how their child influences their daily routines or everyday living may initiate discussion regarding the parents' inability to spend time together as a couple and may raise concerns regarding the availability of respite resources in their extended family. The service provider then would explore why the parents felt that these sources of potential informal supports were not available. The parents may indicate that they do not feel comfortable or know how to ask for support when they need it. This opens the door to the professional talking with the parents about their past experiences and helping the parents identify and articulate service objectives. The service provider may need to play a large role in assisting in the identification of needs by asking the right questions, but optimally the family should be the ones who identify and rank their child and family's service needs.

There will be instances when the service provider notes a potentially important need for a family but one that may be difficult for parents to acknowledge. In these situations, it is important to be sensitive to the way that the need is identified, discussed, and addressed. For example, if it is observed that a father has a distant relationship with his son with a disability and he verbally affirms this situation, he may be asked questions such as "What are your hopes regarding your relationship with your son?" and "What do you think needs to happen in order to develop that desired relationship?" In one such case, the father recognized that he would need to seek counselling in order to resolve his inability to develop a close relationship with his child; however, he was not ready or willing to take this step. The service provider did not aggressively pursue this matter, but affirmed that the father would know what to do when he was ready. During a later meeting involving the service provider and the father, the father noted that he would like to address his need for counselling so that he could become closer to his son. Although the service provider believed that counselling was important for this parent, she waited for the parent to come to this decision on his own through asking gentle and respectful questions, and did not pressure him to take immediate action.

Moving from identified needs to plans. Once parents have prioritized their needs, they should be assisted in translating those needs into goals with expected outcomes and action plans. Outcome statements generally address both process (i.e., the interventions) and outcomes (i.e., the expected results). The statement of objectives must include a list of specific procedures and activities that, if employed, will assist the child or family to meet the perceived needs and achieve a desired outcome (Fewell et al., 1991).

Wording outcomes in the active voice, which specifies what the child or family will do as a result of the intervention, is a helpful strategy (McWilliam et al., 1998). When global outcome statements are made, they need to be more narrowly defined as specific activities or concrete expectations (Moroz & Allen-Meares, 1991). Notari and Drinkwater (1991) suggest that many families will tend to identify broad outcomes for their child. Professionals can provide assistance to better focus and develop short-term goals and to help articulate the series of steps that might be required to achieve those goals. The development of a small number of immediate goals is usually advised. This may give the family a sense of greater participation and invite more optimism that those goals can be achieved (Katz & Scarpati, 1995). McWilliam and colleagues (1998) remind us, however, that although goals should be written in the active voice and be specific, necessary, context-appropriate, inclusive, and have realistic target achievement dates, there are some families who prefer non-specific or general goals that offer flexibility regarding the family's needs.

Attention should be given to writing the FCSP in language that is comfortable and easily understood by parents. Parents appreciate when the FCSP goals are written in their own language rather than in professional jargon (Gallagher & Desimone, 1995). McWilliam et al. (1998) suggest that IFSPs that are written in clear language without the use of jargon tend to be more strengths-focused and highlight the positive aspects of the child and family. Pizur-Barnekow, Patrick, Rhyner, Folk, and Anderson (2010) assessed IFSPs from seven agencies for readability, and found that none prepared IFSP documents at or below the recommended grade 5 level. This finding suggests that service providers are not always sensitive to the fact that many parents will have low literacy levels. Although parents may be highly involved in the assessment and planning sessions, it is not uncommon for them to be disinterested in actually writing out the FCSP or service plan themselves. Some parents may not seem particularly interested in how expected outcomes and action plans are worded, particularly if the support plan is not written in "parent-friendly" language. For example, instead of writing that a child "requires more age-appropriate peer interaction opportunities in order to facilitate social skills development," parents prefer to see outcome statements such as, "Jane will go to preschool two mornings per week so that she has the chance to play with children her age who can stimulate her learning and development." Using language that is understandable and accessible to parents will encourage greater participation by parents and make the plan relevant and meaningful to them.

Although parents often take the lead in articulating their desired goals, service providers can suggest potential plans of action to reach stated goals. An important component of the service provider's role is to offer families information that will assist them in identifying ways to meet the goals that they endorse for their child and family. This role requires that service providers have knowledge that spans the school system, community services, and hospital or medical resources that may be available to the family (Malone, McKinsey, Thyer, & Straka, 2000).

The written FCSP serves as a valuable record of the plan of action for parents. Parents are often overwhelmed after initial meetings with professionals and may have difficulty remembering what they have agreed to do. Furthermore, some parents appreciate when the specific responsibilities of their service provider (or providers) are written in detail on the FCSP; this serves to enhance professional accountability and promotes parental empowerment.

The FCSP is usually recorded in a standardized, written format; examples that illustrate the organization and layout of the IFSP are available that can be directly applied to a FCSP (e.g., Bennett, Lingerfelt, & Nelson, 1990; Pletcher, 1995). Some provinces in Canada have formalized the process for developing a support plan for families that receive provincial family support services. For example, the Nova Scotia government created a support plan procedure for children with autism spectrum disorder (see Province of Nova Scotia, 2002).

Identification of the service coordinator. The FCSP should identify a service coordinator who will be responsible for the monitoring
of the plan set out in the FCSP and who, in some situations, will take
a leadership role in coordinating the activities of other agencies and
their staff members (Fewell et al., 1991). The role of service coordinator may be filled by a professional or a parent. The role of service coordinator is distinct from the role of case coordinator. Dunst, Trivette,
and Deal (1994) suggest that designating professionals as case coordinators, which involves implementing the plan and acting as a liaison
with other agencies, is actually in basic conflict with the philosophy of
family-centred practice, which advocates that families play a lead role
in selecting and securing needed resources. Replacing the role of case
coordination with service coordination is more appropriate for family-
centred services. The service coordinator is typically responsible for assisting with the FCSP process, which includes ensuring that adequate
assessments of the child and family are completed, identifying initial
implementation strategies, and drafting and monitoring the support
plan (Notari & Drinkwater, 1991).

The FCSP may be seen as having three separate components: FCSP
design, followed by FCSP implementation, and then, ongoing evaluation of the FCSP progress. Each component may require varying
degrees of parent and professional leadership, depending on the resources, needs, and knowledge that exist in the parent-professional
partnership.

Facilitating Parent Involvement in Service Planning and Delivery

Although family-centred practice emphasizes a parent-directed process, each family will respond differently regarding their role and
decision-making preferences. Factors that can impact family responsiveness and preferences for involvement include familes' cultural and
educational backgrounds, their views of professionals as partners, and
the emotional and physical health status of the parent (Woods & Lindeman, 2008). Families' prior experiences with service provision may also
affect their beliefs about their role; many families are not accustomed
to playing an active role when receiving services and come to expect
professionals to take the lead. Although we endorse and encourage a
partnership model, consensus has not been reached in the professional
literature regarding the ideal degree of parental involvement in the decision-making process. Recommendations have ranged from parents

fully directing their services, to being equal partners in decision-making, to being consulted regarding service decisions. Families are not always accustomed to being asked to actively participate in their relationships with health care, education, and social service professionals. It is apparent that families do, in fact, differ in their desires and abilities to participate in service planning and coordination. However, it is also apparent that families are capable of determining their own needs and making decisions regarding suitable services when given the opportunity. Minke and Scott (1993) recommend that each parent or "set of parents" be given an option regarding how active they would like to be in developing the support plan.

Notwithstanding that there will be differences among parents about their preferences and abilities to be involved, there are steps that can be taken to facilitate parental involvement in the FCSP process. These approaches often involve explaining the family-centred philosophy and the FCSP process, emphasizing family strengths, facilitating the identification of parent-identified goals, summarizing assessment information gathered to date, and facilitating parent-directed family plans.

Provide information about the process. Parents' willingness to engage with service providers can be enhanced by communicating that they are respected as the experts on their child and that they will work in partnership with professionals to decide on a plan that responds to their needs. It can be helpful for the service coordinator to explain to parents that a family-centred approach emphasizes the strengths of families, the knowledge that families have of their own children and family, the abilities of families to direct their own services, and the need for services to extend beyond the child to family members who may be involved in the life of the child with a disability or complex health challenge. Providing information about family-centred services, including the role of parents, is particularly effective for families who have had negative experiences with service providers in the past that have resulted in a tendency for them to mistrust professionals.

In addition to providing information about family-centred practice, specific interventions that educate parents about FCSPs can be important in encouraging parental participation. Parents are not likely to engage in developing a FCSP if they are unclear about what is involved in the process. It is vital that professionals explain the philosophy that guides the FCSP and the steps involved in the process. Parents need to be aware of the areas that are typically explored during the assessment. Any FCSP documents such as family functioning and support assessments should be shown to the parent early in the engagement and an explanation should be given regarding how these forms are used. The hope is that parents will actively participate early in the service planning process as the roles that are established between parents and professionals in the early stages of service planning will likely set the stage for future collaborative action. Information about the FCSP process may be provided informally through interaction with the service provider or through more formal interventions. For example, Campbell, Strickland, and Forme (1992) found that parents who attend informational workshops on developing service plans feel more confident and are more likely to write their own service plan (see Chapter 8 for further discussion of parent preparation for participation in family-centred services).

Focus on family strengths. Families usually respond positively when they are asked to review the strengths of their family. The service provider can list various strengths that are demonstrated or reported by the parents during the assessment and through observation of family functioning and interaction styles. Some of the strengths that will be identified in this way may not have been seen as "strengths" by the family as they will often see these as "normal" in most families. Many resilient, strong families with children with special needs do not see themselves as being exceptional but consider their own family patterns as normal (Trute & Hauch, 1988). It can be affirming and encouraging to parents when positive family behaviours or beliefs are framed as "patterns of strength" by a professional. Further, some areas that are described as needs by a parent can be reframed into areas of potential strength. As a case example, a mother perceived her tendency to worry about her child as an area in which she required some support. Although the service provider affirmed her concern, her tendency to worry was listed as a strength, as this worry actually demonstrated her love for her child and her desire to be a good parent.

The emphasis on strengths also facilitates an atmosphere of openness and comfort that creates a context in which families are more likely to discuss family concerns and beliefs. Once strengths have been identified and formally noted and the focus turns to family needs, many families will view their needs as less overwhelming and will appear more open to discuss their concerns than they might have been earlier in the process. For example, in a meeting with a family newly opened to service, the parents began disclosing their initial reaction to their child's diagnosis following a conversation about family strengths. This had been a sensitive topic of discussion for them that had not arisen during initial discussions. Although previously these parents had presented as somewhat guarded about discussing needs, they appeared to be relaxed when questions relating to family strengths were introduced by the service provider. This review of family strengths built trust and invited more detailed sharing of information by the parents that included a candid discussion of their early fear and pain regarding the long-term family implications of their child's diagnosis.

Summarize key assessment information. Presenting families with a summary of all assessment information also facilitates parent involvement in the process of developing the FCSP. Parents should be given an opportunity to express whether the professional's understanding of their family's strengths and needs is consistent with their own perceptions of their situation. Parents then should have an opportunity to decide how to proceed with the FCSP session by prioritizing each need that has been identified. Families can be asked to rank the items or to choose the top two or three needs that they feel they would like to address first. This practice ensures that family priorities are the focus of the plan. It is common for only a few needs to be addressed at initial FCSP sessions, as some needs consist of various components, and developing plans of action for several different areas of work may be seen as too overwhelming for some families.

Facilitate parent-directed plans. There are a variety of ways to ensure that the plans that are developed are driven by the families' needs and priorities. Service providers should inform parents of their rights as parents, including their right to lead the decision-making process. Families can be encouraged to steer the assessment process by sharing family concerns and priorities, emphasizing child and family strengths, and being involved in carrying out action plans to get needs met. It is also the responsibility of the service provider to assist families to develop new competencies that will more adequately enable them to participate in service planning and service activation. Families must be fully informed about available education, social service, and health care programs so that they can become more effective advocates for their child and family and can assert their priorities and preferences during the planning process.

Regardless of the capabilities initially exhibited by families, parents know their children better than service providers, as each child is unique and develops within a unique family system. Although families differ in their preferences in developing child and family plans,

all families respond more positively to the process when they are informed and encouraged to actively participate, and when they have a
voice in the development of service goals that are concise, realistic, and
responsive to their changing needs.

Barriers to Effective Implementation of FCSPs

Despite the potential benefits of the FCSP process in operationalizing
family-centred practice with families, such structured approaches to
service planning have been found to be no more effective than other
alternative service planning models when not implemented correctly
(Farel, Shackelford, & Hurth, 1997). There are a number of common barriers to developing effective FCSPs that must be addressed if the FCSP
process is to have its intended effects.

First and foremost is the lack of professional training in family-centred assessment and intervention. Most professionals in childhood disability, child health, child mental health, and child protection services
have not had an adequate educational grounding in family-centred
theory, assessment, and practice. There is evidence that professionals
who have worked in their field for many years and who are more comfortable with traditional practice methods are less likely to write family-centred FCSPs (Jung & Baird, 2003). There is a tendency for some
professionals to want to preserve a child-focused orientation in services when this was what they were trained to do (Katz & Scarpati,
1995; Lawlor & Mattingly, 1998). We have found that many professionals employed in children's services are essentially afraid to work with
families and feel more comfortable working with an individual child
or a parent. Some professionals are unsure of how to assist parents to
become more involved while still maintaining their role as a professional who meets their professional responsibilities to directly assist
the child (Lawlor & Mattingly, 1998). Gallagher and Desimone (1995)
suggest that if professionals can see themselves as consultants instead
of experts, family participation is likely to increase.

Farel and colleagues (1997) found that when service providers did not
perceive a formal service planning process as useful, its potential impact upon children and family well-being was reduced. When service
providers do not have the appropriate training and knowledge about
the support planning process, they may view the process as an extra responsibility as opposed to an essential aspect of the development of a
working alliance with families (Zhang, Fowler, & Bennett, 2004).

It seems that many professionals hold serious concerns about whether most parents possess the skills to effectively participate in the service planning process (Minke & Scott, 1995). These reservations and persistent beliefs may result in a tendency to allow families to depend too much upon professionals (Minke & Scott, 1995). Furthermore, these negative assumptions may result in a lack of information sharing and a lack of consideration for family-developed goals (Katz & Scarpati, 1995).

Although it may be "politically correct" in contemporary children's services to espouse family-centred values, it seems that many professionals still do not implement this perspective in their practice. Staff may view qualities such as parental assertiveness and family decision-making as threatening, even though these same qualities reflect the family's potential for a functional partnership with service providers (Minke & Scott, 1995). Despite espousing philosophies that recognize parents as the optimal decision-makers when planning children's services, professionals have admitted that it can be difficult to relinquish their power and control, as this acts to devalue their knowledge and expertise (Gallagher & Desimone, 1995; Minke & Scott, 1993).

Parents' lack of understanding of the family-centred practice model may be another hurdle in effectively implementing a FCSP process. Parents who are unfamiliar with this orientation in children's services will have difficulty understanding the purpose of the FCSP and its place in service planning and coordination. A partnership model requires informed partners. There is a need for comprehensive training for both professionals and parents regarding the purpose and procedures of the FCSP. Furthermore, opportunities for parents to obtain information about the service delivery system and develop the skills required to engage in the process are needed to ensure that parents participate in the process to the full extent that they desire.

In addition to barriers at the level of individual professionals and parents, there are also structural challenges to family-centred practice such as high caseloads, time pressures, extensive job responsibilities, and scheduling difficulties with parents and various service providers that can impede work with families (Farel et al., 1997; Gallagher & Desimone, 1995; Zhang et al., 2004). When professionals express scepticism about the utilization of FCSPs with families, a primary concern that is often raised is the anticipated increase in time required to implement a planning process that results in a formal FCSP. It must be acknowledged that the development of a FCSP does require a commitment of time to meet with families and jointly author the plan. Although the initial amount of time spent with families may increase at times due to more in-depth child and family assessment, the goal of family-centred practice is to assist parents to gain the knowledge and skills to direct or coordinate their own services. Thus, over time in their work with many families, the service provider will spend increasingly less time initiating service referrals and supports. As parents become more informed and confident, they will be able to act more often as their own "service coordinators" and be better able to respond themselves to the shifting needs of their child and family.

Concluding Comments

Most experienced practitioners will acknowledge that the preparation of an initial FCSP is not an end in itself, but only one beginning step in what may be a long and ongoing process of engagement and planning. The preparation of the FCSP is not a simple procedure with an easy set of steps, but is an emerging process that is based on a shared vision of what will be a collaborative venture involving parents and professionals. The working alliance between the parent and professional is paramount in the process of moving forward with an FCSP. As has been explained in Chapter 4, a mutually positive, trusting, and hopeful working relationship must be established if the assessment and planning involved in developing an FCSP is to result in interventions that will be effective in meeting the needs of children and their families.

REFERENCES

Bailey, D.B., Jr, McWilliam, P.J., Winton, P.J., & Simeonsson, R.J. (1992). *Implementing family-centered services in early intervention: A team-based model for change.* Cambridge, MA: Brookline Books.

Beckman, P.J., & Bristol, M.M. (1991). Issues in developing the IFSP: A framework for establishing family outcomes. *Topics in Early Childhood Special Education, 11*(3), 19–31. http://dx.doi.org/10.1177/027112149101100304

Bennett, T., Lingerfelt, B.V., & Nelson, D.E. (1990). *Developing individualized family support plans: A training manual.* Cambridge, MA: Brookline Books.

Boone, H.A., Moore, S.M., & Coutler, D.K. (1995). Achieving family-centred practice in early intervention. *Infant-Toddler Intervention, 5*, 395–404.

Brown, W., Thurman, S.K., & Pearl, L.F. (1993). *Family-centred early intervention with infants & toddlers: Innovative cross-disciplinary approaches.* Baltimore, MD: Paul H. Brooks Publishing Co.

Campbell, P.H. (1991). Evaluation and assessment in early intervention for infants and toddlers. *Journal of Early Intervention, 15*(1), 36–45. http://dx.doi.org/10.1177/105381519101500106

Campbell, P.H., Strickland, B., & Forme, C.L. (1992). Enhancing parent participation in the individualized family service plan. *Topics in Early Childhood Special Education, 11*(4), 112–24. http://dx.doi.org/10.1177/027112149201100410

DeGangi, G.A., Wietlisbach, S., Poisson, S., Stein, E., & Royeen, C. (1994). The impact of culture and socioeconomic status on family-professional collaboration: Challenges and solutions. *Topics in Early Childhood Special Education, 14*(4), 503–20. http://dx.doi.org/10.1177/027112149401400409

Dunst, C.J., Trivette, C.M., & Deal, A.G. (Eds.). (1994). *Supporting and strengthening families: Methods, strategies and practices.* Cambridge, MA: Brookline Books.

Farel, A.M., Shackelford, J., & Hurth, J.L. (1997). Perceptions regarding the IFSP process in a statewide interagency service coordination program. *Topics in Early Childhood Special Education, 17*(2), 234–49. http://dx.doi.org/10.1177/027112149701700207

Fewell, R.R., Snyder, P., Sexton, D., Bertrand, S., & Hockless, M.F. (1991). Implementing IFSPs in Louisiana: Different formats for family-centered practices under Part H. *Topics in Early Childhood Special Education, 11*(3), 54–65. http://dx.doi.org/10.1177/027112149101100306

Gallagher, J., & Desimone, L. (1995). Lessons learned from implementation of the IEP: Applications to the IFSP. *Topics in Early Childhood Special Education, 15*(3), 353–78. http://dx.doi.org/10.1177/027112149501500307

Gowen, J.W., Christy, D.S., & Sparling, J. (1993). Informational needs of parents of young children with special needs. *Journal of Early Intervention, 17*(2), 194–210. http://dx.doi.org/10.1177/105381519301700209

Joanning, H., Demmitt, A., Brotherson, M.J., & Whiddon, D. (1994). The individualized family service plan: A growth area for family therapy. *Journal of Family Psychotherapy, 5*(3), 69–81. http://dx.doi.org/10.1300/j085V05N03_04

Johnson, L.J., Gallagher, R.J., LaMontagne, M.J., Jordan, J.B., Gallagher, J.J., Huntinger, P.L., & Karnes, M.B. (1994). *Meeting early intervention challenges: Issues from birth to three* (2nd ed.). Baltimore, MD: Paul H. Brookes Publishing Co.

Jung, L.A., & Baird, S.M. (2003). Effects of service coordinator variables on individualized family service plans. *Journal of Early Intervention, 25*(3), 206–18. http://dx.doi.org/10.1177/105381510302500305

Kalyanpur, M., & Rao, S.S. (1991, October). Empowering low-income black families of handicapped children. *American Journal of Orthopsychiatry, 61*(4), 523–32. http://dx.doi.org/10.1037/h0079292 Medline:1836108

Katz, L., & Scarpati, S. (1995). A cultural interpretation of early intervention teams and the IFSP: Parent and professional perceptions of roles and responsibilities. *Infant-Toddler Intervention, 5,* 177–92.

Lawlor, M.C., & Mattingly, C.F. (1998, April). The complexities embedded in family-centered care. *American Journal of Occupational Therapy, 52*(4), 259–67. http://dx.doi.org/10.5014/ajot.52.4.259 Medline:9544351

Malone, D.M., McKinsey, P.D., Thyer, B.A., & Straka, E. (2000, August). Social work early intervention for young children with developmental disabilities. *Health & Social Work, 25*(3), 169–80. http://dx.doi.org/10.1093/hsw/25.3.169 Medline:10948456

McGonigel, M.J., & Garland, C.W. (1988). The individualized family service plan and the early intervention team: Team and family issues and recommended practices. *Infants and Young Children, 1*(1), 10–21. http://dx.doi. org/10.1097/00001163-198807000-00004

McWilliam, R.A., Ferguson, A., Harbin, G.L., Porter, P., Munn, D., & Vandiviere, P. (1998). The family-centredness of individualized family service plans. *Topics in Early Childhood Special Education, 18*(2), 69–82. http://dx.doi. org/10.1177/027112149801800203

Minke, K.M., & Scott, M.M. (1993). The development of individualized family service plans: Roles for parents and staff. *Journal of Special Education, 27*(1), 82–106. http://dx.doi.org/10.1177/002246699302700106

Minke, K.M., & Scott, M.M. (1995). Parent-professional relationships in early intervention: A qualitative investigation. *Topics in Early Childhood Special Education, 15*(3), 335–52. http://dx.doi.org/10.1177/027112149501500306

Moroz, K.J., & Allen-Meares, P. (1991). Assessing adolescent parents and their infants: Individualized family service planning. *Families in Society, 72,* 461–8.

Notari, A.R., & Drinkwater, S.G. (1991). Best practices for writing child outcomes: An evaluation of two methods. *Topics in Early Childhood Special Education, 11*(3), 92–106. http://dx.doi.org/10.1177/027112149101100309

Pizur-Barnekow, K., Patrick, T., Rhyner, P.M., Folk, L., & Anderson, K. (2010, August). Readability levels of individualized family service plans. *Physical & Occupational Therapy in Pediatrics, 30*(3), 248–58. http://dx.doi. org/10.3109/01942631003780869 Medline:20608861

Pletcher, L.C. (1995). *Family-centered practices: A training manual.* Chapel Hill, NC: ARCH National Resource Center.

Province of Nova Scotia. (2002). *The individual family service plan (IFSP): Guidelines for practice, enhanced services for families with children birth to six years of age with autism spectrum disorder.* Halifax, NS: Child and Youth Action Committee, Department of Community Services.

Ridgley, R., & Hallam, R. (2006). Examining the IFSPs of rural, low-income families: Are they reflective of family concerns? *Journal of Research in Childhood Education, 21*(2), 149–62. http://dx.doi.org/10.1080/02568540609594585

Sexton, D., Snyder, P., Rheams, T., Barron-Sharp, B., & Perez, J. (1991). Considerations in using written surveys to identify family strengths and needs during the IFSP process. *Topics in Early Childhood Special Education, 11*(3), 81–91. http://dx.doi.org/10.1177/027112149101100308

Trute, B., & Hauch, C. (1988). Building on family strength: A study of families with positive adjustment to the birth of a developmentally disabled child. *Journal of Marital and Family Therapy, 14*(2), 185–93. http://dx.doi.org/10.1111/j.1752-0606.1988.tb00734.x

Turbinville, V., Lee, I., Turnbull, A., & Murphy, D. (1993). *Handbook for the development of a family-friendly individualized family service plan* (2nd ed.). Lawrence, KS: Beach Centre on Families and Disability.

Woods, J.J., & Lindeman, D.P. (2008). Gathering and giving information with families. *Infants and Young Children, 21*(4), 272–84. http://dx.doi.org/10.1097/01.IYC.0000336540.60250.f2

Zhang, C., Fowler, S., & Bennett, T. (2004). Experiences and perceptions of EHS staff with the IFSP process: Implications for practice and policy. *Early Childhood Education Journal, 32*(3), 179–86. http://dx.doi.org/10.1023/B:ECEJ.0000048970.35673.b2

10   A Case Study of Family-Centred Practice

KATHRYN LEVINE

Introduction

Family-centred service encompasses both a conceptual framework and action elements that translate family-centred theory into practice. The conceptual framework provides workers with an informed approach that builds on the key aspects of family-centred theory; it emphasizes that practice must be respectful, relational, congruent, planned, and specific. Although the process may appear linear, in reality the implementation of family-centred practice can be complex and dynamic, and the boundaries between the theoretical knowledge base of the worker and how this is connected with practice (action components) are fluid. Family-centred practice represents a paradigm shift regarding conceptualizations of how to respond to family needs, moving from what has historically been a child-centred approach to one that acknowledges the importance of the family that surrounds the child. The key components of family-centred practice include the establishment of a collaborative relationship, identification of specific family needs, assessment of formal and informal supports, the implementation of supports and interventions based on family need, and the ongoing evaluation of family-centred practices.

How can service providers implement the principles of family-centred practice in their work in children's service organizations? Can service providers go beyond understanding the ideas in theory and integrate them into daily practice? This chapter describes the application of family-centred theory and its practice framework to a family that is headed by a single mother. Using a case example as the basis for analysis, this review will consolidate and characterize the major issues in the implementation of family-centred practice and the implications of these issues for service provision and support within children's services.

Simply put, the goal of family-centred practice is to facilitate the achievement of the family's goals. Service provision is a means to assist families to first identify their needs that would facilitate their goals for their child and then begin to collaboratively work to identify resources that would meet these needs. Service provision is done in a context in which parents are able to acknowledge their strengths and recognize that help-seeking is not an admission of inadequacy but, rather, a movement towards family empowerment.

The beginning point for family-centred practice is the relationship between family members and the service provider. For many families, the need for intervention services arises out of an unanticipated change in family circumstances. Requesting or accepting services can be difficult in the best of situations. "Independence" continues to be upheld as a dominant value, and needing assistance for oneself can be viewed in a negative manner. Independence, however, does not imply that families should be completely self-reliant. It is through connections between and among families and community institutions, including the informal networks of friends, family, and neighbours as well as the broad range of support services, that many families are able to meet their diverse needs. A central theme in family-centred practice is the ability of workers to support the position that when provided with accurate information and resources, families are capable and competent to manage the myriad of challenges they may encounter, particularly families with children with special needs.

How do service providers establish relationships? Role clarification, shared understanding of service procedures, and use of personal disclosure along with an appreciation of what each can contribute have a positive influence on relationship development. Being a person who appreciates being with and working with people also assists the service provider develop a strong alliance with families. As well, it is important to acknowledge the connection between agencies' policies and procedures and how these can facilitate or act as a detriment to developing effective helping relationships. Further, it is important to recognize that self-esteem influences how individuals perceive relationships.

From the perspective of the service provider, there is a need to balance the available information about the family in order to be prepared and, at the same time, remain aware of any preconceived ideas or beliefs about models of family functioning. For example, in the absence of an awareness of one's own perceptions, images of single mothers can connote particular stereotypes: young, poor, welfare-dependent, and overwhelmed. It is clearly important that professionals engage in a self-reflective process to identify their feelings regarding any family system that may trigger some negative feelings. From a family-centred perspective, good practice invites workers to reflect on their own attitudes and how they are socially constructed as well as to develop the capacity to foster relationships based on ideas of personal empowerment.

Family Situation

Lisa, age 46, is the mother of Ryan, her 8-year-old son, who was diagnosed with autism at age 6 by a child development specialist. The diagnosis was given after Lisa had experienced many difficulties with Ryan in the daycare and kindergarten systems. Although for several years Lisa had thought that Ryan was having some developmental problems (minimal language development, limited range of interests, difficulty with change and transitions), she had consistently been advised that she was "worrying" too much and that Ryan would "grow out" of these issues. At times, various suggestions had been made by professionals for her to connect Ryan with a Big Brother in order for him to have an appropriate male role model, enrol him in sports activities, or become a better disciplinarian. Lisa had attended numerous meetings with daycare staff and appointments with a variety of specialists prior to being referred to a screening clinic for child behaviour problems. It was at this clinic that Ryan was given the diagnosis of autism. Although this was not perceived as "good news," Lisa did feel somewhat reassured that her concerns about her son's behaviour were valid.

Lisa is employed as a paralegal with a small law firm and resides in a large urban community. She relocated from another province back to the urban area in which she was raised in order to access a more comprehensive range of services for her son. A second reason for returning to her home province was to foster stronger relationships between her son and her family, including her parents, siblings, and their children.

Lisa encountered several stressors in the past 7 years that had made life challenging. She left a long-term relationship after several increasingly difficult years, including relocating to a new province in order for her partner to attend school. One year after moving, her partner was diagnosed with severe depression that left him unable to work or attend school. This placed a significant strain on their financial resources;

Lisa became the sole income earner and thus the family was completely dependent upon her earnings from her position as a paralegal. Since their separation, her ex-partner has not paid child support as he is receiving a small disability pension and therefore is not in a position to provide financial support to their son. As well, his mental health issues minimize his capacity to connect with their son at an emotional level, leaving Lisa to assume the roles of both father and mother to their son. Although Ryan's father is not available, Lisa did express that she wants her son to remain connected with her ex-partner's extended family.

Lisa moved to an urban centre in order to access specialized school programming for her son. However, it was only through coincidence (by speaking with another parent whose child is in the same school program) that Lisa became aware that there is a department of the government that provides support services to families with children with special needs. The parent gave Lisa the contact information for the program. The parent further expressed that the program had been really helpful to her and her family and recommended that Lisa contact them, even just to talk about what the program could offer. Lisa's previous involvement with other helping agencies made her somewhat sceptical about the "helpfulness" of the service system, but she was curious about the other parent's positive recommendation. Lisa thought about it for a while and then began to think it might be helpful. Lisa telephoned the number of the agency and was told that she should expect to receive a phone call in approximately one week.

Building a Foundation of a Respectful, Collaborative Relationship

Family-centred practice is facilitated by the relational abilities of the service provider to emotionally engage with the family in a supportive and non-judgmental manner. Positive parent-provider relationships are essential to engaging with families, and first impressions can be an important predictor of the future success of the relationship. Kelly Stephens, who was assigned Lisa's file, contacted Lisa by telephone to introduce herself as the family support worker who would assist Lisa's family. Lisa was somewhat surprised that she had received a phone call so quickly (although she had been advised that she could expect a phone call in a week, she had been anticipating a much longer waiting period). Kelly enquired whether Lisa had a few minutes to speak on the telephone. When Lisa indicated that she did, Kelly talked about the agency that she worked for as one that provides supports to families with children with special needs. Kelly advised that, if Lisa wished, she could send out a package of information and then arrange to meet with Lisa about a week later to review it. She said that some families prefer to receive the information prior to meeting as it helps them understand the services offered by the agency, and thus, they can decide whether they wish to pursue the referral. Alternatively, if Lisa wished, they could simply arrange to meet and Kelly would bring the information with her. Lisa said that she would prefer the information prior to the visit and then the opportunity to meet with Kelly. Kelly asked if there were particular days or times of the day that were best for Lisa. She replied that her work schedule was not very flexible, but that perhaps she could extend a lunch hour by a few minutes. Kelly replied that she was very flexible and mentioned that her agency prioritized time with families over the technicalities of work schedules and "office hours." Therefore, if after work suited Lisa, she was available. Again, somewhat surprised, Lisa indicated that generally Wednesdays around 5 p.m. could work as her parents picked up her son from school on those days for dinner and an activity (bowling, a movie, etc.). Kelly indicated that 5 p.m. the following Wednesday worked well for her and confirmed that she would send out the information package. Lisa began to ask for directions to the office and, at this point, Kelly advised that where the two of them met was up to Lisa – she could come to Kelly's office if she chose, they could meet at Lisa's home if she felt comfortable doing so, or they could also meet in a neighbourhood coffee shop if that suited her. All options were available. With some relief, Lisa indicated that it would be easiest to meet at her home and gave Kelly directions.

First Impressions and Worker Qualities

The family's first impressions of the service provider are a critical step in establishing the relational climate for service that will follow. A key characteristic of family-centred practice is universally noted to be the personal attributes/qualities of the service provider and how these are central to the success of family-centred service. At their first contact, Kelly arrived at the agreed-upon time at Lisa's house. She parked in the driveway and rang the doorbell. Lisa greeted her at the door and invited her inside. Kelly took off her boots as Lisa apologized for the disarray in the front hall – coats were piled everywhere, along with toys, a collection of newspapers and flyers, and numerous boots, shoes, and runners. Kelly replied that apologies were not necessary – and added that her front hall looked much the same as Lisa's, even though she herself did not have young children. Kelly further acknowledged that she appreciated that Lisa had invited her to her home, recognizing that not everyone feels comfortable having a service provider come to their house. At this point, Lisa realized that although she had received the package of information from Kelly, she had not had the opportunity to read it. Kelly responded that was certainly okay, and that, if Lisa wanted, they could go over it together.

Lisa led Kelly to the kitchen and asked if she wanted anything to drink. Kelly said that a glass of water would be much appreciated. She then went on to introduce herself, explaining that she is the worker from Children's Special Services and that the purpose of this first meeting was to provide information about the program's mandate and her role within the program. As a family support worker, she is employed by the government agency responsible for connecting families with children with disabilities with the supports and resources that they would find helpful. Part of her role is to assist the family in learning about the range of services and supports that are available and whether any would fit with the family's needs. Kelly emphasized that it was important to acknowledge that Lisa's preferences regarding the roles of the "helper" were fundamental in terms of their relationship and encouraged Lisa to inform Kelly if there was anything that was not helpful to her.

Kelly described that Children's Special Services is located within the Department of Family Services and is a voluntary program. Not only do parents have the right to choose to participate in the program, but the level at which they involve themselves is entirely at their discretion. Having a child with a disability is different for every family, and part of the program's philosophy is to work with families based on their understanding of what the diagnosis means. Kelly also introduced the idea that many families think that Children's Special Services functions as a child protection agency and emphasized that she is not a child welfare worker but a family support worker. Lisa felt some sense of relief; although she had been somewhat aware of the difference, she felt reassured that Kelly raised the issue directly.

Kelly explained the process of how she prefers to work with families. Unfortunately, difficult experiences that families sometimes have with previous workers may contribute to apprehension when meeting a new service provider. Therefore, taking the time to have a discussion about the family's history of involvement with previous services is valuable in understanding and engaging families. Kelly began the discussion by introducing the subject of how some families with children with disabilities have historically felt "blamed" by the social service system in a manner that suggested that they were somehow responsible for their children's disabilities and family circumstances. Although she indicated that this feeling of blame was likely not intentional, it had often contributed to an adversarial or mistrustful relationship between families and service providers. Kelly asked if that had ever been Lisa's experience. Lisa was surprised to hear Kelly speak so openly and honestly about what she had always considered to be her individual experience because of being a single mother. Lisa talked about some of her past experiences, how some professionals had labelled her as "over-involved" with her son, how childcare staff and other professionals including educators had suggested that Ryan's difficulties were related to her returning to work full-time and consequently "neglecting" her son's needs, and how the offer of "help" at times seemed based on professionals' perceptions of her inadequacy as a parent rather than as an authentic expression of assistance in managing the multiple demands of childcare, employment, and household responsibilities. Kelly listened attentively as Lisa relayed her prior experiences. She responded by emphasizing that if she inadvertently sent that type of message, she would hope that Lisa would feel free to discuss it with her.

Kelly then asked if Lisa would like to review the information package. Lisa opened the package and found several pamphlets and several other forms. The first pamphlet described the program and its philosophy of service; Lisa noted that the term "family-centred" was used rather than referring to children's needs. Kelly pulled out a form that was entitled "Family Needs Survey."[1] Kelly explained that this form had been developed as a way of identifying the information and support needs that families would like additional information about. She talked about how as a service provider, it was important for her to learn about Lisa's information needs from Lisa's perspective, rather than assuming she knew what Lisa's needs were. She explained that although there may be items that Lisa would not consider relevant to her situation, she may find some of the identified needs would fit for her. However, as with all services, it was a choice whether to complete the survey or not.

At this point, it was 6:30 p.m. When she realized the time, Lisa felt uncomfortable and expressed how sorry she was for keeping Kelly way past office hours. Kelly indicated that personally, and from the organizational standpoint, there were no "office hours." She clarified that the program is based on the assumption that all workers are doing their best and do not need to "prove" that they are working; therefore, they are encouraged to set their own schedules based on family availability. She went on to say that although she herself is not a parent, she suspects that for most single parents, time is never considered an excess commodity, and she was appreciative that Lisa had taken the time out of her schedule to meet with her. Kelly then enquired as to whether Lisa would like to meet again. The idea that Lisa had a "choice" to meet again was surprising. It was a different experience to be asked whether she would like to meet, as previous service providers had simply assumed that she would be available (and always during the daytime!). She agreed to a second meeting, and Kelly suggested that perhaps prior to the second meeting, if she wished, Lisa could complete the Family Needs Survey and that it could serve as their starting-off point. She also asked if she could meet Ryan, to which Lisa agreed.

Lisa's Perspectives

Lisa's first impressions of Kelly were very positive and different from many of Lisa's prior contacts with "helpers" who she experienced as either condescending or needing to "counsel" her. Lisa was especially impressed with how Kelly was sensitive to her situation as a single mother. A key distinction in family-centred practice is the recognition of families as unique groups of people rather than cases. The social construction of "good mother" rarely includes an acknowledgment that this term can describe families headed by single women. Historically, mothers have held the primary responsibility for children's emotional and physical well-being along with other responsibilities in the family domain. Consequently, when the family experienced challenges, mothers were frequently blamed for their children's issues.

When Lisa described her separation to Kelly, she commented: "I know I'm a terrible person for leaving Ryan's father when he was ill. I'm the selfish witch who only thought of herself. But it was not good for anyone; there had been problems in our relationship before Ryan was born, and we simply were not able to overcome these problems in order to make the changes that Ryan needed. I couldn't be responsible for both David and Ryan, and Ryan is not the adult! As hard as this move was on me, I think this situation is much better for Ryan – he seems a bit more settled."

Kelly's response was thoughtful and emphasized how it is important for parents to acquire a sense of control over their family life. As well, she attributed the positive changes seen in Ryan to Lisa's own strengths, abilities, and actions. Lisa felt good that Kelly had both sensed and acknowledged that not all two parent families are by definition better than single mother families. Unlike other relationships with service providers, Kelly did not judge Lisa as someone who was responsible for a "failed marriage" but as someone who had chosen to put the needs of her son ahead of her own.

The Second Meeting – Helping Parents Identify Family Needs

Family-centred practice is grounded in the belief that service provision is best managed when organized around family-identified goals and needs. However, clients may not know how to respond to a question about needs, and difficulties may surface when providers act as perceived "gatekeepers" to information or services. Consequently, there is often a large gap between the information that service providers have and the information that families receive. It is important for workers to begin from the position that many families enter the social service system with the belief that they're not sure what they want and don't know how to get it or that they don't know enough to know what they don't know.

As the second meeting approached, unlike some of her previous experiences, Lisa did not feel apprehensive. In the two week interim, she had taken the time to review the Family Needs Survey and found it to be a helpful process, as it identified some issues that she had not previously considered. As well, it was easy to identify the items that she considered important:

- Information about services that are presently available for my child
- Information about the service my child might receive in the future
- Explaining my child's condition to my parents or my spouse's parents
- Locating babysitters or respite care providers who are willing and able to care for my child (not sure)
- Finding recreational activities for my child to participate in
- Locating a dentist who will see my child

When Kelly arrived, both Lisa and Ryan greeted her at the door. After Kelly came in, they went into the living room. Kelly spent the next 15 minutes interacting with Ryan. She sat on the floor with him and engaged with the toy trains that he could play with for hours on end. Lisa's parents then arrived and took Ryan for an evening of bowling and dinner. Lisa presented the completed Family Needs Survey. She felt that the form was a helpful way for her to share with Kelly the areas on which she needed additional information and provided a good structure for their conversation. When they came to the item on locating babysitters or respite care providers (to which Lisa had responded "not sure"), Lisa indicated that her response was partially a result of her dislike of the term "respite." She said it implied that she experienced her son as a "burden" and that she needed relief from the "hardship" of being with him. Lisa described that this was not at all how she viewed her relationship with her son, and by this definition, she did not need "respite" from him. However, when Kelly enquired further about childcare arrangements, Lisa was able to identify that an area she did struggle with was her reduced ability to leave home for errands like shopping for groceries and other needed things due to Ryan's need for supervision and potential for behavioural difficulties. She also added that she thought it would be helpful for Ryan to have someone outside the family with whom he could participate in community activities. In response, Kelly indicated that she appreciated Lisa's perspective and described that the roles of respite workers varied considerably, depending upon the family's need. Kelly agreed to review the list of available workers and provide Lisa with the names of three whom she could meet in order to share her expectations, prior to committing to the service.

Kelly noted that Lisa had not indicated that "talking with other parents" was one of her information needs. When asked about this, Lisa replied that although she understood that other parents may appreciate the benefits of parent support groups, she did not. She talked about how she had attended a group at the time that Ryan was first diagnosed that was not specific to children with autism but, rather, focused on children with disabilities in general. Although she recognized that some parents could find them useful, she herself did not as she found there was a certain degree of "alarmist" thinking that was promoted in terms of potential negative emotional reactions that she personally did not find beneficial at that time. Kelly replied that she understood and indicated that although the goal of most groups is to help facilitate supportive connections between parents, some of the group discussion can focus on negative aspects of parenting children with special needs.

Kelly suggested that if, in the future, Lisa was willing and interested in attending another one, she should let Kelly know, and she would try to locate one that was focused on practical rather than emotional support.

After their discussion of the Family Needs Survey, Kelly enquired as to whether Lisa had gone through any of the other forms. Lisa replied that in fact, she had been curious about one entitled "Family Implications of Childhood Disability," and subsequently completed it. She asked what the purpose of the form was. Kelly indicated that it is one way of helping workers learn more about the meaning that having a child with disabilities holds for different families. Kelly asked if Lisa wished to share her form with her, to which Lisa agreed. Kelly reviewed the form and noted that although Lisa had indicated that Ryan's disability had placed some limitations and restrictions on her family, she had also indicated a number of positive responses. Kelly explained that from her perspective, Lisa is clearly managing the additional demands of parenting a child with special needs, and she is also able to acknowledge the positive aspects of her situation. Lisa agreed and responded that completing the form had caused her to reflect upon her current situation in a much different way than she had previously. She indicated that other parents often expressed sympathy or pity for her and did not appear to understand that, at times, Ryan gave Lisa immense pleasure. She said that she felt really good that the program, via Kelly, understood that having a child with disabilities was not always perceived as a "tragedy," and that there are many positive emotions that parents experience as well.

The construction of an eco-map[2] is a process that can be used to show the range of support sources available to families, as well as the nature of the relationships with these sources of support, both positive and negative. At the second meeting, Kelly asked if she and Lisa could develop an eco-map together, to give Kelly a sense of the supports and systems with which she and Ryan were involved. Although Lisa was surprised at some of Kelly's questions (she had not previously considered whether her relationship with Ryan's school was stressful or whether her employer was supportive), Kelly asked the questions in a respectful manner, and Lisa interpreted the process as being thorough rather than intrusive.

Through the eco-map, Kelly identified a critical dilemma for Lisa, one that she had previously not spoken about. Although relationships with extended family can be important sources of support for single parents, they can also come with emotional costs. Kelly enquired as to how Lisa felt returning to her home community after having lived away for many years. Lisa related how it had not been an easy decision and one that she experienced as "failure" at times. Lisa talked about how wanting to be closer to her family was her way of protecting Ryan in the future, believing that Ryan's relationships with her siblings and their children would ideally extend beyond the time that she was able to care for him. At the same time, her family's support and connection with her and Ryan came at a cost. She indicated that her family sometimes suggested that she "coddled" Ryan by maintaining his routines rather than expecting him to accommodate to change. She asked if Kelly could help her find a way to communicate to her extended family that Ryan was different from children without autism and that her perceived "coddling" was a means of mitigating some of the "meltdowns" he had when stressed. She expressed some guilt over these feelings – her parents had a close relationship with Ryan, and she did not want her family to perceive that she was ungrateful, but she also wanted them to maintain a "grandparent" role and to respect her way of managing Ryan's behaviour.

Kelly listened attentively to Lisa and enquired as to whether Lisa would find it helpful to speak with another worker from Kelly's office who had extensive experience working with multigenerational families. Lisa considered this and thought that it could be an option, if not now, then in the future. Kelly agreed to forward the contact information for the other worker to Lisa when she returned to the office.

The Third Meeting

Prior to the third meeting, Kelly emailed Lisa and asked if they could use the upcoming meeting to develop a Family-Centred Support Plan (FCSP). According to Kelly, the FCSP is a way for families to identify their goals for their family (for their children as well as for themselves), consider their immediate and future service needs, and outline the "next" steps in the process. Lisa replied to the message and asked if the FCSP was the same as an Individualized Education Plan (IEP) that the school staff had talked about. Kelly replied that although they are similar processes, the FCSP is a "whole family" plan that extends beyond the child's individual needs to consider needs of other family members as well, while the IEP focuses solely on the child's educational program at school. Kelly further suggested that some parents choose to have their extended families participate in this process and that Lisa should feel free to include a family member or friend in the meeting if she wished. Lisa agreed to consider whether she wanted anyone else to participate.

Lisa invited her brother, Mark, to attend the FCSP meeting. After introductions were made, Kelly began the meeting by asking Lisa what kinds of aspirations she had for herself and Ryan in the next 6 months. Lisa indicated that she hoped that Ryan could become more comfortable in the community. Although initially reluctant to try something new, when he is with someone familiar, he appears to relax and enjoy himself. For example, Lisa had discovered a playground in the neighbourhood that had wonderful play structures. Lisa described that after several visits, Ryan was now able to play by himself on the swings and the climbing structure. However, given the other demands on her time (work, grocery shopping, laundry, cooking, cleaning), this was not something that she could do as often as she would have preferred. Kelly wrote on the plan – "Ryan is an active boy and would like to become more comfortable in the community." This is a goal that the respite worker could address, by locating different activities in the community that Ryan would enjoy.

Kelly then turned to Lisa and asked "This is a great goal for Ryan – what about yourself?" Lisa replied that she was fine, and that any service should be for Ryan, not for her. At this point, Mark interjected and said, "You have wanted to start that Human Resources program." He explained to Kelly that Lisa's workplace was prepared to provide her with both tuition costs and an educational leave for the program, but she had not been willing to take the next step because of Ryan. Kelly asked Lisa if that was something that she would like to do. Lisa replied, "Of course, but now is not the time." Kelly then asked what Lisa would need in order to consider entering the program. Lisa said that it would take at least one evening a week that she did not have. At this point, Kelly asked if there was anyone in her family or other source of support that could assist her. Mark replied before Lisa had the chance to respond: "Yes, there's my wife and myself. We would love to help you out with this, but you have never asked for help – you are so darned independent, but we really want to support you in achieving this goal. We would be happy to either come over here and stay with Ryan while you are in class, or have Ryan come to our house – whatever works."

Kelly asked if that would be helpful to Lisa. Lisa appeared surprised and pleased at her brother's words and indicated that yes, this would certainly allow her to pursue this option. Kelly then wrote on the FCSP –

"Lisa will explore the possibility of enrolling in the Human Resources program at the downtown campus." Lisa and Kelly then went through the remaining items on the Family Needs Survey (which Lisa had previously completed) and finished the plan. Kelly asked Lisa to review it and then indicated that she would take it back to the office for typing, and Lisa would be sent a copy.

At the end of the FCSP meeting, Kelly asked if there were any other issues that Lisa would like to address. Lisa asked if Kelly could attend the school meeting with her, as someone who is knowledgeable about children with special needs. Lisa indicated that although she knew the school staff had Ryan's best interests in mind, there were times when she felt intimidated by the school team but felt unable to disagree or refuse their recommendations. Kelly responded that Lisa is the expert on her child with special needs, but agreed to attend the IEP meeting with Lisa.

The School Meeting

As promised, Kelly attended the IEP meeting with Lisa at Ryan's school. Present at the meeting were the classroom teacher, the resource teacher, the speech and language pathologist, the occupational therapist, and the educational assistant who was assigned to work with Ryan. The school psychologist was not present but had submitted a report. After introductions were given, the classroom teacher explained that the purpose of the meeting was to update Lisa on the assessments that had been completed and subsequent goals that each of the specialists had developed. At this point, Kelly turned to Lisa and said: "Before hearing from the team, it would be really helpful for all of us to hear your thoughts about Ryan's progress, what his strengths are, what areas you feel are important for him to develop, and where he may benefit from additional support."

Lisa appreciated that Kelly created this opportunity for her. She identified that in her daily interactions with Ryan, communication was an important issue. As the person who spent the most time with him, she was aware of what he was trying to express; however, others struggled to understand his needs. This clearly created frustration for Ryan, and simple requests frequently escalated into major "meltdowns" due to his limitations in communication. For Lisa, this was a critical issue. The team listened as Lisa described her goal for Ryan as being an ability to tell her and others what he wants and needs. In response, the speech

and language pathologist suggested that for children who have language delays, one means of facilitating their communication is through
the use of picture symbols. Based on the child's individual needs, a
communication book is developed that includes pictures of food, activities, and people who are familiar to the child. For example, when
children are thirsty, they would identify the picture of the juice box.
She further explained that some parents had expressed concern that if
children became reliant on picture symbols, then it may prevent them
from learning to communicate verbally. In her experience, this has not
occurred. In fact, she had read recent research (which she offered to
share with Lisa) that suggested that the recognition and use of pictures
symbols was an important preverbal skill. Lisa responded that this appeared to be an excellent idea that would help Ryan to learn how to
communicate with others. The speech and language pathologist asked
if Lisa could write down all the familiar items that Ryan used on a daily
basis in order to develop the pictures, to which Lisa eagerly agreed. The
pathologist indicated that she would create two books, one for school
and one for Lisa and others to use at home.

The classroom teacher then raised the issue of Ryan's social skills.
She described how the school psychologist could also create a program
that would reinforce Ryan's social skills, modelled on positive behavioural reinforcement. She described that one way that children with
autism can develop social skills is to reinforce them with food or other
enjoyable items when they demonstrate eye contact or other social initiatives. She went on to say that she would contact the school psychologist after the meeting to set up a program for Ryan. At this point, Kelly
interjected and asked if this was something that Lisa was comfortable
in pursuing. Lisa hesitated, but then replied that, although she understood the importance of social skill development, she did not feel comfortable "rewarding" Ryan for specific behaviours. She understood that
this was an important area for some parents, but it was not currently
one of her priorities. Kelly then suggested that perhaps this could be
discussed at some point in a future meeting, once the team has focused
on Ryan's communication.

Five Months Later

Several months passed after Kelly attended the school meeting with
Lisa. One day, Kelly telephoned Lisa to enquire about how she and
Ryan were doing. Lisa replied that, for the most part, everything was

going well. She felt very positive about Carly, Ryan's respite worker, and was very appreciative of how this relationship gave Lisa some free time on the weekends. Lisa laughed when she described how on Saturday, she had met a friend for coffee: "In the afternoon!! On a Saturday!!" Six months ago, that would never have been possible. She further reported that she had developed much stronger working relationships with the school staff. Kelly asked if any other issues had arisen since they had last spoken. Lisa indicated that there had been one issue but that she had dealt with it herself. The teacher had again suggested the intensive behavioural program for Ryan, but Lisa still did not feel that it was the appropriate time. This time, however, she felt that they respected her position. "I don't feel that they are judging me anymore – they seem to respect my decisions with regard to Ryan's school program." She also talked about how her brother had become an important support for her. She described an incident the previous Sunday when the family had been at her parents' home for dinner, and she had allowed Ryan to eat his meal by himself in the family room. He had spent the afternoon interacting with the family and his cousins and had approached Lisa with his "train" picture, which she knew represented "alone" time. When her parents mentioned that Ryan had been doing so well and that perhaps he should learn to eat with the family, Mark had responded that Lisa understands Ryan's needs best, and that the family should respect Lisa's decisions as to when Ryan could be encouraged to take on new behaviours and when it was acceptable to maintain his routines. Lisa told Kelly that it had felt really good to have her brother advocate for her and that he likely would not have known to do so if he had not been at the FCSP meeting with her. She had also completed the first course of her Human Resources program and was excited about what she was learning. Mark and his wife had been very helpful in spending time with Ryan when Lisa was in class. Kelly replied that it was good to hear that Lisa and Ryan were doing well. She asked if there were any other issues that had arisen, and Lisa indicated that, at this time, the services that were in place were working well for her and Ryan. She laughed and said that things could change – she has learned life is certainly not predictable! Kelly asked if it would be okay if she kept in touch with Lisa and Ryan, something like a "maintenance" phase. Kelly indicated that if anything changed prior to her call, however, Lisa should feel free to contact her at any time. Lisa replied that Kelly would definitely be the first person she contacted if anything came up. She then went on to say how much she had appreciated Kelly's guidance over the past few months: "I really appreciated how you respected my position as a single parent and did not see me and Ryan as a 'less-than' family. You did not see our difficulties as the result of my being a single parent – you could see the problems as being outside of Ryan and me. You helped me see where my supports are, and you gave me the opportunity to identify what I saw as the important goals for Ryan and myself, which I experienced as incredibly validating. If it wasn't for your encouragement and support, we probably wouldn't be doing as well as we are today. Thank you so much!"

Analysis of Family-Centred Practice

In this situation, there are several examples of effective family-centred practice at the relational and service provision levels.

1 First, the agency recognized the importance of timely follow-up with intakes and referrals; Kelly's initial contact with Lisa occurred shortly after she had received the assignment, within the timelines that had been outlined to Lisa in her first phone call.
2 The implementation of family-centred practice can be challenging for some service providers, as their relationships with parents will often extend beyond traditional professional boundaries. Kelly ensured that she, rather than the client, was flexible in terms of scheduling the initial appointment as well as the location and gave Lisa choice about the "when" and the "where."
3 It is important for the worker to display an awareness of the different frames of reference held by families. Kelly acknowledged the potential risks in terms of public perceptions of having a "professional" from a children's service agency come to the home.
4 Kelly openly introduced some of the stereotypical assumptions regarding single motherhood that may be internalized by women in Lisa's position. The worker's capacity to openly acknowledge, reflect, and refute Lisa's worries about being labelled a "bad mother" greatly contributed to Lisa's trust that she would not be blamed for her child's difficulties nor made to feel inadequate as a function of asking for help.
5 While clearly knowledge and skills are essential for service providers, the relationship that developed between Lisa and Kelly was a

key factor in Lisa's choice to continue to meet with Kelly and receive services that she found helpful.

6 The willingness of Kelly to be flexible in terms of scheduling, assuming some activities that went beyond Lisa's expectations, spending additional time with Lisa, and meeting her son all strengthened their initial relationship.

7 Kelly took the time to explore with Lisa the meaning of her identified priorities for herself and Ryan. Although many parents find parent-to-parent support helpful, at the present time, Lisa did not, and this decision was respected by Kelly.

8 A key principle of family-centred service is the understanding that parents will make the best decisions for their families when in possession of accurate, comprehensive information. Although Lisa was initially apprehensive about respite service, her ability to meet potential respite providers to share her expectations regarding the intent of the respite relationship facilitated her ability to make an appropriate decision.

9 There was recognition of the importance of Kelly effectively using her professionally acquired knowledge when providing information to the family on the service, supports, and resources available to Lisa. For example, the suggestion of a counsellor who specializes in multigenerational family issues was perceived to be helpful to Lisa.

10 The inclusion of Lisa's needs both for herself and her son as part of the FCSP process is a key indicator of family-centred practice. Lisa's ability to return to school was facilitated by her brother's support, as well as additional respite hours provided by Kelly. Family-centred practice helps families identify sources of support that exist within their informal networks as well as in the formal service system.

11 Family-centred practitioners assume an advocacy role when necessary. At the initial school meeting, Kelly ensured that Lisa's educational priorities for her son took precedence over the school team's priorities.

12 In her interactions with Lisa, Kelly used all opportunities to help Lisa develop the competencies and skills she needed to be able to identify her needs and acquire the supports required to address those needs. In this way, the practice was empowering as it was based on the belief that families will move towards self-sufficiency when they feel empowered to do so themselves.

NOTES

1   For information on the Family Needs Survey, see Bailey, D.B., Jr, & Sime-
    onsson, R.J. (1988). Assessing needs of families with handicapped infants.
    Journal of Special Education, 22, 117–27.
2   For information on the eco-map, see Hartman, A., & Laird, J. (1983). *Fam-
    ily-centered social work practice.* New York, NY: Free Press.

PART FOUR

Special Themes in Family-Centred Practice

11   Considering Fathers of Children with a Disability in Family-Centred Practice

DAVID B. NICHOLAS

Introduction

The concept of fatherhood is undergoing shifts in Canadian and other western societies. Earlier models largely relegated fatherhood to bread-winning and child discipline. As a result, fatherhood was seen as peripheral to the nurturing and daily care of children. In recent years, there has been greater recognition of the important roles that fathers play in the lives of their children. We are beginning to ask important questions such as "what important impacts do fathers have on their child's development?" and "how is fatherhood meaningful and re-warding to men?" Images of fatherhood are shifting from a view of fathers as stoic and detached to more recent perspectives of fathers as relational and integral to family well-being.

Yet, despite these shifts, there continues to be counterbalancing per-spectives and portrayals that depict fathers in terms of aloofness, irre-sponsibility, and disengagement. Common expressions or terms used comprise negative ideas such as "absent fathers," "deadbeat dads," and other pejorative terms. While not wanting to gloss over the heartache that is caused by irresponsible fathering in the lives of families, ste-reotypes that overemphasize exceptions to the norm of fathering may distort a common understanding of fatherhood and discourage recog-nition and celebration of the fact that fathers make a profound differ-ence in the lives of their children.

Accordingly, it appears that we are at crossroads with conflicting im-ages and perspectives on fatherhood. To add to this complexity, little is known about fathering a child with a disability. This form of fatherhood confounds the experience and enactment of fathering, yet relatively little is known about fathering a child with a disability. This chapter grapples with fathering a child with a disability with the aim of reflecting on, and adding to, the discussion of family-centred practice. Family-centred models invite us to examine ways in which fatherhood can be understood and supported as it contributes to the well-being of the family as a whole as well as its constituent parts: the child with a disability, siblings without disabilities, mother, father, grandparents, et cetera.

Fathers' Role in Parenting a Child with a Disability

Parental hands-on care may be increased and changed when a child has a chronic health condition or disability. However, to date, we have relatively few models upon which to base our understanding of fathering a child with a disability. Clearly, more has been written about the impact of disability on the experience of mothers than on fathers. While mothers generally report more time in caregiving roles than fathers, both mothers and fathers are profoundly affected by their child's disability, and hence may be in need of supportive professional services (Heller, Hsieh, & Rowitz, 1997).

The literature increasingly supports the notion that fathers' involvement is critical to a child (Cowan, Cowan, Pruett, Pruett, & Wong, 2009; Caldwell, Rafferty, Reischl, Loney, De Loney, & Brooks, 2010), and specifically to a child with a disability (Quinn, 1999). Childhood disability imposes added stress and anxiety on parents. The literature is mixed in comparing maternal and paternal experiences of stress and anxiety related to their child's disability. On balance, however, a child's disability yields substantial parental worries related to the child's present needs and anticipated future – worries that are often projected beyond the parents' lifetime as the parents must plan for the eventual dependent care for their adult child with a disability. While these worries associated with child disability are experienced by both mothers and fathers, fathers may receive less support (Nicholas, 2010; Nicholas, McNeill, Montgomery, Stapleford, & McClure, 2003), potentially rendering fathers at heightened risk for unaddressed chronic anxiety and psychoemotional strain.

Fathers demonstrate a wide array of roles in the lives of their children with disabilities. A recent study suggested that fathers tend to be most involved in playing with their child, nurturing, disciplining, and decision-making about services and less involved in teaching, therapy, and issues of daily hygiene, dressing, and feeding (Simmerman,

Blacher, & Baker, 2001). In a recent study examining paediatric asthma, differences were found between mothers and fathers in their perception and experience of their child's condition (Cashin, Small, & Solberg, 2008). Mothers and fathers differed in their opinion of what comprised the most difficult aspect of care; fathers were most concerned about physical exacerbations of asthma such as an asthma attack. Relative to mothers, fathers provided care from less of a protective stance and, as such, felt that caregiving needs were less demanding.

Fathers describe their role as an advocate, resource gatherer, and supporter of the family through paid employment. Beyond providing resources to the families, two thirds of fathers in a recent study were actively involved in their child's learning and development, such as helping with school work (Carpenter & Towers, 2008). Synergistic and tag team roles between mothers and fathers of children with disabilities were described whereby many mothers and fathers – as co-parenting dyads – "covered off" similar caregiving roles and worked synergistically to support one another and meet the caregiving needs of their child (Nicholas, Zwaigenbaum, McKeever, MacCulloch, & Roberts, 2009a). Patterns of parental roles emerged, and couples or co-parents worked to develop complementarity in how each of them could contribute to the well-being of their child.

Clearly, the diagnosis of disability requires a substantial proportion of parental attention and energy, shifting relationships between parents, among family members (e.g., with healthy children), and between family members and individuals outside the family (e.g., frequently reduced parental time spent with friends). Often, intensive caregiving results in less dense and/or severed "non caregiving-related" relationships, leaving parents and families increasingly socially isolated.

Parents invariably need to develop tenable lifestyle patterns that address their child's care needs. Extensive financial costs are often incurred, in some cases with substantial impacts on family resources (Azar & Badr, 2010). Employment options may diminish due to one parent needing to remain at home to care for the child with a disability, often resulting in shifting roles, substantially decreased income (Goble, 2004; Nicholas, Zwaigenbaum, McKeever, MacCulloch, & Roberts, 2009b), and/or uneven workforce patterns in the home such that one parent may juggle multiple jobs to offset the caregiving spouse's lack of employment income.

In a recent study examining the support needs of fathers of children with spina bifida, fathers identified parenting challenges and blessings, epitomized by paternal sorrow over their child's struggles, yet deep appreciation and admiration for the child (Nicholas, 2003; Nicholas et al., 2004). Fathering thus held layers of complexity, including the opportunity to appreciate life in new ways and reconcile priorities and what fathers determined to *really* matter. Inherent in fathers' depictions of their lives was the uniqueness of their experience represented by barriers and, in many cases, marginalization of the disabled child and family within the community. As an example, mobility and access comprised ongoing barriers for children as their parents struggled to ensure equitable access to various venues in daily life. Challenges confronting fathers and their families, outlined in Table 11.1, highlight multilayered difficulties at macro, mezzo, and micro levels.

Fathers' Experience in the Workplace

Fathers of a child with a disability frequently experience insufficient workplace flexibility to attend to their child's care needs and appointments. Workplace barriers appear to result from employers' lack of understanding about, or responsiveness to, the extraordinary needs of children with disabilities (e.g., care demands, clinic visits). Fathers and their families reap the consequences of unsupportive workplace requirements and employment policies, leading to fathers continually missing clinic education and support and being less present than mothers at key moments of daily care and child development. Carpenter and Towers (2008) address fathers' challenging vocational experiences and identify a "loss of opportunities and earnings, and the struggle to get the flexibility ... [fathers need] to combine employment and providing care" (p. 120). This lack of work-related flexibility renders fathers vulnerable to outcomes including (a) un/under-employment; (b) extensive daily absence from the home as a result of extensive and/or inflexible working hours (e.g., lack of options for workplace absence due to childcare needs, need for multiple jobs) required due to heightened cost for disability services; (c) lost opportunities for career advancement (e.g., geographic immobility due to long waitlists in regions for disability services, reduced flexibility that may preclude managerial roles); (d) inner turmoil over the insensitivity of workplace supervisors, colleagues, or systems; and (e) employment and financial vulnerability. By default, mothers often leave the workforce (or work part-time) due to extensive caregiving demands, with negative implications on personal career advancement and families' financial well-being. For both mothers and fathers, the lack of workplace options as well as insufficient

Table 11.1. Challenges Confronting Fathers and Their Families

Level of imposed challenge	Experience of fathers and families
Macro-level challenge	Marginalizing attitudes related to disability (e.g., less worthy of community access)
	Lack of existing fathering models and images relevant to childhood disability
	Insufficient health, financial, and employment support policies for families in which a child has a disability
Mezzo-level challenge	Insufficient public funding and resources for the child with a disability and their family
	Lack of resource coordination resulting in a complex maze of disability resources
	Services often delivered in the home, potentially resulting in para-professional intrusiveness in personal spaces (e.g., the home) and family life
Micro-level challenge	Child's missed developmental milestones, which incur chronic or recurring parental grief
	Ongoing focus on the child's needs permits less time and energy for other family needs (e.g., healthy siblings, parental relationship)
	Rigid eligibility criteria and unfriendly resource systems amid intense child need result in tension, frustration, and anger yet dependence
	Disability issues (e.g., difficult child behaviours, alternative treatment possibilities) may heighten confusion and/or disagreement between parents
	Family and individual exclusion in the community; social isolation
	Extraordinary care requirements; parental exhaustion; extraordinary financial costs
	Unsupportive workplace environments may result in parent un/under-employment and financial instability

disability-related provincial and federal employment policies, impede individual and family choices and quality of life.

Overall Impact on Fathers

The fact that fathers persevere amid multiple layers of challenge and stress is a testament to paternal and family commitment and resilience. Keller and Honig (2004) report that acceptance of the child and her/his disability and family harmony can serve to buffer against stress. MacDonald, Hastings, and Fitzsimons (2010) reported that "psychological acceptance was related to father's psychological adjustment. Specifically, fathers who reported more acceptance of difficult emotions and thoughts associated with their child with intellectual disability also reported more positive gain or benefits from this child, less stress associated with the impact of the child on the father and the family and fewer symptoms of anxiety and depression. Psychological acceptance was also found to act as a mediator of the impact of children's behaviour problems on paternal stress, anxiety and depression" (p. 33).

Despite elements that buffer stress for fathers, the literature increasingly recognizes that fathers' "lived experience" includes unresolved frustration (Carpenter & Towers, 2008; Nicholas, Gearing, et al., 2009) and, in some cases, simmering or periodic anger and/or sorrow (Nicholas, Gearing, et al., 2009). Fathers further carry these difficult emotions in relative isolation and, in some cases, grapple with feelings of being peripheral to the daily care of their child. Care demands and stresses further shift over time and child development. For instance, puberty imposes unique dilemmas for fathers, such as personal care needs for an adolescent daughter or reported difficulties finding male attendants for an adolescent or adult son, thereby often requiring a father's accompaniment in the community (e.g., potentially needing attendant care in a gender-specific facility such as a restroom). In summary, fathers and their families navigate a complex and shifting terrain, often with insufficient resources and a lack of existing "fatherhood models" to guide these men. Clearly, fathers and their families may be at risk for emotional and adjustment issues, potentially needing and benefiting from professional support.

Implications for Service Delivery

Fathering a child with a disability appears to manifest a unique form of fatherhood; however, we know little about how that experience is internalized or formulated and how support can be most effectively provided. Current interventions tend to reflect a traditional support orientation towards emotive sharing, yet this approach may generally not fit as readily for men as women. Creativity and relevance in reshaping support programs for fathers emerge as pressing priorities in advancing pro-father resources.

The growing fatherhood literature increasingly advocates an interventional paradigm fostering fatherhood adaptation and recognition of fathers' strengths and parenting capabilities (Hawkins & Dollahite, 1997). In contrast to earlier pathological or deficit-oriented perspectives, fatherhood interventions are increasingly framed as empowering, strengths-based, and resilience-oriented. Fatherhood narratives are being explored in interventions whereby fathering a child with a disability may be seen in terms of an "eclipse" of both struggle and celebration, with much in the narrative that may not readily add up to what has traditionally been upheld as "fathering." Innovative family-centred approaches entail supporting fathers as they grapple with caring for and protecting their families in ways that weave together notions of disability, masculinity, love, father identity, and family life. Narrative approaches to therapy offer promise as they offer means for fathers to define and characterize their stories in ways that go beyond traditional ways of "telling" and reconciling truths about fatherhood and family experience.

There is a current lack of services for fathers of children with a disability, and existing services often appear ill-suited to fathers' unique needs and to men's communication styles in general. These gaps leave fathers at risk for insufficient parenting education and support. Finding accessible and meaningful supports for fathers merits increased effort, as the literature demonstrates that men's peer networks often diminish over time (Tudiver & Talbot, 1999). Relative to women, some men may have greater difficulty talking about health concerns or issues (Tudiver & Talbot, 1999) and are less comfortable openly expressing emotion (Gearing, 2002; Tudiver & Talbot, 1999). These potential differences and difficulties invite us to enhance both intervention content and processes in optimizing effectiveness.

Developing targeted supports for fathers has been a slow-growing process in clinical practice for families impacted by paediatric disability (e.g., Nicholas, Gearing, et al., 2009). Gearing (2002) argues that gender is a consideration relative to interventions for men. This invites the development of models that carefully consider men's communication styles, ways in which men relate to others, and methods by which sharing can be supported. Such considerations likely will have a bearing on the therapeutic encounter with fathers. Accordingly, sequencing and proportionality of affect, depth of experiential description prior to affect exploration, and interventional aim will engender important elements in potentially eliciting favourable outcomes.

Examples of specific strategies include technology- or activity-oriented interventions that may offer greater appeal to men as viable means of engagement, targeted and purposeful therapeutic activity, and "paced" opportunities for relationship formation and emotion exploration. These approaches would seemingly be more "hands-on" relative to traditional support resources, such that fathers could incrementally build rapport and, as comfortable, share personal struggles or family concerns. For instance, through technology-based activities such as developing a blog for fathers or contributing to the development of an electronic care "manual" for families as they navigate the care system, fathers could be facilitated in engaging in personal stories with the potential for cathartic exploration in online writing. Other examples of hands-on activity that may appeal to men's potential affinity for "doing" rather than initial "emoting" include activity-oriented tasks of relevant community or "civic" engagement, tasks that yield tangible, needed outcomes and in so doing, foster community benefits. For participating fathers, personal and family outcomes also might include peer support, self- and family awareness, health education, self-esteem, mastery, and coping. Specific engagement activities could entail community- or facility-based strategies for improving process mapping in navigating care for children with disabilities, fund development for resource infusion in the community, et cetera.

Given that little is known about fathers' experiences related to disability, engaging fathers in the development of a resource exploring fathering experiences would be an excellent initial engagement opportunity for fathers. This would inherently invite fathers to reflect on their own journeys, potentially resulting in personal gain as well as benefits for program enhancement. These examples invite consideration of new ways for service delivery practitioners and programs to partner with fathers in hearing their voices and facilitating meaningful opportunities for engagement towards understanding and authentic change.

Notwithstanding sensitivity to fathers' ways of being and the need for relevant interventions, caution is recommended to not narrowly presume a stereotypical view of fatherhood, and thereby gloss over the vast diversity among fathers with a "one size fits all" interventional response (McNeill, 2001). This inherent tension invites critical reflection and flexibility, potentially yielding interventions that grapple with men's commonalities and differences as well as contemporary understanding about disability and family-centred practice. Flexibility in how services reflect and respond to fathers' experiences and needs constitutes a pressing priority for clinical and empirical development in paediatric disability. An example of an intervention for fathers, as outlined below, illustrates the potential for attending to the needs of fathers of a child with a disability – in this case, spina bifida.

A Peer Support Intervention for Fathers of Children with Spina Bifida

Given emerging literature demonstrating that fathers are profoundly affected by childhood spina bifida, a therapeutic group specifically for fathers was implemented in Ontario, Canada. The group was initiated following clinical recognition that existing supports tended to be insufficient in addressing fathers' needs. It was also noted that fathers were often absent from clinical support, in part, it was presumed, because clinical services were offered during daytime office hours when most fathers were at their jobs. Beyond this apparent lack of resource flexibility to provide services when fathers were available, there was a growing awareness among the clinical team that, relative to other family members, fathers were more isolated and systemically overlooked. Fathers were observed to generally rely on their wife/partner for information and support related to spina bifida, often with little or no other outlets to gain or share disability-related concerns and worries. Most fathers knew no other fathers who also had a child with spina bifida; hence, they lacked similar peers, role models, and mentors.

Given these gaps in care for fathers, an intervention was sought that would build upon family-centred sensitivities, including meaningful and accessible support for all in the family – in this case, fathers. Such an intervention would necessarily require an alternative model that could both attend to fathers' needs and overcome barriers related to their limited time availability, employment commitments, and geographic disparity.

A support group for fathers was thus piloted. It was decided that a group offering information and support "for fathers, by fathers" was desirable in ascertaining and addressing fathers' support needs. A priority that the intervention be accessible to as many fathers as possible resulted in the decision to facilitate the group using online technology (for more details about the intervention and outcomes, see Nicholas, 2003; Nicholas et al., 2004).

The Intervention

Fathers of children and adolescents (18 years of age or younger) with spina bifida participated in the online group, a network entitled "Just for Dads." Facilitated by a social worker, the network comprised both information and support, with a focus on mutual aid and social support. Participating fathers identified experiences, needs, and solutions associated with their child's condition, its impact on family life, and the parenting journey for fathers. The initial pilot ran for 6 months, and based on its successful implementation, the online network emerged as an ongoing family support resource facilitated within the community.

Fatherhood Narratives: Hearing the Voices of Fathers in Child Disability

With the permission of participants, verbatim transcripts of fathers' dialogue in the "Just for Dads" network were analysed. Findings identified that prior to the group, fathers had seldom communicated their struggles and worries regarding their child's spina bifida. With a viable means of peer sharing offered by the network, fathers appeared to collectively find their voice in claiming, articulating, and in some cases, shifting or reframing their experience. Several fathers stated, often with sadness, that their involvement with their child was insufficient and, in varying degrees, they longed for more involvement in their child's life, school, and disability/health management. For many, information sharing with other fathers in similar circumstances appeared to be a conduit for conveying challenging realities and articulating lessons learned. Accordingly, the online format not only served as a practical means of giving and receiving information, but also reduced fathers' isolation and, for several, reportedly heightened personal engagement in their child's care.

The peer support model in this intervention appeared beneficial. For instance, personal information shared by fathers in the group located each participant as an expert in his own experience as a father and family member. Their commentary allowed for emergent narratives reflecting shared experiences of fathering in a disability context, experiences that often contradicted stereotypical perspectives or expectations of what several had earlier envisioned of fatherhood. The group concluded that existing models of fathering in media, social discourse, and families of origin often were irreconcilable with elements of their lived reality of fathering a child with a disability.

In this process of reflection and discovery, fathers supported one another in redefining and delineating elements of their unique fathering experience and of how much their child and family meant to them. Accordingly, the group provided participants with the opportunity to refine understanding and/or articulate their realities, which included considering resistance strategies in instances of perceived resource inequities or unacceptable clinical care or communication. As a result of exploring their experience, some fathers conceded feeling incompetent in issues relating to their child's disability or care. With greater awareness of this as a common experience, fathers reclaimed the importance of learning about spina bifida and its impact on their child and family, supporting their partner/wife in the caregiving endeavour, and asserting themselves with health care professionals and resource brokers for greater professional information and support. Finally, some fathers concluded that the group heightened their commitment to their families, and their realization of the value that their family brought to them.

These findings support the advancement of narrative approaches in supporting experiential, relational, and affective experiences for fathers (Dienhart & Dollahite, 1997; Dollahite, Hawkins, & Brotherson, 1996). Interventions that heighten fathers' understanding and nurturing are linked to greater mastery and empowerment in fathering (Nicholas et al., 2004).

Outcomes of the Fatherhood Intervention

Pre- and post-intervention questionnaires were administered to participants in the fathers' spina bifida network. Consistent with observation and qualitative data collected about fathers' experiences, outcome measures revealed a statistically significant positive difference in elements of empowerment: sense of challenge, positive attitude, motivation, and hope ($p = 0.01$) based on Meaning of Illness Questionnaire items (Browne et al., 1988). Emergent findings suggest important interventional processes, including relationship building among participants, clarity of intervention aims, examination of concrete issues prior to expectations for affective expression, and attention to logistics such as individual participant accessibility to the intervention.

Consistent with the literature, this intervention appears to support the potential of targeted approaches for fathers of children with a disability. Emergent approaches increasingly appear to invite fathers to share their experience, recognize the value of paternal involvement in their child's care, and celebrate the role of fatherhood in the life of the child – all important aims in nurturing father involvement and family-centred practice.

Emergent Features of Clinical Support for Fathers

In recent work with fathers within social support contexts, observations have been reported with implications for clinical care. In the therapeutic encounter, the use of a story or narrative genre has demonstrated outcomes that appear to overcome some challenges identified in traditional services that rely largely on affect expression and exploration of feelings. While the counsellor or facilitator may invite participant feelings associated with fathering and/or disability experience, men may initially be more attuned to concrete or storied accounts from which affective content and expression can later emerge. Too quickly inviting affective responses from men in the clinical encounter may thwart engagement and ultimately limit therapeutic gain. Rather, a focus on the concrete such as information sharing, storytelling, mutual aid, and lessons learned may open doors for relational points of connection and idea generation, affirmation, and change readiness. Fathers' commitment to "whatever it takes" to help their child may invite opportunities for task-oriented strategies that ultimately advance affective exploration related to fathering, child disability, and family life.

As part of the articulation of stories relating to fathers and families in which a child has a disability, fathers' description of their nuanced struggle and achievements, including contradiction, irony, paradox, et cetera, becomes critical in plot development. Supporting fathers in grappling with how their experience may *not* fit with what they had envisioned or desired of fatherhood warrants clinical acumen and the development of fatherhood- and disability-based models of clinical support. For instance, what may be presented as a tragedy, and thus is tinged with sadness or anger, may also offer simultaneous growth or insight from which gratitude can be found. Weaving affect and humour into fathers' stories appeared to resonate with fathers in the spina bifida group, and emerged as a moderator of intense emotions (Nicholas et al., 2004). In that group, fathers periodically infused humour in their narrative as a means of managing the emotions that accompanied their experience. A skilled clinician's support for these apparently important functions of men's use of humour and affect modulation seems crucial. Also important are clinical assessments of family-based experiences, the possible need for renegotiation of ways to support fathers and others in the family such as mothers and children, and the accommodation of culturally mediated considerations.

A variety of suggestions have been made, often by fathers themselves, for ways to improve current support resources. All fathers (including those who do not have a child with a disability) may need certain kinds of support. In a study examining support for family members in general, fathers expressed varying needs for support in the following areas: mental health (e.g., mood), reduced intoxicant use, management of emotions (e.g., expression of feelings, self-esteem), employment, physical health, parenting, child care, and social relationships (Tanninen, Häggman-Laitila, & Pietilä, 2009). Carpenter and Towers (2008) argue that to effectively facilitate discussion with fathers and engage them in decision-making about their child, practitioners need to consider fathers' work patterns when arranging appointments and meeting times. They further suggest that fathers seek to be respected as equal partners and recognized for what they have contributed to family life.

Beyond support for fathers in coping, Davis and May (1991) suggest that fathers "need assistance and information on ways to discuss their child with relatives, co-workers and strangers who may stare, compare, and make inappropriate remarks" (p. 88). They further argue that professionals need to believe that fathers need to be part of the decisions made regarding their child's care, and thereby provide fathers with a variety of ways to be involved in that care. Peer support, as has been illustrated in this chapter, is recommended as an important resource for fathers, as well as activities that encourage mothers and fathers to explore assumptions regarding gender roles and stereotypes (Davis & May, 1991; Quinn, 1999). In the aim of advancing support to fathers, Davis and May (1991) suggest fathers' engagement in the training of professionals and in program and policy development as well as further education for students and professionals.

Waite-Jones and Madill (2008) identify five content areas upon which to focus in support for fathers: (a) *comparison* in which fathers can contrast how their child and family are different from what they consider to be "normal," (b) *loss* associated with the child's condition, (c) *constraints* such as barriers to engaging with the child or acquiring needed services, (d) *concealment* associated with fathers potentially disguising their feelings in the aim of appearing strong, and (e) *social and emotional adjustment*. MacDonald et al. (2010) suggest that "psychological acceptance may act a mediator variable [which would] support the exploration of acceptance and mindfulness-based interventions to help reduce psychological distress for parents of children with intellectual disabilities" (p. 34).

To effectively support fathers' adaptation to childhood disability, practitioners need to communicate in ways that are relevant to fathers. While seeking to be sensitive to male-based communication, fathers may not be as unemotional as they are often stereotyped to be. Davis and May (1991) report that many men value independence and an ability to take care of themselves and their families. As such, directly "opening up" to sources of support and becoming vulnerable may not be as palatable a coping strategy for men as it is for women. Notwithstanding this caution, Davis (2007) suggests that conventional forms of support, such as support groups, are underused by men. More innovative ways to engage men in dialogue invite creativity and perhaps activities with a recreational or concrete focus (Davis, 2007).

Heiman (2002) suggests that finding effective means for supporting parental resilience requires three key components: "(a) an open discussion and consultation with family, friends, and professionals; (b) a positive bond between the parents, that supports and strengthens them; and (c) a continuous and intensive educational, therapeutic, and psychological support for family members" (p. 169). Practitioners are well-positioned to facilitate in each of these areas for and with fathers and their families.

Sensitivity to fathers' realities and their family's disability-related experiences and concerns is critical to effectively supporting their adaptation to the child's disability and the resulting need for navigation of care. Developing clinical approaches that incorporate gendered communication may offer insight for service development for fathers, with ultimate benefits for the family as a whole. This invites new models for clinical innovation within assessment and intervention frameworks including theoretical development and evaluation in ultimately seeking best practice.

Conclusion

These are exciting and challenging times for practitioners and program planners working with fathers of children with disabilities. It is a time in which we are beginning to explore fatherhood as it both contributes to and reflects family nurturance. Yet, there continue to be critical gaps in service relevance, effectiveness, and accessibility for fathers. Davis and May (1991) conclude that it "is imperative that adequate assistance be developed for fathers and their needs. They need to regain personal control through coming to terms with their grief, gaining emotional support, and becoming active participants in the decisions affecting their children's lives. To do so may open lines of communication for all family members and accelerate the healthy rebalancing of the family" (p. 88).

Such advances in services to fathers invite the development of strategies to engage, nurture, and co-create growth and family sustenance. While it is important not to single out or isolate one member of the family, what we are proposing here are relevant approaches to supporting fathers in their care and connection within the family unit. This invites greater attunement to fathers' nuanced ways of being, thinking, engaging, and problem solving. Practitioners and researchers face tremendous opportunity yet challenge in pursuing this important area of practice development. To the extent that meaningful, flexible, and responsive resources are available, fathers can be supported as they care for their children and families, and thereby advance the important aim of family-centred practice.

REFERENCES

Azar, M., & Badr, L.K. (2010, February). Predictors of coping in parents of children with an intellectual disability: Comparison between Lebanese mothers and fathers. *Journal of Pediatric Nursing, 25*(1), 46–56. http://dx.doi.org/10.1016/j.pedn.2008.11.001 Medline:20117676

Browne, G.B., Byrne, C., Roberts, J., Streiner, D., Fitch, M., Corey, P., & Arpin, K. (1988, November-December). The meaning of illness questionnaire: Reliability and validity. *Nursing Research, 37*(6), 368–73. Medline:3186480

Caldwell, C.H., Rafferty, J., Reischl, T.M., De Loney, E.H., & Brooks, C.L. (2010, March). Enhancing parenting skills among nonresident African American fathers as a strategy for preventing youth risky behaviors. *American Journal of Community Psychology, 45*(1-2), 17–35. http://dx.doi.org/10.1007/s10464-009-9290-4 Medline:20082239

Carpenter, B., & Towers, C. (2008). Recognizing fathers: The needs of fathers of children with disabilities. *Support for Learning, 23*(3), 118–25. http://dx.doi.org/10.1111/j.1467-9604.2008.00382.x

Cashin, G.H., Small, S.P., & Solberg, S.M. (2008, October). The lived experience of fathers who have children with asthma: A phenomenological study. *Journal of Pediatric Nursing, 23*(5), 372–85. http://dx.doi.org/10.1016/j.pedn.2007.08.001 Medline:18804018

Cowan, P., Cowan, C., Pruett, M., Pruett, K., & Wong, J. (2009). Promoting fathers' engagement with children: Preventive interventions for low-income families. *Journal of Marriage and the Family, 71*(3), 663–79. http://dx.doi.org/10.1111/j.1741-3737.2009.00625.x

Davis, C. (2007, May 23–9). Don't forget dad: Fathers of children with a disability often feel excluded from support networks but want to feel as respected as mothers. *Nursing Standard, 21*(37), 22–3. Retrieved from http://nursingstandard.rcnpublishing.co.uk/resources/archive/browse.asp?JournalId=9&VolumeNumber=21&IssueNumber=37 Medline:17549999

Davis, P., & May, J. (1991). Involving fathers in early intervention and family support programs: Issues and strategies. *Children's Health Care, 20*(2), 87–92. http://dx.doi.org/10.1207/s15326888chc2002_3

Dienhart, A., & Dollahite, D.C. (1997). A generative narrative approach to clinical work with fathers. In A.J. Hawkins & D.C. Dollahite (Eds.), *Generative fathering: Beyond deficit perspectives* (pp. 183–99). Thousand Oaks, CA: Sage Publications.

Dollahite, D.C., Hawkins, A.J., & Brotherson, S.E. (1996). Narrative accounts, generative fathering, and family life education. *Marriage & Family Review, 24*, 333–52.

Gearing, R.E. (2002). Gender diversity: A powerful tool for enriching group experience. In S. Henry, J. East, & C. Schmitz (Eds.), *Social work with groups: Mining the gold* (pp. 89–104). Binghamton, NY: Hawthorne Press.

Goble, L.A. (2004, July-September). The impact of a child's chronic illness on fathers. *Issues in Comprehensive Pediatric Nursing, 27*(3), 153–62. http://dx.doi.org/10.1080/01460860490497787 Medline:15371113

Hawkins, A.J. & Dollahite, D.C. (Eds.). (1997). *Generative fathering: Beyond deficit perspectives*. Thousand Oaks, CA: Sage Publications.

Heiman, T. (2002). Parents of children with disabilities: Resilience, coping, and future expectations. *Journal of Developmental and Physical Disabilities, 14*(2), 159–71. http://dx.doi.org/10.1023/A:1015219514621

Heller, T., Hsieh, K., & Rowitz, L. (1997). Maternal and paternal caregiving of persons with mental retardation across the lifespan. *Family Relations, 46*(4), 407–15. http://dx.doi.org/10.2307/585100

Keller, D., & Honig, A.S. (2004, July). Maternal and paternal stress in families with school-aged children with disabilities. *American Journal of*

Orthopsychiatry, 74(3), 337–48. http://dx.doi.org/10.1037/0002-9432.74.3.337 Medline:15291710

MacDonald, E.E., Hastings, R.P., & Fitzsimons, E. (2010). Psychological acceptance mediates the impact of the behaviour problems of children with intellectual disability on fathers' psychological adjustment. *Journal of Applied Research in Intellectual Disabilities, 23*(1), 27–37. http://dx.doi.org/10.1111/j.1468-3148.2009.00546.x

McNeill, T. (2001). *Holistic fatherhood: A grounded theory approach to understanding fathers of children with juvenile rheumatoid arthritis (JRA).* Unpublished doctoral dissertation, University of Toronto, Toronto, ON.

Nicholas, D.B. (2003). Participant perceptions of online groupwork with fathers of children with spina bifida. In N. Sullivan, E.S. Mesbur, N.C. Lang, D. Goodman, & L. Mitchell (Eds.), *Social work with groups: Social justice through personal, community and societal change* (pp. 227–41). Binghamton, NY: The Haworth Press, Inc.

Nicholas, D.B. (2010, June). *The experience of family care for autism over the course of pediatric development: Perspectives of mothers and fathers.* Paper presented at the Canadian Association of Social Work Education Conference, Montreal, QC.

Nicholas, D.B., Gearing, R.E., McNeil, T., Fung, K., Lucchetta, S., & Selkirk, E. (2009). Experiences and resistance strategies utilized by fathers of children with cancer. *Health & Social Work, 48*(3), 260–275. http://dx.doi.org/10.1080/00981380802591734

Nicholas, D.B., McNeill, T., Montgomery, G., Stapleford, C., & McClure, M. (2004). Communication features in an online group for fathers of children with spina bifida: Considerations for group development among men. *Social Work with Groups, 26*(2), 65–80. http://dx.doi.org/10.1300/J009v26n02_06

Nicholas, D.B., Zwaigenbaum, L., McKeever, P., MacCulloch, R., & Roberts, W. (2009a, April 15–17). *Evaluating the experience of maternal and family care of children with autism over the course of pediatric development.* Paper presented at the International Conference on Innovative Research in Autism, Tours, Loire Valley, France.

Nicholas, D.B., Zwaigenbaum, L., McKeever, P., MacCulloch, R., & Roberts, W. (2009b, October). *The lived experiences of fathers of children with autism: Preliminary findings.* Paper presented at the 15th Annual Qualitative Health Research Conference, International Institute for Qualitative Methodology, Vancouver, BC.

Quinn, P. (1999). Supporting and encouraging father involvement in families of children who have a disability. *Child & Adolescent Social Work Journal, 16*(6), 439–54. http://dx.doi.org/10.1023/A:1022349321767

Simmerman, S., Blacher, J., & Baker, B.L. (2001). Fathers' and mothers' perceptions of father involvement in families with young children with a disability. *Journal of Intellectual & Developmental Disability, 26*, 325–38. http://dx.doi.org/10.1080/13668250120087335

Tanninen, H.M., Häggman-Laitila, A., & Pietilä, A.M. (2009, October). Resource-enhancing psychosocial support in family situations: Needs and benefits from family members' own perspectives. *Journal of Advanced Nursing, 65*(10), 2150–60. http://dx.doi.org/10.1111/j.1365-2648.2009.05080.x Medline:20568320

Tudiver, F., & Talbot, Y. (1999, January). Why don't men seek help? Family physicians' perspectives on help-seeking behavior in men. *Journal of Family Practice, 48*(1), 47–52. Medline:9934383

Waite-Jones, J., & Madill, A. (2008). Concealed concern: Fathers' experiences of having a child with juvenile idiopathic arthritis. *Psychology & Health, 23*(5), 585–601. http://dx.doi.org/10.1080/08870440802036911

12 Culturally Sensitive Family-Centred Practice

DAVID ESTE

Introduction

During the past two decades, human service professionals have been challenged to ensure the programs and services offered by their organizations are responsive and effective to the changing racial, ethnic, linguistic, and cultural composition of today's diverse population in Canada. An extensive body of literature exists, based both in theory and prescriptive research, which practitioners can utilize in their efforts to provide effective programs for service users from varied backgrounds.

Several factors have contributed to the growing volume of literature focused on practices to address increasing diversity. A major force driving both health and social service organizations to engage in culturally sensitive practice in North American society is the rapidly changing demographics (Este, 2007). For example, Canada's population is becoming more diverse in the dimensions of race, ethnicity, culture, and linguistics (Statistics Canada, 2008). Canada's immigration policy is viewed as the major reason for the increasing diversity in Canadian society. According to the Annual Report to Parliament on Immigration 2010, between 240,000 and 265,000 immigrants would be admitted into Canada. The same figure was expected for 2011 (Citizenship and Immigration Canada, 2010). According to the 2006 Census (Statistics Canada, 2008), an estimated 5,068,100 individuals belonged to a visible minority, which accounted for 16.2% of Canada's total population. This figure is up from 13.4% in 2001 and 11.2% in 1996. Between 2001 and 2006, the visible minority population in Canada increased by 27.2%, five times faster than the 5.4% growth rate of the total population. This was largely the result of the high proportion of immigrants and refugees who belonged to the visible minority groups. In 2006, 75% of the recent immigrants who arrived since 2001 were visible minorities. This compared with 72.9% of visible minority newcomers in 2001 and 74.1% in 1996. It is anticipated that the percentage of newcomers who belong to a visible minority group will continue to represent a strong majority of those who will be allowed to migrate and settle in Canadian society. For the first time, South Asians supplanted the Chinese as the largest visible minority, followed by Chinese and Blacks, respectively. Geographically, visible minorities had a strong presence in Canada's largest census metropolitan areas. Almost all (95.9%) resided in these areas as compared with 68.1% of the country's total population (Statistics Canada, 2008).

The increasing demand from diverse populations for service providers to be more sensitive and responsive to their issues and needs as well as the desire to become full partners in the planning and delivery of services represent two more factors for the increased attention to diverse service users. Members of diverse communities also contend that mainstream intervention approaches do not always address the unique needs of their communities. The codes of ethics of professional associations such as social work, nursing, and psychology strongly state that all clients are entitled to competent professional services (Canadian Association of Social Workers, 2005; Canadian Nurses Association, 2008; Canadian Psychological Association, 2000). Hence, from both a professional and moral perspective, it is incumbent upon service providers who engage in family-centred practice to provide services in a culturally sensitive manner that respects the values of diverse families. These codes serve as another significant factor propelling health and social service organizations to become culturally sensitive in all of their practices.

This chapter focuses on the knowledge, competencies, and values required by health care and human service professionals engaged in family-centred practice to effectively work with young children with disabilities and their families from diverse backgrounds, particularly immigrants and refugees. More specifically, the chapter is focused on culturally sensitive practice in the context of family-centred practice. Initially, key concepts that are critical to any discussion of culturally sensitive practice are presented, followed by a description of the knowledge, skills, and values required by practitioners in their quest to be responsive to diverse populations. Finally, a brief discussion is provided on the role family-centred organizations that provide services to children with disabilities and their families must play to promote and sustain environments where culturally sensitive practice is truly valued and embraced.

Key Concepts

Defining what is meant by culture is essential to any discussion focused on cultural sensitivity. Merriam-Webster (2009) defines culture as "the customary beliefs, social forms, and material traits of a racial, religious, or social group," while Olandi (1992) describes it as "the shared values, norms, traditions, customs, arts, history, folklore, and institutions of a given people" (p. vi). Perry and Tate-Manning (2006) maintain that culture "can be broadly understood as a social group that among many other similarities can share values, beliefs, customs, and worldviews" (p. 737). Finally, Henry, Tator, Mattis, and Rees (1995) view culture as "the totality of ideas, beliefs, values, knowledge, and way of life of a group of people who share a certain historical, religious, racial, linguistic, ethnic, or social background" (p. 326). These definitions leave the impression that culture is static. Some writers, however, contend that cultures are fluid. James (2003) states that "changes within a culture are due to global influences, the movement of people from one country and/or region to another, and the interaction of various racial, ethnic, and social groups" (p. 202). Yee (2003) makes the same assertion related to the fluid nature of the term: "this approach reduces 'culture' to a static concept and reduces people to celebrations of dress, customs, and behaviours. This reification of the concept culture further mystifies people's social relations and allows one to make generalizations about people's behaviour without considering their material, lived experiences of racism, classism, sexism, ableism, and heterosexism" (p. 99).

Culture may be used to acknowledge characteristics of groups such as immigrants and refugees, or it may be used to identify and use the strengths of individuals, families, or communities (Kirmayer & Minas, 2000). Typically, information on culture presented to human service professionals is in the form of texts that summarize the patterns of behaviour in specific population groups. This may lead to the general tendency to form stereotypes that result in interventions that may not address the issues confronting a particular client. Cultures are not unified, harmonious, seamless wholes that speak out with one narrative voice (James, 2003, p. 201), and it is therefore incumbent on health and human service professionals to recognize the inherent uniqueness of individuals and families. Failure to adhere to this dimension of culture may result in stereotyping or negative labels being attached to families coming from diverse communities. Such behaviour may result in another barrier or stigma for these families, making it difficult for them to have a sense of belonging in Canadian society.

Family-centred service providers who as part of their practice do not pay attention to the cultural backgrounds of their clients may experience negative consequences. A lack of understanding about the culture of families and its impact on their situations may serve as an obstacle in the professional's ability to engage with these clients in a meaningful way. By not attempting to understand their cultural reality and distinctive views, practitioners may force their own beliefs on families, which may diminish the desire of families to work with helping professionals.

Culturally Sensitive Practice

There are several terms and concepts that describe the processes practitioners and organizations undertake when dealing with the needs of diverse client systems including ethnically sensitive practice, managing diversity, cultural competency, and diversity competency. Culturally sensitive practice is another term that has captured attention in professions such as nursing, psychology, social work, and medicine (Calvillo et al., 2008; Josipovic, 2000; Leishman, 2006).

Within the literature, various definitions of the term "cultural sensitivity" exist. An early conceptualization was provided by Westermeyer (1976), who stated that "cultural sensitivity is understanding and respecting the values, worldviews, attitudes, and preferred behaviour patterns of the client" (p. 315). Moore (1992) stated that it "reflects a concern for comprehending the interaction of persons of different backgrounds giving deliberate attention to their differences and similarities. Often, this understanding focuses on differences in living patterns, belief systems, and normative values of a culture" (p. 250). In a more expansive definition, Resnicow, Soler, Braithwaite, Ahluwalia, and Butler (2000) maintain that cultural sensitivity is "the extent to which ethnic/ cultural characteristics, experiences, norms, values, behavioural patterns and beliefs of a target population as well as historical, environmental, and social forces are incorporated in the design, delivery, and evaluation of targeted health promotion materials and programs" (p. 272). Finally, Foronda (2008) stresses that cultural sensitivity "is employing one's knowledge, consideration, understanding, respect, and tailoring after realizing awareness of self and others and encountering a diverse group or individual. Cultural sensitivity results in effective communications, effective interventions, and satisfaction" (p. 210).

Consistently, several themes appear to dominate the literature on cultural sensitivity and professional practice. The general consensus is that practitioners (a) need to be aware of their specific cultural, racial, and ethnic identity and experiences; (b) need to be informed about different racial, cultural, ethnic, and diverse groups; (c) must possess strong empathy and skills in order to work with clients from diverse backgrounds and experiences; and (d) must have intrinsic values that truly reflect their willingness and commitment to work in an ethical manner with different client systems. These themes will be illustrated in this chapter using immigrants and refugees as the illustrative populations. The following section presents descriptions of practice perspectives that family-centred practitioners need to understand in their practice with immigrant and refugee families.

Relevant Practice Perspectives

The ecological perspective. When working with immigrant and refugee children and their families, it is critical for the family-centred practitioner to utilize the perspective known as ecological theory (Segal & Mayadas, 2005) as developed and presented by Germain and Gitterman (1996). This perspective focuses on the reciprocal relationships between the person and her/his environment, with an emphasis on the consequences of the exchanges between the two entities. As part of the assessment process, practitioners need to explore not only the settlement and adaptation processes the families experience in their new country but also explore questions that focus on the reasons for leaving one's homeland, experience of migration, resources that are available to function in unfamiliar environments, and the receptiveness of the new host country (Segal & Mayadas, 2005).

Segal and Mayadas (2005) maintain that it is important for family-centred professionals to use a person-in-environment perspective when dealing with newcomers. It is also imperative that family-centred practitioners apply a macro perspective when working with immigrants and refugees. By only focusing on individual or family functioning, there is a strong probability that the messages being imparted to newcomers are negative in nature with the tendency of blaming these individuals for their circumstances. This position ignores structural and systemic barriers that contribute to the array of issues newcomers encounter in trying to adapt to life in Canadian society. Typical problems include language barriers, role reversal in families, changes in socio-economic status, challenges in adjusting to the educational system, and loss of support systems.

Drachman (1992), who developed the "Stage of Migration Framework," asserts the critical importance of practitioners' use of a person-in-environment perspective when working with newcomers. The framework explicitly identifies the types of information and knowledge required to help newcomers adjust and adapt. Writers such as Pine and Drachman (2005) and Earner and Rivera (2005) contend that helping professionals must understand the migration process from pre-migration to resettlement. Pine and Drachman developed a broader conceptual framework that can serve as a tool for assisting practitioners who work with immigrant refugees and families. Building on Drachman's earlier model, this latest framework once again recognizes the intersection between the newcomers' experiences in their country of origin and the settlement process in Canada.

The strengths perspective. The strengths perspective is also helpful for family-centred practitioners in their assessment and ongoing work with immigrant and refugee children and their families. Weick, Rapp, Sullivan, and Kisthardt (1989) maintain that the perspective serves as a corrective for the imbalance caused by preoccupation with the deficits and liabilities of people. A strengths perspective rests on an appreciation for the positive attributes and capabilities that individuals possess and the social resources that can be developed and sustained. When encountering the various challenges and barriers faced by newcomer children and their families, family-centred professionals may be overwhelmed and, as a result, they must clearly appreciate that individuals will do better in the long run when they are able to identify, recognize, and use their strengths and resources in their environment.

One of the basic concepts associated with the strengths perspective is that people have survived to this point – certainly not without pain and struggle – through employing their will, their vision, their skills, and as they have grappled with life, what they have learned about themselves and their world. Practitioners need to understand these capacities and make alliance with this knowledge in order to help (Saleeby, 1997, p. 302).

Culturally Sensitive Practice

One of the prevailing themes in the literature describing culturally sensitive practice is the assertion that for professionals such as family-centred practitioners, the journey to become a "culturally sensitive practitioner" is a lifelong process. There is also the strong belief that professionals need to possess specific knowledge, skills, and values along with a strong commitment by their organizations to both value and support the delivery of culturally sensitive services (Butler & Molidor, 1995; Este, 1999).

There is strong consensus within the literature that practitioners require different types of knowledge (College of Nurses of Ontario, 2009; Dewees, 2001). For example, these individuals need to be aware of the characteristics of specific groups such as racialized minorities and immigrants and refugees, have an understanding of phenomena such as discrimination, racism, and integration, and be familiar with different concepts such as social class.

The starting point for family-centred service providers who aspire to practice in a culturally sensitive manner is to become aware of their own culture. Each person has particular beliefs, values, and biases s/he has learned, and these elements affect the way individuals view and respond to their world and other people in it. Hence, it is imperative for practitioners to engage in the process of self-reflection to help identify values and biases that influence not only their approach and interventions but also how they may impact clients. By not being aware of their beliefs, values, attitudes, and feelings about working with individuals who are different from themselves, family-centred care practitioners may inadvertently engage in destructive and oppressive care. Such awareness requires a measure of introspection and sensitivity to one's own biases, stereotypes, and values. Equally important is the need for culturally sensitive practitioners to identify their membership in different social groups based on gender, class, race, sexual orientation, physical/psychological ability, religion, and age and how these memberships may impact their practice with clients from diverse backgrounds.

Anderson et al. (2005) provide the following as sample questions that may assist practitioners in the process of reflecting on how their personal values, beliefs, and experiences may influence the nature of their practice with families from different cultures: (a) What are my own beliefs about newcomers or other cultural groups in Canada and how might these enter how I interact with individuals from these communities; (b) What assumptions am I making about this person, and about this particular group; (c) Why do I think (or feel) this way; (d) Where did I get my information; (e) What might I learn if I talk to the person; and (f) What may we have in common? (p. 340).

Professionals wishing to employ family-centred practice must become knowledgeable about the world view of clients (Jeff, 1994; Sue, 2006) in order for them to become culturally sensitive in their practice. Schiele (2000) defines world views as follows: "A world view can be defined succinctly as the overarching mode through which people interpret events and define reality. It is a racial or ethnic group's psychological orientation toward life. It provides a group with a structure expressing its own cultural truths, a way to organize its experiences and interpretation into a logical and fairly stable conceptual scheme" (p. 1).

Edwards (1994) describes the value of understanding world views from a practice perspective and identifies the following contributions: assessing the client's cultural background and fundamental orientation towards life; diagnosing problems and planning treatment; empowering cultural and ethnic families and individuals; and finally, designing innovative programs and interventions (p. 22). Commenting on the dangers of not understanding the world view of clients from diverse backgrounds, Brown and Barrera (1999) state that "whenever we look at reality through only one lens, we significantly increase the probability that our perceptions and interpretations will be biased and stereotypic" (p. 36).

Acculturation status. When working with immigrant and refugee families, family-centred practitioners need to assess what Bennett and colleagues describe as the family's acculturation level. Acculturation consists of social and psychological exchanges that take place between individuals of different cultures (Berry, 1998). More specifically, Berry (1997, 1998) maintains that the acculturation process entails the learning of new behaviours, attitudes, and values that the individual needs to incorporate into her or his everyday existence to function in a new environment. This learning process can produce levels of stress to which an individual or a family needs to adapt. How family members cope with stressors is theorized to determine how they adapt. Within the family context, practitioners need to be sensitive to the different acculturation rates of family members. Typically, children and youth acculturate at a faster rate than their parents, and this may lead to the emergence of intergenerational conflict.

Beliefs. This section is composed of two parts. The first part of the discussion is focused on the importance of family-centred practitioners gaining an understanding of the family's beliefs related to health and illness. The second part is centred on the value of exploring with the family the beliefs and feelings of having a young child with a disability as well as determining the ways in which the family deals with this particular situation.

As noted by several writers (Hancock & Perkins, 1985; Kleinman, 1980; Vaughn, Jacques, & Baker, 2009), all cultural and ethnic groups hold beliefs related to health, illness, and disability as well as practices for maintaining well-being or receiving treatment when it is required. As part of her/his interaction with immigrant/refugee and other culturally diverse families, it is important for the family-centred professional to gain an understanding of the beliefs held by these clients. This may provide insights to the practitioner related to the family's relationship with the practitioner. For example, a family-centred practitioner should explore questions such as "what is health" and "what is good health from the family's perspective."

However, it is also important for family-centred practitioners to go beyond understanding the meanings associated with good health and find out from families what strategies or methods they use in maintaining good health. Another area that should be explored is the barriers and challenges that newcomer families encounter in their efforts to achieve "good health." This information may assist the practitioner in developing interventions that hopefully will address some of the barriers faced by these families.

Previous experience with health/social service systems. Another important dimension of the assessment process involves understanding what kind of health and social service agencies and organizations families have encountered in the past. Some immigrants and refugees, for example, come from countries where the health and social service systems are limited or non-existent. An important role that family-centred professionals may have is educating family members about the health and social service systems in Canada and, in particular, identifying families with a child with a disability and helping them get connected with needed resources in the community. Hence, these practitioners may find themselves performing service coordination activities.

Family constitution. Having knowledge of what constitutes a "family" is an important dimension family-centred practitioners should understand when working with families from diverse backgrounds. As Anderson and Fenichel (1989) state, the concept of what constitutes a family differs from one cultural group to another. For example, in many African immigrant and refugee communities, the concept of the extended family prevails, which includes direct family members as well as friends and neighbours. The extended family plays an important role, such as assisting in the rearing of children as well as serving as an important source of support. They also may be contributors to the decision-making process in some newcomer families (Este & Tachble, 2009).

The lack of family support typically provided by the extended family in the country of origin is frequently cited as a major adjustment that immigrant and refugee families experience in their efforts to adapt to life in Canada (Este & Tachble, 2009; Simich, Beiser, & Mawani, 2003; Stewart et al., 2008). For example, as a result of limited extended family, immigrant and refugee fathers may be placed in the position where they must take on more household responsibilities such as caring for their children. For practitioners working with diverse families with a child with a disability, having an understanding of the family's composition may help in the development of support plans for the child with special needs and, in particular, in the identification of who in the family are the main caregivers.

Child-rearing. There is consensus within the literature that human service professionals such as family-centred practitioners should have some understanding of the child-rearing practices of groups such as immigrants and refugees. Lin and Fu (1990) emphasize the need for helping professionals to enquire about the child-rearing practices that will enable service providers to become more knowledgeable "about the patterns of socialization among immigrants who have to accommodate to the social expectations of their culture of origin and their culture or relocation" (p. 249). As well, a number of writers (Chao, 1996; Sethi, Este, & Charlebois, 2001; Swick, 1985) contend that child-rearing practices are influenced by cultural orientations and that the cultural context is central to parenting styles and parent-child interactions. A major finding of the study conducted by Sethi et al. (2001), which examined the child-rearing practices of recently migrated South Asian and Chinese women with children from infancy to age 6, stressed the following: "It is clear that child-rearing practices have both universal and unique aspects across cultures. The universal aspect of child-rearing is that all parents, regardless of their cultural orientations, wish their children to become valued members of the society. However, to accomplish this goal, parents use unique beliefs, values, and practices of their cultural group" (p. 18).

One of the most important pieces of knowledge that helping professionals must obtain when working with families from diverse communities is the families' beliefs and attitudes related to disability (Rogers, Ochoa, & Delgado, 2003). Practitioners should not assume there is a universal view associated with the concept "disability." Bennett, Zhang, and Hojnar (1998) contend that "perceptions of disability are important dimensions of the history and traditions of many cultures" (p. 233). These same writers maintain that in some cultures the family with a child with a disability is believed to be cursed by God and the disability is a form of punishment for past sins (p. 233).

Failure to understand that there are different meanings associated with the term "disability" may limit the practitioner's ability to effectively work with the child and the family and may in turn result in inappropriate interventions. Practitioners need to be cognizant that a family's perception of a disability may influence parental decisions related to child-rearing practices, whether to seek services, and if so, what services are going to be used and from whom. Based on a family's beliefs about a disability, helping professionals may find themselves in the position of adjusting service delivery to not only meet the needs of the child but also the family's beliefs associated with disability.

Closely related is the need for family-centred professionals to have some knowledge related to beliefs and practices regarding parenting. Cultural groups have values and norms that dictate child-rearing practices. For example, a primary value in Sudanese families is the belief that children need to respect their parents as well as other adults within the family and the larger community. Mothers typically play a dominant role in raising children along with other female relatives and community members. Sudanese fathers often take the lead role as financial provider for their families.

Help-seeking behaviour represents another important piece of knowledge for a culturally sensitive family-centred professional. Cartledge, Kea, and Simmons-Reed (2002) contend that immigrant and refugee families typically do not seek help for their children with emotional and behavioural difficulties for reasons such as language barriers, lack of knowledge about availability of services, cultural taboos, and beliefs that services will not be helpful (p. 10). Family-centred practitioners also need to be aware of how immigrant and refugee families cope with a child with a disability. For example, who in the family is the primary caregiver? How do families deal with the stress that may exist (Harry, 2002)?

Refugees. Family-centred practitioners also need to be aware of a specific group of newcomers who are designated as refugees. According to

Canada's immigration policies, conventional refugees represent a class of individuals who have left their country and cannot return because of a well-founded fear of persecution for reasons of race, religion, nationality, group membership, or political opinion (Fleras & Elliot, 2000, p. 267). The second major group are sponsored refugees who are preselected abroad by government officials or by private agencies, individuals, clubs, or church groups with private sponsors obligated to provide support for 10 years.

It is imperative that family-centred practitioners who work with refugees determine the circumstances that led to the departure of their clients from their countries. It is not uncommon for these individuals to have suffered some type of persecution or to have witnessed severe forms of violence. As a result of the violence experienced or witnessed by these individuals, they may suffer from post-traumatic stress disorder (PTSD). Symptoms of PTSD may include recurring recollections of past trauma, dreams/nightmares, feelings of sadness, restricted affect, social numbness/withdrawal, memory impairment, and avoidance of activities that may trigger flashbacks of events. Individually and collectively, these symptoms may impact on the ability of refugees to successfully integrate into their new society (Chambers & Ganesan, 2005).

Skills

Skills acquisition is another requirement for family-centred service providers who aspire to be effective in their practice with diverse families (Bennett et al., 1998). The key skill for culturally sensitive practice is the ability to develop a positive working alliance with these families. An important aspect of this process is to make serious efforts to understand the social reality of these clients. Empathy is critical in the development of trusting relationships with clients. Heinonen and Spearman (2001), in commenting on the term, remark that empathy "refers to the ability to understand clients in their situations and from their perspectives" (p. 113). Empathic practitioners who accept their clients regardless of cultural heritage, values, or belief systems may be well positioned to develop a meaningful and trusting relationship. If families feel they are heard and respected by the practitioner, this indeed may be a key marker of the individual's ability to practice in a culturally sensitive manner.

A critical component of work with diverse clients such as immigrants and refugees is the assessment process. Culturally sensitive practitioners must conduct thorough assessments and must take into consideration how cultural factors may impact the situation. As part of the assessment process, Edwards (1994, p. 53) maintains that the following questions be posed to clients who are immigrants or refugees: (a) when and how did the clients or families migrate to their current community, (b) what prompted the move from their country of origin, (c) what has been the easiest thing to adjust to, and (d) what things have been most difficult for the client?

In addition to questions based on Drachman's (1992) framework (discussed earlier), questions focused on the families' beliefs about children with a disability, the supports that exist in helping them cope with this situation, and how they manage are additional areas to explore in the assessment process. In addition, an analysis of the specific needs of these families requires attention by the family-centred practitioner.

Culturally sensitive interviewing, an important aspect of the assessment process, is another critical skill required by family-centred professionals working with diverse families. It is important for these professionals to be aware of their level of intrusiveness and directness, social distances, formality, and ways of addressing families. Consideration also needs to be given to the types of questions posed to families, as there may be issues that are considered taboo for families to discuss with professionals.

Helping professionals must be aware of, and sensitive to, their clients' verbal and non-verbal communication. Having an understanding of the specific meanings of non-verbal communication imparted by different culturally diverse families and being observant in practice should contribute to greater understanding of particular client systems.

The ability to form relationships with individuals and communities across cultures is becoming increasingly important as individuals in some cultures rely on traditional healers to deal with health-related concerns. Commenting on the role traditional healers may play with clients of Arab background, Al-Krenawi and Graham (2003) state that "among traditional healers are amulet writers, the Dervish, Koranic healers and others who provide tangible support, advice, and consultation during such life events as mourning, distress, crises, traumas or various mental or physical illness" (p. 188). Consulting with traditional healers and spiritual leaders as well as practitioners who have worked with culturally diverse clients may be very helpful.

Working with Interpreters

Given the increasing linguistic diversity, the ability to work with interpreters is rapidly becoming an important skill required by professionals.

In the past, typically, family members were asked to serve as interpreters; however, if health care facilities or social service agencies have access to professionally trained interpreters, it is highly recommended that these individuals provide interpretation and translation services. One of the limitations of using someone who is not a professional interpreter is that the individual may have a limited vocabulary to converse in the professional domain. Anderson et al. (2005) comment on this situation: "Family members may be willing to translate, but there are often shortcomings with their fluency in English … Family members may be placed in uncomfortable situations when asked to communicate personal information or may only selectively relay information back to the patient" (p. 347).

Anderson and Fenichel (1989) stress that it is essential to have well-trained, skilled interpreters "who are able to make conceptual transfers, including transfers of idiomatic usages and meanings of information" (p. 12). For family-centred practitioners working with families whose mother tongue is not English, accessing professionally trained interpreters may contribute to the development of a relationship with the family and result in the most appropriate intervention for the young child and his/her family.

Value Base

Knowledge and skill are only two of the requirements of a culturally sensitive practitioner in the field of family-centred practice. Within the literature, it is emphasized that these individuals must have a value base or attitudes congruent with the goals of culturally sensitive practice. Service providers are faced with the challenge to ensure all clients, regardless of their backgrounds, are treated in an equitable manner and that the systemic barriers families with children with disabilities encounter are addressed.

Acknowledging and accepting that cultural differences exist and impact the delivery and utilization of services represent another salient value premise (Este, 1999). If family-centred professionals approach their clients with the belief they are all equal, these individuals will negate the lived realities of clients from diverse communities. For example, if professionals working with racialized immigrant clients adopt this stance, in essence, these practitioners will be applying a "colour-blind" approach. Dominelli (1998) maintains that this approach stresses the notion that all people are the same – that members of one race [or population] will have similar problems, needs, and objectives. From a service delivery perspective, programs and services will be provided without taking into consideration the racial characteristics of those who are service users. If practitioners work with clients in this manner, it is highly likely their effectiveness with individuals and families will be extremely limited.

Another critical value premise is cultural relativism, which stresses that no specific world view is superior, better, or more correct than another; the perspective is simply different. Like an individual, groups possess unique world views. By understanding this concept, practitioners can situate themselves to learn other world views and creatively approach their work with families and children from diverse communities.

Finally, professionals who aspire to practice in a culturally sensitive manner must recognize that heterogeneity within cultures is as important as the diversity between cultures. Waxler-Morrison and her colleagues (2005) comment on this value: "While there are usually shared beliefs, values, and experiences among people from a given ethnic group, quite often there is widespread intra-ethnic diversity. Factors such as social class, religion, level of education and area of origin in the home country (rural or urban) make for major differences" (p. 246). Being knowledgeable about this reality will prevent practitioners from stereotyping clients.

Possessing the values presented does not ensure professionals working with children and parents from diverse communities are or will become culturally sensitive practitioners. It is imperative that these individuals have the relevant knowledge and acquire the skill set previously discussed.

Organizational Context

The process of culturally sensitive practice is not limited to practitioners engaged in family-centred service with diverse clients. Within the literature, there is a strong consensus that the organizations in which these individuals work must also adopt processes and policies that clearly support and value this practice. For example, Sue (2006) maintains that institutions which employ health and social service employees are monocultural in the policies and practices that are used. As a result, problems that service users such as immigrants and refugees encounter may often be the result of organizational or systemic factors.

Hence, organizations that engage in family-centred service are challenged to ensure the programs and care they provide meet the needs of diverse communities, that the staff complement within these organizations reflects the changing diversity in the local geographic areas, and finally, that the organization values and supports culturally sensitive practice.

Another important theme associated with a culturally sensitive organization is the critical role that senior administrators play in fostering an environment where culturally sensitive practice is sustained and becomes part of the organization's culture (Este, 1999). Bate, Kahn, and Pye (2000) recommend that leadership be viewed as a process as organizations engage in the process of becoming culturally sensitive. Tangible signs of leadership provided by senior administration include (a) supporting staff in their development to become culturally sensitive practitioners, (b) developing and implementing a vision around the "place" where the organization would be if it functioned as one that strives to be culturally sensitive, and (c) engaging in constant communication related to the importance and significance of culturally sensitive practice to the managing and governing of the organization. Collectively, the implementation of these initiatives is a solid indicator that the leadership is highly committed to culturally sensitive practice.

Conclusion

Given the diversity that exists in Canadian society, family-centred practitioners need an education that will enable them to work with all Canadians regardless of their backgrounds and life experiences. It is imperative that this education provides the knowledge and skills required to work effectively with diverse families, as possessing just the necessary knowledge base and skills for working with families with young children with disabilities is deemed insufficient in the process of developing culturally sensitive practitioners. As part of this education, it is extremely important that family-centred practitioners embrace the value of practicing in a culturally sensitive manner. It is also absolutely necessary for these service providers to treat their clients in a respectful manner and to be completely open to learn from families.

From an agency perspective, the creation of a work environment that fosters excellence in services provided to diverse communities such as immigrants and refugees must be a major organizational goal. Writers such as Hyde (2004), Sue (2006), and Gallop and Este (2006) maintain that it is critical for administrators of health and social service agencies to create climates in their organizations that promote culturally sensitive practice and integrate it throughout the entire organization. In essence, health and social service organizations must be at the vanguard of cultural sensitivity philosophy and behaviour. This is another clear indication that they indeed are family-centred entities.

REFERENCES

Al-Krenawi, A., & Graham, J. (2003). Social work practice with Canadians of Arab background. In A. Al-Krenawi & J. Graham (Eds.), *Multicultural social work with diverse ethno-racial communities in Canada* (pp. 174–201). Toronto, ON: Oxford University Press.

Anderson, J., Kirkham, S., Waxler-Morrison, N., Herbert, C., Murphy, M., & Richardson, E. (2005). Delivering culturally responsive health care. In N. Waxler-Morrison, E. Richardson, J. Anderson, & N. Chambers (Eds.), *Cross-cultural caring* (pp. 323–52). Vancouver, BC: University of British Columbia Press.

Anderson, P., & Fenichel, E. (1989). *Serving culturally diverse families of infants and toddlers with disabilities.* Washington, DC: National Center for Clinical Infant Progress.

Bate, P., Kahn, R., & Pye, A. (2000). Towards a culturally sensitive approach to organization structuring: Where organization design meets organization development. *Organization Science, 11*(2), 197–211. http://dx.doi.org/10.1287/orsc.11.2.197.12509

Bennett, T., Zhang, C., & Hojnar, L. (1998). Facilitating the full participation of culturally diverse families in the IFSP/IEP process: Infant-toddler intervention. *Transdisciplinary Journal, 8,* 227–49.

Berry, J. (1997). Immigration, acculturation and adaptation. *Applied Psychology: An International Review, 46,* 5–34.

Berry, J.W. (1998). Acculturation and health: Theory and research. In S.S. Kazarian & D.R. Evans (Eds.), *Cultural clinical psychology, theory, research and practice* (pp. 29–57). New York, NY: Oxford University Press.

Brown, W., & Barrera, I. (1999). Enduring problems in assessments: The persistent challenges of cultural dynamics and family issues. *Infants and children, 12*(1), 34–42. http://dx.doi.org/10.1097/00001163-199907000-00007

Butler, L., & Molidor, C. (1995). Cultural sensitivity in social work practice and research with children and families. *Early Child Development and Care, 106*(1), 27–33. http://dx.doi.org/10.1080/0300443951060104

Calvillo, E., Clark, L., Ballantyne, J.E., Pacquiao, D., Purnell, L.D., & Villar-
ruel, A.M. (2008, April). Cultural competency in baccalaureate nursing
education. *Journal of Transcultural Nursing, 20*(2), 137–45. http://dx.doi.
org/10.1177/1043659608330354 Medline:19129519

Canadian Association of Social Workers. (2005). *Code of Ethics 2005.* Ottawa,
ON: Canadian Association of Social Workers. Retrieved from http://www.
casw-acts.ca/en/what-social-work/casw-code-ethics

Canadian Nurses Association. (2008). *Code of ethics for registered nurses* (Cen-
tennial ed.). Ottawa, ON: Canadian Nurses Association. Retrieved from
http://www2.cna-aiic.ca/CNA/documents/pdf/publications/Code_of_
Ethics_2008_e.pdf

Canadian Psychological Association. (2000). *Canadian code of ethics for psychologists* (3rd ed.). Ottawa, ON: Canadian Psychological Association. Retrieved from http://www.cpa.ca/cpasite/userfiles/Documents/Canadian%20
Code%20of%20Ethics%20for%20Psycho.pdf

Cartledge, G., Kea, C., & Simmons-Reed, E. (2002). Serving culturally diverse children with a serious emotional disturbance and their families. *Journal of Child and Family Studies, 11*(1), 113–26. http://dx.doi.
org/10.1023/A:1014775813711

Chambers, N., & Ganesan, S. (2005). Refugees in Canada. In N. Waxler-Morrison, J. Anderson, E. Richardson, & N. Chambers (Eds.), *Cross-cultural caring: A handbook for health professionals* (2nd ed., pp. 289–322). Vancouver, BC:
University of British Columbia Press.

Chao, R.K. (1996). Chinese and European American mothers' beliefs about the
role of parenting in children's school success. *Journal of Cross-Cultural Psychology, 27*(4), 403–23. http://dx.doi.org/10.1177/0022022196274002

Citizenship and Immigration Canada. (2010). *Annual report to parliament on immigration 2010.* Ottawa, ON: Minister of Public Works and Government Services Canada.

College of Nurses of Ontario. (2009). *Practice guideline: Providing culturally
sensitive care.* Retrieved 22 October 2010, from http://www.cno.org/Global/
docs/prac/41040_CulturallySens.pdf

Culture. (n.d.). In Merriam-Webster Online Dictionary. Retrieved from http://
www.merriam-webster.com/dictionary/culture

Dewees, M. (2001). Building cultural competency for work with diverse families: Strategies from the privileged side. *Journal of Ethnic & Cultural Diversity
in Social Work, 9*, 33–51. http://dx.doi.org/10.1300/J051v09n03_02

Dominelli, L. (1998). *Anti-racist social work: A challenge for white practitioners and
educators.* London, UK: Macmillan.

Drachman, D. (1992). A stage of migration framework for service to immigrant populations. *Social Work, 37*, 68–72.

Earner, I., & Rivera, H. (2005). Introduction. *Child Welfare, 8*, 531–6.

Edwards, V. (1994). Understanding culture as a process. In R. Surber (Ed.), *Clinical case management: A guide to comprehensive treatment of serious mental illness* (pp. 42–54). Thousand Oaks, CA: Sage.

Este, D. (1999). Cultural competency and social work: An overview. In G. Yong-Lie & D. Este (Eds.), *Professional social services in a multicultural world* (pp. 27–48). Toronto, ON: Canadian Scholars Press.

Este, D. (2007). Cultural competency and social work practice in Canada: A retrospective examination. *Canadian Social Work Review, 24*, 93–105.

Este, D., & Tachble, A. (2009). Fatherhood in the Canadian context: Perceptions and experiences of Sudanese refugee men. *Sex Roles, 60*(7-8), 456–66. http://dx.doi.org/10.1007/s11199-008-9532-1

Fleras, A., & Elliot, J.L. (2000). *Unequal relations: An introduction to race, ethnicity, and Aboriginal dynamics in Canada* (3rd ed.). Scarborough, ON: Prentice Hall.

Foronda, C.L. (2008, July). A concept analysis of cultural sensitivity. *Journal of Transcultural Nursing, 19*(3), 207–12. http://dx.doi.org/10.1177/1043659608317093 Medline:18411414

Gallop, C., & Este, D. (2006). Multicultural organizational development (MCOD): The fundamental transformation of Canadian social work education. *International Journal of Diversity in Organisations, Communities, and Nations, 6*, 107–18.

Germain, C., & Gitterman, A. (1996). *The life model of social work practice: Advances in practice and theory* (2nd ed.). New York, NY: Columbia University Press.

Hancock, T., & Perkins, T. (1985). The mandala of health: A conceptual model and teaching tool. *Health Promotion (Oxford, England), 24*, 8–10.

Harry, B. (2002). Trends and issues in serving culturally diverse families of children with disabilities. *Journal of Special Education, 36*(3), 132–40. http://dx.doi.org/10.1177/00224669020360030301

Heinonen, T., & Spearman, L. (2001). *Social work practice: Problem solving and beyond*. Toronto, ON: Irwin.

Henry, R., Tator, C., Mattis, W., & Rees, T. (1995). *The colour of democracy: Racism in Canadian society*. Toronto, ON: Harcourt Brace.

Hyde, C.A. (2004, January). Multicultural development in human services agencies: Challenges and solutions. *Social Work, 49*(1), 7–16. http://dx.doi.org/10.1093/sw/49.1.7 Medline:14964514

James, C. (2003). *Seeing ourselves: Exploring race, ethnicity and culture* (3rd ed.). Toronto, ON: Thompson Educational Publishing.

Jeff, M.F.X. (1994). Afrocentrism and African American male youths. In R.B. Mincy (Ed.), *Nurturing young black males* (pp. 99–118). Washington, DC: Urban Institute Press.

Josipovic, P. (2000, June). Recommendations for culturally sensitive nursing care. *International Journal of Nursing Practice, 6*(3), 146–52. http://dx.doi.org/10.1046/j.1440-172x.2000.00201.x Medline:11249413

Kirmayer, L.J., & Minas, H. (2000, June). The future of cultural psychiatry: An international perspective. *Canadian Journal of Psychiatry, 45*(5), 438–46. Medline:10900523

Kleinman, A. (1980). *Patients and healers in the context of culture: An exploration of the borderland between anthropology, medicine, and psychiatry.* Los Angeles, CA: University of California Press.

Leishman, J.L. (2006, May). Culturally sensitive mental health care: A module for 21st century education and practice. *International Journal of Psychiatric Nursing Research, 11*(3), 1310–21. Medline:16776439

Lin, L.Y., & Fu, V. (1990). A comparison of child-rearing practices among Chinese, immigrant Chinese, and Caucasian American parents. *Child Development, 61*(2), 429–33. http://dx.doi.org/10.2307/1131104

Moore, S.E. (1992). Cultural sensitivity treatment and reach issues with black adolescent drug users. *Child & Adolescent Social Work Journal, 9*(3), 249–60. http://dx.doi.org/10.1007/BF00755864

Olandi, M. (1992). Defining cultural competence: An organizing framework. In M. Olandi (Ed.), *Cultural competence for evaluations: A guide for alcohol and other drug abuse prevention practitioners working with ethnic/racial communities* (pp. i–viii). Rockville, MA: Department of Health.

Perry, C., & Tate-Manning, L. (2006). Unravelling cultural constructions in social work education: Journeying toward cultural competence. *Social Work Education, 25*(7), 735–48. http://dx.doi.org/10.1080/02615470600905986

Pine, B.A., & Drachman, D. (2005, September-October). Effective child welfare practice with immigrant and refugee children and their families. *Child Welfare, 84*(5), 537–62. Medline:16435650

Resnicow, K., Soler, R., Braithwaite, R., Ahluwalia, J., & Butler, J. (2000). Cultural sensitivity in substance abuse prevention. *Journal of Community Psychology, 28*(3), 271–90. http://dx.doi.org/10.1002/(SICI)1520-6629(200005)28:3<271::AID-JCOP4>3.0.CO;2-I

Rogers, D.L., Ochoa, T.A., & Delgado, B. (2003). Developing cross-cultural competence: Serving families of children with significant developmental needs. *Focus on Autism and Other Developmental Disabilities, 18*(1), 4–8. http://dx.doi.org/10.1177/108835760301800102

Saleeby, D. (1997). *The strengths perspective in social work practice* (2nd ed.). New York, NY: Longman.

Schiele, J. (2000). *Human services and the Afrocentric paradigm*. Binghamton, NY: Haworth Press.

Segal, U.A., & Mayadas, N.S. (2005, September-October). Assessment of issues facing immigrant and refugee families. *Child Welfare, 84*(5), 563–83. Medline:16435651

Sethi, S., Este, D., & Charlebois, M. (2001). Factors influencing the child-rearing practices of recently migrated East Indian and Chinese women with children from infancy to age six. *Hong Kong Nursing Journal, 37*, 14–20.

Simich, L., Beiser, M., & Mawani, F.N. (2003, November). Social support and the significance of shared experience in refugee migration and re-settlement. *Western Journal of Nursing Research, 25*(7), 872–91. http://dx.doi.org/10.1177/0193945903256705 Medline:14596184

Statistics Canada. (2008, April 8). 2006 Census: Ethnic origin, visible minorities, place of work and mode of transportation. *The Daily*. Retrieved from http://www.statcan.gc.ca/daily-quotidien/080402/dq080402a-eng.htm

Stewart, M., Anderson, J., Beiser, M., Mwakarimba, E., Neufeld, A., Simich, L., & Spitzer, D. (2008). Multicultural meanings of social support among immigrants and refugees. *International Migration (Geneva, Switzerland), 46*(3), 123–59. http://dx.doi.org/10.1111/j.1468-2435.2008.00464.x

Sue, D.W. (2006). *Multicultural social work practice*. Hoboken, NJ: John Wiley & Sons.

Swick, K. (1985). Cultural influences on parenting: Implications for parent educators. *Journal of Instructional Psychology, 12*, 80–5.

Vaughn, L.M., Jacques, F.M., & Baker, R.C. (2009). Cultural health, attributions, beliefs, and practices: Effects on health care and medical education. *Open Medical Education Journal, 2*, 64–74.

Waxler-Morrison, N., Anderson, J., & Richardson, E. (2005). *Cross-cultural caring: A handbook for health professionals*. Vancouver, BC: University of British Columbia Press.

Weick, A., Rapp, C., Sullivan, W., & Kisthardt, W. (1989). A strengths perspective for social work practice. *Social Work, 34*, 350–4.

Westermeyer, J. (1976). Clinical guidelines for the cross-cultural treatment of chemical dependency. *American Journal of Drug and Alcohol Abuse, 3*(2), 315–22. http://dx.doi.org/10.3109/00952997609077200 Medline:1032745

Yee, J. (2003). Whiteout: Looking for face in Canadian social work practice. In A. Al-Krenawi & J. Graham (Eds.), *Multicultural social work in Canada: Working with diverse ethno-racial communities* (pp. 98–121). Don Mills, ON: Oxford University Press Canada.

PART FIVE

Administration Issues

13 Supervision to Enhance Family-Centred Practice

ALEXANDRA WRIGHT

Introduction

This chapter aims to provide direction for supervisors who are responsible for overseeing practitioners providing services within the context of an organization whose mandate is to create family-centred policy and deliver family-centred service. While the chapter does not present a new model of supervision and relies substantially on the writings of experts in the supervision field (e.g., Kadushin & Harkness, 2002; Shulman, 1993, 2006) to summarize critical components of the supervision context and process, the chapter does offer a different perspective on supervision with an emphasis on the application of supervision within a family-centred context of service planning, delivery, and evaluation. This model of supervision from a family-centred perspective can be applied within multiple contexts including, for example, health, mental health, and child welfare.

Research examining services for families with disabilities has found a link between positive family outcomes and supervision. For example, Sloper, Greco, Beecham, and Webb (2006) reported key workers (i.e., service providers) who had ongoing and regular supervision focusing on their work positively impacted outcomes for families. In addition, Wright, Hiebert-Murphy, and Trute (2010) found that professionals perceived regularly scheduled supervision to positively impact their ability to implement family-centred services and that supervisors were considered leaders in family-centred practice as they "set the tone" for its implementation (p. 121). Hiebert-Murphy, Trute, and Wright's (2011) findings suggest that practitioners required further training in general practice skills as well as, in particular, family-centred practice skills when providing family-centred services to families. Supervision provides an excellent opportunity to develop knowledge and skills for family-centred practice, and supervisors occupy a unique role in the implementation of family-centred services.

Supervision within a family-centred context can be conceptualized as a reflection of three different knowledge and skill axes. The first axis is the supervision axis. This axis consists of issues related specifically to supervision and the supervisor's role, generally considered transferable to different clinical supervision settings. Topics in this first axis include the supervisor's administrative, educational, and supportive roles with a particular focus on the "parallel process" (the similarity between the supervisor–service provider relationship and the service provider–family relationship), the working alliance between the supervisor and the supervisee, and evaluation of the performance of supervisees. Other topics considered in the first axis include the stages of the supervisory process and content specific to the supervisory context. The second axis comprises the four stages of service provision in which the supervisee is engaged with a family, and that the supervisor oversees: intake and assessment, intervention, evaluation, and transfer/closure. Each of these stages has direct service and administrative matters that should be addressed in the supervisory setting and are generally transferable to various social or health care contexts. The third axis relates specifically to key family-centred practice elements that the supervisor should ensure the supervisee uses when providing services (e.g., enabling, empowering, and engaging with the family). An important aspect of the supervisory role is to work with a service provider to develop the necessary skills and knowledge for the implementation of family-centred practice. Sound supervision reflects a balance of the three key interconnecting axes. By conceptualizing the three axes (the supervisory process and content, the service stages, and the fundamentals of family-centred practice) as the basis of family-centred supervision knowledge and skills, a fuller understanding emerges of supervision from a family-centred perspective.

This chapter begins with a definition of supervision and provides a summary of critical components of the supervision process and content. The chapter continues with a discussion of supervision from a family-centred perspective within the context of practice stages and highlights key elements of family-centred practice that should be incorporated as part of ongoing supervision (i.e., engagement, respect, and partnership with families). A summary of issues related to ethics and evaluation follows, highlighting the supervisor's role in addressing ethical issues related to families receiving services as well as issues concerned with staff and the organization. The final section of the chapter concentrates on challenges to supervision in a family-centred context.

A General Discussion of Supervision

The definition of supervision. In a review of literature on social work supervision, Bogo and McKnight (2006) note that supervision refers to a variety of functions with the objective of attaining efficiency in service provision. Supervision is most often considered an administrative task linking staff's professional activities to the organization's mandate. Supervision provides a process for accountability in which the organization assigns the supervisor authority and responsibility to oversee service providers' work. In addition to the administrative function, Kadushin and Harkness (2002) identify two additional supervisory functions, educational and supportive, and define a supervisor as someone who is "an agency administrative-staff member to whom authority is delegated to direct, coordinate, enhance, and evaluate the on-the-job performance of the supervisees for whose work he or she is held accountable" (p. 23). Successful and effective supervision should result in increased competence for the service provider as well as the supervisor, and improved services for families (Kadushin & Harkness, 2002; Munson, 2002).

Supervisors have many administrative responsibilities including the assignment of eligible families to service providers, monitoring of service provision (i.e., assessment, intervention, and evaluation), and regular oversight of service delivery to ensure organizational policies and procedures are implemented (Shulman, 1993). Kadushin and Harkness (2002) list specific administrative tasks that supervisors must perform:

1 Staff recruitment and selection
2 Inducting and placing workers
3 Work planning
4 Work assignment
5 Work delegation
6 Monitoring, reviewing, and evaluating work
7 Coordinating work
8 Communication (p. 47)

Other administrative tasks include providing an opinion on staff promotions and pay increases (Shulman, 1993), remediation, reassignment, and at times, termination (Kadushin & Harkness, 2002). In addition, family-centred administrative functions can include allocating funding for special projects (e.g., projects related to assessed family need or for a team initiative), committee work, and teamwork with other professionals and family members. Supervisors must ensure that the service provided meets legal requirements and responsibilities as well ethical principles. Supervisors must also address the administrative needs of the agency. Thus, supervisors must ensure that service providers complete necessary forms and abide by agency policies. Kadushin and Harkness (2002) also identify advocacy, administrative buffering, and acting as a change agent as additional supervisory functions. Hopkins and Austin (2004) note that supervisors link the micro practices of the organization to the larger macro policies and practices and can influence the establishment of a positive organizational climate (i.e., a reduction in perceived stress and burnout).

Educational supervision is "concerned with teaching the worker what he or she needs to know to do the job and helping him or her learn it" (Kadushin & Harkness, 2002, p. 129). This supervisory responsibility focuses on identifying the necessary knowledge and skills service providers require to fulfil their position, and determining the means and content necessary to ensure this is realized. At times, supervisors themselves provide the necessary instruction or knowledge, and at other times, supervisors plan with the service provider to select other professional development opportunities such as staff training. Austin and Hopkins (2004) note that supervisors perform a vital role in facilitating the collection, dissemination, and sharing of learning within the organization as well as on an inter-organizational level.

The third supervisor function, supportive supervision, refers to the context in which the supervisor provides assistance to service providers when dealing with challenging issues through the use of encouragement, reassurance, and autonomy (Kadushin & Harkness, 2002; Shulman, 1993). Supportive supervision also includes activities that promote a positive working environment and staff morale and require "people-centred" skills to meet the expressive needs of service providers (Kadushin & Harkness, 2002, p. 218).The function of supportive supervision is important, as the supervisor enables the service provider to constructively deal with feelings that have the potential to negatively impact service provision. For example, if a service provider is experiencing anxiety when providing services to a particular family, these feelings may be challenging the service provider's ability to develop rapport with family members. In supportive supervision, the supervisor acknowledges the service provider's feelings and enables the service provider to address these issues in order to promote growth, development, professional autonomy, and ultimately, service effectiveness (Kadushin & Harkness, 2002).

Supervision can occur in various modalities: for example, in a one-to-one setting (in which the supervisor and the service provider meet to discuss workload issues) and in a group-based supervision context (in which there is one supervisor with multiple service providers; Bogo & McKnight, 2006). Peer group supervision involves peers who consult and problem solve together, without the participation of a supervisor. This approach is not included in the discussion in this chapter. Supervision can occur face-to-face, via the telephone, through some other electronic means (e.g., online), or even through correspondence. The most effective supervision formats include group supervision, individual case consultation, the use of videotapes or live supervision with feedback, the demonstration of practice skills by the supervisor, and the use of one-way mirrors (Kadushin & Harkness, 2002).

The supervisory relationship itself can vary in intensity and structure depending on the experience and knowledge of the service provider (Shulman, 2006). Kadushin and Harkness (2002) suggest that planned, weekly individual supervision sessions are necessary for new workers. Munson (2002) suggests that effective supervision requires that the (a) structure of supervision be explicit and known to the service provider, (b) supervision occur regularly, (c) supervision be consistent in terms of the supervisor's style and approach, (d) focus of supervision be case-oriented, with all learning connected to the case, and (e) supervision be evaluated. Regular, planned meetings between the supervisor and the service provider create an opportunity for the supervisor to meet administrative, educational, and supportive functions.

Falender and Shafranske (2007) list 12 best practices recommended for competency-based supervision. This list provides a helpful guideline for supervisors to direct supervisory tasks and responsibilities. What is clear from this list is the expectation that supervisors are prepared, active, responsible, organized, and very importantly, role models and mentors in their approach to supervision. The 12 recommendations are paraphrased in the following section. Competent supervision requires that

1 The supervisor self-assesses on clinical and supervision expertise and competency issues.

2 The supervisor engages with the supervisee to facilitate the emergence of a working alliance.

3 The supervisor commits to the practice of supervision integrating integrity, ethics, appreciation of diversity, and evidence-based practice.

4 The supervisor delineates supervisory expectations, including standards, rules, and general practice as well as goals and competencies the supervisee must attain and the tasks necessary to achieve them.

5 The supervisor collaborates with the supervisee to develop a supervisory contract and links the original competencies document to the contract and to evaluation procedures.

6 The supervisor reviews supervisee work and facilitates inquiry leading to supervisee self-awareness and reflective practice as features of the evaluation process.

7 The supervisor models and engages the supervisee in self-assessment and development of metacompetence from the onset of supervision and throughout.

8 The supervisor provides ongoing feedback, verbal and written, and encourages and accepts feedback from the supervisee.

9 The supervisor maintains communication and responsibility for observing problems in the supervisory relationship. (p. 238)

Supervision requires that supervisors have sufficient education and training to enable them to be effective in their work (Falender & Shafranske, 2007; Munson, 2002). This includes knowledge and skills related to service provider needs, as well as knowledge and skills related to the organization and the broader political environment (Hopkins & Austin, 2004). In addition to the knowledge and skills a supervisor brings to the position based on formal education and work experience, supervisors also need an orientation to the supervisory role and ongoing professional development opportunities (Kaiser & Barretta-Herman, 1999). Supervisors themselves require regular supervision (including performance evaluations) to enhance their growth and effectiveness (Kadushin & Harkness, 2002).

The phases of supervision. There are at least three phases of supervision (although Shulman adds a fourth phase that precedes the beginning phase): the beginning, the middle (also referred to as the work phase), and the ending or transition phase (Kadushin & Harkness,

2002; Shulman, 1993, 2006). Within each supervision session, there is also a beginning, middle, and ending or transition phase. Each of these phases requires different types of engagement, skill, and knowledge from the service provider and the supervisor.

In the beginning phase, the supervisor is responsible for scheduling supervision, setting the session's structure, and preparing for the meeting (Kadushin & Harkness, 2002; Munson, 2002). The supervisor must ensure that the meeting is scheduled in advance and that the location and time are convenient for the service provider. A supervision contract between the supervisor and the service provider creates a formal means to structure the supervision process, although it is important to note that without follow-up, a contract can be meaningless (Munson, 2002). The supervision contract provides an understanding of expectations for the supervisor-supervisee relationship (Shulman, 1993). This includes "the basis for the supervisory alliance, enhanced articulation of expectations, informed consent, and definition of parameters of the relationship and the process" (Falender, n.d., p. 40). The contract should address the following:

- Content and context of supervision
- Scope of practice under supervision
- Length of contract period
- Roles and expectations of supervisee and supervisor
- Learning activities, processes, supervisor and supervisee responsibilities, feedback, and mutually defined goals and tasks
- Legal/ethical parameters
- Informed consent and confidentiality
- Agency/practice requirements and rules
- Ethical codes, licensing statutes, and laws
- Agency/site personnel practices
- Performance expectations
- Specific knowledge, skills, values
- Modes of formative and summative evaluation. (Falender, n.d., p. 42)

In practice, competency-based supervision requires the supervisor and supervisee to understand and respect each other's rights and responsibilities, including the legal and ethical contexts of the work provided; to be clear on boundaries between the supervisor, supervisee, and service recipient; to clarify that personal issues can be a part of the supervisory agenda (and if necessary, a referral for support services may be made); to know that supervision sessions are documented; to be clear on the self-assessment requirements as well as the specifics of performance evaluations (i.e., what method of evaluation is used, when, and how often); to be aware that certain cases may be transferred and that the supervisor may become involved with a family should the supervisee be limited in her/his capacity; to review limits to confidentiality; and to understand the complaint process. The use of a supervision contract provides the supervisor and the service provider a basis on which to develop a working alliance through the identification of mutually determined goals and tasks (Falender, n.d., p. 45).

In order to prepare for the supervision session, the supervisor should review the service provider's documentation and form completion to ensure administrative requirements are met. Incomplete documentation should be noted and raised during the session. The supervisor should engage in clarifying and teaching in order to support the service provider in the fulfilment of the service provider's responsibilities. As well, the supervisor should assess the educational needs of the supervisee and identify ways in which these needs may be addressed. An educational plan for all service providers should be created to devise opportunities for knowledge and skill development (Friedman & Poertner, 1995). For example, should the service provider demonstrate a lack of knowledge regarding the importance of developing rapport with families, the supervisor could provide the service provider with an article identifying the importance of relationship building in family-centred practice and prepare some suggestions regarding specific skill development, which the supervisor could then model for the service provider. All phases of supervision provide important opportunities for knowledge transfer; by setting an expectation of learning during the beginning stage of supervision, the blueprint is set for effective learning to occur throughout the supervisory relationship and for professional growth, development, and increased autonomy to result.

In the preliminary phase of supervision, both the supervisor and supervisee focus on the work of "tuning in" and develop empathy about their issues related to the supervisory process (Shulman, 1993, p. 36). This process allows both the supervisor and the service provider to discover similar feelings or thoughts and to become sensitized to the other's issues. The beginning phase of supervision also requires the service provider to determine whether s/he will "engage meaningfully" with the supervisor, also known as the "first decision" (Shulman, 2006, p. 26). In order to commit to supervision, the relevance of the supervisory process to the service provider's work must be explicit. The supervisor is an authority figure, and thus the service provider may be cautious during the preliminary phase. Issues related to authority should be addressed in this phase as the supervisor's role is inherently a position of authority (Munson, 2002). Shulman (2006) argues that any response to questions or comments related to authority should contain the following: genuineness in the supervisor's response (which reflects hearing what the service provider is saying), supervisor empathy (which has to be accepted by the service provider), encouragement for the service provider to find her/his "own voice," and integration of the personal with professional selves (p. 31). Finally, the supervisor has to ensure that the service provider feels safe to express herself/himself within the supervisory context.

In the middle or work phase of supervision, the focus of supervision is on the work of the service provider, and the supervisor and service provider must ensure that work is not avoided and that work goes beyond superficial issues and the "illusion of work" (Shulman, 2006, p. 27). Shulman explains that facilitative confrontation is used to deal with complex or emotionally demanding factors. This process results in the "second decision," which involves a commitment by the service provider to engage with more complex issues (Shulman, 2006, p. 27). This is considered the work implementation phase.

In the ending or transition phase, the supervision relationship between the supervisor and the service provider is stopping, usually due to one person accepting a new position or leaving the organization due to a changing life circumstance. During this phase, the importance of "door knob therapy" must be addressed (when the most important issues of the work are raised at the end of a supervision session; Shulman, 2006, p. 27). The parallel process may also be evident during this stage and the supervisor should support the service provider in dealing with feelings or thoughts regarding endings (or transitions) with the supervisor and/or families. It is important to address issues in this phase, as poor or negative endings and transitions can affect service and supervision effectiveness. The supervisor must ensure that steps are identified to successfully complete necessary work.

Supervision from a Family-Centred Perspective

Dunst, Trivette, and Deal (1988) emphasize that family-centred practice is characterized by three key tenets related to the service provider's role with the family: the service provider's approach to service is proactive, her/his involvement with families is enabling, and the practice is empowering. Enabling refers to "creating opportunities," empowering refers to "meeting needs and achieving aspirations in a way that promotes a clear sense of intra-family mastery and control over important aspects of family function," and competence refers to the family's "ability to negotiate its course of development" (p. x). Dunst et al. (1988) highlight the importance of other characteristics of family-centred practice that service providers should apply when working with families. Parents are considered the experts on the family and should be given the right to make decisions regarding their needs and how to meet their needs (with the understanding that family members' rights and well-being are protected). Furthermore, the focus of family-centred practice is strengths-based. Positive functioning is a focus of the intervention process and negative outcomes may be associated with help-giving behaviour that is not enabling or empowering.

These basic family-centred practice principles are highly applicable to supervision. When providing supervision to service providers, supervisors should be proactive in the supervisory process and seek to enable and empower service providers to successfully complete their work. Supervisors should focus on service providers' strengths and positive functioning. As with help-giving to families, if supervisors undermine the competence and control of service providers, learned helplessness, low self-esteem, passivity, or dependency may result (Dunst et al., 1988). In addition, family-centred service providers are expected to assume multiple roles when working with families, including being an empathetic listener, teacher, therapist, consultant, resource, enabler, mobilizer, mediator, and advocate (Dunst et al., 1988, pp. 91–3); these roles parallel the supervisor's role when working with service providers in a supervisory relationship.

Supervisor skills. In the context of family-centred services, the supervisor must work with the service provider and model and facilitate service provider learning (Kadushin & Harkness, 2002). As with family-centred practice, relationship is a key concept in supervision. Shulman (2006) stresses the importance of the "supervisor-practitioner working alliance" or "working relationship" (p. 23). Similarly, from a family-centred perspective, supervision emphasizes the development of a strong relationship between the supervisor and the service provider. This relationship is described as interactional and "reciprocal," with both the supervisor and service provider contributing to supervisory outcomes (Shulman, 1993, p. 16). Shulman's parallel process is relevant for supervision in a family-centred context. While common-alities exist between the supervisor–service provider relationship and the service provider–family relationship (the parallel process), the su-pervisory relationship is not a therapeutic relationship, as the intent of supervision is not to provide an analysis of the service provider. When evidence of the parallel process arises, the supervisor strives to assist the service provider in developing awareness of patterns or issues and encourage discussion and learning.

Family-centred practice emphasizes building rapport and develop-ing trust with families. Supervision provides an occasion for the super-visor to model the development of a strong supervisor–service provider working alliance (or working relationship) through communication, re-lationship, and problem-solving skills. The working alliance is defined by rapport, trust, and caring and provides the basis for the supervisor to influence the service provider in an interactional relationship (Shul-man, 1993). Shulman (1993) notes some variables that affect the work-ing relationship such as age, modality of practice, degree of authority, experience, and the service setting (e.g., school psychologist or nurse in a hospital or social worker in a family counselling clinic). However, regardless of the variations, the "core dynamics and skills" of the su-pervision process remain the same, and supervision effectiveness is the product of the supervisor's and service provider's contribution to the process (Shulman, 2006, p. 26).

Shulman's (2006) seven supervision skills necessary for the devel-opment of a working relationship are applicable to supervision in a family-centred context. First, supervisors need to use honesty and ap-propriate self-disclosure in the supervisory relationship. The second skill that supervisors use to promote the working relationship is the ability to articulate the service provider's feelings "a half step ahead" of her/him. The third and fourth supervisory skills focus on the ser-vice provider and require that the supervisor be interested and con-cerned about the service provider's feelings and able to validate those concerns and feelings. Listening, showing concern, and validating the service provider's feelings encourage a discussion of issues that may be otherwise difficult. The fifth skill is the ability of the supervisor to share her/his feelings. This skill requires the supervisor to model the appro-priate sharing of feelings to benefit the service provider's professional development (Shulman, 1993). Congruent with the parallel process, the service provider learns how and when to share feelings with families to benefit the family receiving services and to provide effective services.

The supervisor must also ensure that the service provider's life experiences are validated and that the service provider is recognized as the expert on her/his life. Finally, the supervisor must contract to work with the service provider in a reciprocal relationship, and not "on" the service provider. In this way the work of supervision is shared and the supervision relationship is effective (Shulman, 2006).

While the supervisor must be skilled in core elements of supervision, the supervisor must also be knowledgeable of general practice stages of direct service delivery: intake, assessment, intervention, evaluation, and closure (Falconer & Swift, 1983; Maidman, 1984). Throughout the service provider's involvement with a family, the supervisor should ensure that the five practice stages are addressed and that specific family-centred content and appropriate tools (e.g., genograms, eco-maps) are synchronized with each stage. The supervisor should ensure that in each supervisory session the service provider locates the stage of practice and identifies specific objectives or goals and the tasks necessary to meet the stated and agreed-upon goals and objectives.

During the intake and assessment stage of service provision, the supervisor should ensure that the service provider is conscious of the importance of putting effort into relationship building. Intake and assessment provide the service provider with the opportunity to begin to build a respectful relationship with the family, one based on partnership and recognition of the parents as experts regarding their children's need. In terms of partnership, the supervisor should encourage the service provider to offer examples of stepping outside of the "expert" role and moving away from paternalistic approaches of service provision, in which the service provider determines the needs and solutions, to a strengths-based approach, in which the service provider works in partnership with the family as it moves towards growth and development. This can occur through practical means, such as the provision of an information flyer on a specific disability, and also through an emotional connection, such as listening and responding to a parent's frustration with prior services received. The supervisor needs to ensure that the service provider is able to describe her/his initiatives to actively engage with the family during this stage and listen empathetically when meeting with family members. In addition, service providers should reflect on their initial methods of engaging with the family to begin to identify resources necessary to support family functioning (Dunst et al., 1988).

Chapter 5 provides the reader with a family assessment model that service providers should employ when working with families. Intake and assessment are critical for the collection of family information upon which a service plan is made. Consequently, the supervisor should determine whether the service provider has sufficient and reliable information regarding the family's needs. The referral source, the family, background documents (e.g., agency files), and other allied service providers can all contribute to the family assessment. In addition, the supervisor may encourage the use of measures or tools to assist in family assessment. For example, the Family Needs Survey (Bailey & Simeonsson, 1988) provides a useful measure of psychosocial support needs in families with children with disabilities. The specific assessment and intervention model used should be discussed during supervision.

Hiebert-Murphy, Trute, and Wright (2008) describe four patterns of service entry (i.e., early entry, prompt entry, delayed entry, and atypical entry) that correspond to different service needs. Service needs range from families requiring the provision of information and little service (early entry), to those families requiring reasonable or prompt service (prompt entry and delayed entry), to some families requiring information, prompt access, and clarification about service providers' roles (atypical entry; p. 427). This typology may be helpful for service providers and their supervisors when they assess family needs to better understand the type of need and the immediacy of the needs.

Although ethical practices should be addressed throughout the stages of involvement with a family, intake and assessment provides an ideal opportunity for the supervisor to ensure that the service provider adheres to ethical standards. For example, the supervisor should remind the service provider to request that parents sign consent forms enabling the service provider to speak with allied professionals or support agencies or to access reports related to the family's needs. This stage also offers the service provider an initial opportunity to clearly state the breadth and limitations of her/his role, expectations regarding her/his work with the family, and the agency's mandate including family-centred policies and practices. While this information should be reviewed on several occasions throughout the service relationship, the supervisor can emphasize the importance of the intake and assessment stage of service delivery as setting the stage for an honest, interested, helpful, and empowering relationship. Positive engagement with families during this stage of service provision can set the base for a future trusting relationship, critical for family-centred practice. Service providers must be clear and honest with families about what they can and cannot do.

During a supervision session, the supervisor should confirm with the service provider that s/he has made efforts to meet with all family members during the intake and assessment stage to ensure that their perceptions and understanding of their needs are heard. The supervisor can question whether the service provider focuses on one family member's needs or attends to the needs of all of the family members when working with the family. Thus, the supervisor should ensure that the service provider's reported assessment of the family includes the identification of strengths and challenges facing the family members. Supervisors should request that the service provider includes information regarding the family's formal and informal support networks (Tracy & Pine, 2000) and ask that service providers provide a genogram and eco-map as visual assessment tools to advance the understanding of the family and the range of its service needs (Dunst et al., 1988). Supervisors should also ensure that service providers respond to families in a timely way, again sending a clear message to the family that its concerns or questions are important to the service provider, thus setting a positive pattern for the relationship.

Throughout all stages of the service provider's work with a family (intake, assessment, intervention, evaluation, and transfer/closure), the supervisor should check that the service provider is engaging the core elements of family-centred practice. For example, as discussed in Chapter 4, the working alliance is of particular importance for service providers to develop and maintain with families. Throughout the phases of supervision and the stages of service provision, supervisors should ensure that the supervisee consciously strives to maintain a relationship-based approach to working with the family. This includes working respectfully and collaboratively with families. During the supervision sessions, the supervisor should ask the service provider for examples of her/his efforts to build rapport and work in partnership with parents and children. In addition, service providers should provide examples of efforts made to create a trusting relationship with families. Examples could include honesty in not knowing all the answers or following through on specified tasks (e.g., a referral for other services). Working respectfully and in partnership also requires that the service provider acknowledge the expertise of parents in knowing their children's needs and in decision-making regarding their children.

During supervision, other key elements of family-centred practice must be addressed and supervisors should routinely request that service providers present relevant information and examples of service activities. For example, the service provider should identify whether and how families were empowered to make informed decisions regarding service options. Service providers should also provide examples of the ways in which they help families to access resources to meet their needs. This involves identifying supports available from both formal systems and informal sources and incorporating these resources into the family's plan. In order for service providers to enable and empower families, social systems must provide families with opportunities to display competence (Dunst et al., 1988). Service providers should work in such a way that family members attribute behaviour change to their own actions. Unless this occurs, families will not gain a sense of control or mastery in their lives, which is essential to empowerment (Dunst et al., 1988). In addition, service providers should demonstrate to supervisors that the intervention plan formulated to address assessed child and family needs is realistic. In practical terms, this requires that service providers determine the accessibility and availability of local community services. If the formal or informal resources are insufficient or inaccessible, the intervention plan will likely result in frustration for both the family and the service provider. Service provider frustration or anger with insufficient, poor-quality, and/or limited quantity of collateral services may be a specific topic to be addressed in supervision.

Based on the assessment, the service provider, in partnership with the family, produces a Family-Centred Support Plan (FCSP, see Chapter 9). During this stage of service provision, regular supervision should include a review of the stated goals and tasks identified to meet the goals (with corresponding responsibilities and timelines). Service providers should provide detailed and up-to-date accounts of the family's functioning and needs. In addition, changing or emerging needs should be presented and reviewed. The supervisor should also review the intervention plan with the service provider to ensure that the assessment plan addresses the concerns of all family members. Throughout the service delivery phase, service providers should demonstrate to supervisors their efforts to enable, empower, build on family resilience with, and work in partnership with families. The service provider should be able to identify to the supervisor how s/he promotes positive family functioning (of all members), enhances efforts to meet needs (through the mobilization of resources) based on the family's functioning style, strengthens the family's social network and utilizes support available from the informal network, and uses helping behaviour to promote the family's development of skills and abilities to access resources (Dunst et al., 1988). During a supervision session, the service provider should refer to the family's FCSP, identifying successes and challenges and planned activities or approaches to overcome obstacles. Where modifications to the FCSP are necessary, the service provider should be expected to articulate changes and the reasons for the changes.

The supervisor also has the responsibility to ensure that the service provider articulates a method to evaluate the success of meeting service goals and objectives (i.e., program effectiveness; Kadushin & Harkness, 2002). Within the context of family-centred services, the FCSP is the basis for evaluating the effectiveness of service provision. Thus, supervisors should ask service providers to reflect on the services they provide in partnership with families and discuss whether further service involvement is necessary or the family no longer requires services. Feedback from collateral service providers is also necessary to determine future service needs, and supervisees should consider the perspectives of other service providers when appropriate. Should there be conflicting or ambiguous views, supervisors should work with supervisees to clarify their opinions and positions to determine a process to positively resolve issues.

When a service provider resigns from her/his position and a transfer to another service provider is required, the supervisor must ensure that a transfer summary is provided by the departing service provider that identifies short-term and longer-term goals and tasks and clearly notes issues of immediacy. In addition, an introduction visit between the family and the new service provider should be arranged by the departing service provider. Issues of loss and grieving may be appropriate as supervision topics during transitions and endings.

Each of the core elements of family-centred practice does not need to be reviewed in every supervision session. However, over the service period of involvement with a family, the supervisor should determine whether or not the supervisee employs the core elements of family-centred practice during the provision of services. If the service provider identifies challenges, the supervisor can use this as an opportunity to re-visit family-centred practice elements.

Ethics and Supervision

Ethical standards are subsumed in performance evaluations and include adherence to legislative requirements, professional standards, agency policies, as well as personal moral standards. Family-centred services must adhere to ethical standards, and the supervisory context provides a formal context in which ethical issues should be discussed. Ethical issues often occur when the supervisor is faced with making a decision concerning conflicting positions (Reamer, 2004). For example, supervisors are required to approve service plans, which may include having to decide when needs-assessed services will be terminated due to capped budgetary requirements. At other times, agency policy may be in conflict with a family's needs (for example, a child transitioning from children's to adult services). In addition, supervisors must ensure that service providers and they themselves are adequately knowledgeable and skilled to meet the requirements of their position. Reamer (2004) posits that supervisors must be knowledgeable about multiple areas of ethical concern that fall under two general categories: service user issues and staff and agency issues. Supervisors must ensure that staff and the wider organization are aware of, and promote, service users' rights. This includes having clear policies and procedures related to confidentiality, records, consent, boundaries, access to information, service termination, and a formal complaints process. With regards to staff and agency issues, documentation of work with families and of supervision sessions, management of records, professional development opportunities, the appropriate use of consultation, fraud, and staff performance are all topics with which supervisors should be familiar.

Two ethical and legal responsibilities are of particular concern for the supervisor. The first relates to the oversight responsibility the supervisor holds in relation to the supervisee's work, "respondent superior ... and vicarious liability," in which the supervisor's negligence of duty is believed to add to the supervisee's negligence (Reamer, 2004, p. 100). Poor supervision or no supervision can create a risk of legal liability for supervisors. Accordingly, the supervisor should ensure that the service given is not negligent due to the service provider's acts of omission or acts of commission. As well, the supervisor has a duty to ensure s/he is qualified and competent to effectively supervise and meet the professional, legal, and ethical responsibility for the service provider. This requires knowledge, skills, ongoing professional development, and accessibility to a supervisor's supervisor or professional consultant to confer with regarding difficult issues.

Ethics and evaluation. Supervisors have an ethical and professional responsibility to evaluate supervisees and ensure that they and their supervisees are competent in their work. For example, the Canadian Association of Social Workers' (CASW) Guidelines for Ethical Practice

Standard 3.4.3 requires that "social workers evaluate supervisees' performance in a manner that is fair and respectful and consistent with the expectations of the place of employment" (CASW, 2005, p. 15). Further, according to the CASW Guidelines for Ethical Practice Standard 3.4.1, supervisors have a duty to supervise "only within their areas of knowledge and competence" and only when they "have the necessary knowledge and skill" to enable them to perform their job effectively (CASW, 2005, p. 14). Falender and Shafranske (2007) advise that supervisors consult when in any doubt on an issue of competency. Kadushin and Harkness (2002) advocate for regular supervisor performance evaluations, including feedback from subordinates.

With regards to supervisor evaluation of supervisees, the evaluation is aimed at ensuring the service provider is adhering to her/his organization's job requirements, as well as to professional requirements. Evaluation in this context has three primary goals. First, evaluation meets one administrative goal in that the outcome of the evaluation process is a written report to be used in managerial decision-making. Second, evaluation provides the opportunity for the supervisor to perform the educational function of her/his role and aims to develop the service provider's professional knowledge and skills. Third, the evaluation process aims to improve the organization's performance (Kadushin & Harkness, 2002). Munson (2002) emphasizes the evaluation of supervisee learning and separates administrative or effectiveness of service provision in evaluation, arguing that increased learning produces increased effectiveness.

Performance evaluations are one means of appraising the service provider's functioning (Kadushin & Harkness, 2002). Formal evaluations should occur at least annually (and at a minimum, every 6 months for those service providers on probation). Formal evaluations provide the supervisor and the supervisee with an opportunity to highlight strengths of the work period, identify growth in specific areas, and note specific challenges to be addressed. This provides the supervisee with an explicit, formally documented record of her/his work, which may be used to assist in career planning, as part of the determination regarding eligibility for promotions or pay raises. In addition, the evaluation process can help to encourage service providers to advance their professional education and provide a setting for clarifying new learning goals (Kadushin & Harkness, 2002).

Service provider competence is of utmost importance for families receiving services and for the employing organization. Supervisors have a responsibility to provide regular and systematic evaluation of the supervisee's work in order to develop the service provider's potential, as well as to be accountable to families receiving services and the organization providing the services (Kadushin & Harkness, 2002; Munson, 2002; Shulman, 1993). Kadushin and Harkness note that the most important benefit for the families receiving services is that they are "more likely to be ensured of effective service and protected from continuation of inadequate services" (p. 334). Regular staff evaluations reflect an organization that promotes accountability to the community through service provider accountability to families (Kadushin & Harkness, 2002).

Supervisors benefit from the evaluation process, as it provides the base on which to build educational supervision and can help with meeting supervisors' administrative tasks (Kadushin & Harkness, 2002). The evaluation process and recording ensures that supervisors meet employment standards through administrative competence. In addition, performance evaluations may provide the organization with feedback regarding problematic policies or practices negatively affecting services for families, or highlight subjects for service provider training. In this context, the supervisor acts as the link between front-line service providers and managers to communicate strengths or limitations to agency policies or practices.

While formal evaluation should occur annually (and at least once during a service provider's probationary period), the assessment of service provider performance is not a one shot endeavour; rather, it is a systematic process in which the supervisor engages with the supervisee to set performance goals, identify expectations, and provide administrative, educational, and supportive direction as needed. Accordingly, regular weekly or monthly supervision sessions should be documented with a list of key tasks to be addressed and concurring timelines, with specific methods to be applied. Issues that require immediate attention or are of a serious nature should be clearly noted for prompt follow-up. When supervisees accomplish the tasks as specified, their efforts should be praised, acknowledged, and encouraged (and when possible rewarded, for example through a performance review or merit award) by the supervisor.

In terms of ensuring general adherence to policy (in the broadest sense), supervisors should ensure that staff read and understand mandated (i.e., legislation authorizing) services to families. Their duties and agency responsibilities should be clearly defined and well understood. Any potentially conflicting legislation must be reviewed through legal consultation to clarify policy and service implications. In addition, supervisors must ensure that services are provided within the remit of professionally ethical codes of conduct. As well, on an agency level, services provided and the staff who implement them must support and reflect a family-centred philosophy. One of the supervisor's tasks is to ensure that this occurs, and when it does not, her/his task is to work in partnership with the service provider to determine the necessary tasks to remediate the situation.

In situations where supervisees do not comply with their formal workplace tasks, supervisors must ensure that due process and documentation occur, respecting all legislative requirements regarding employment standards. If specific administrative, educational, or supportive needs are identified, and if the service provider has failed to comply with agreed-upon or required tasks, the supervisor must ensure the issue is clearly documented, with expectations specified. Supervisors must actively engage their supportive function to determine what options are available for supervisees should they be in violation of, or non-compliant with, agency policy. Mistakes are opportunities for learning, and strategies for improvement should be identified (Munson, 2002). Supervisors must follow-up with all aspects of service provision that do not meet standards (whether program specific, organizational, legal, or ethical). Thus, if a service provider has not proven knowledgeable or skilled in an area that is required, the supervisor in partnership with the supervisee should move to remediation and create a plan to ensure that the expected skill or knowledge area is addressed. Some organizations offer an employee assistance program, which may be an option for meeting the service provider's needs. The role of the supervisor is to assist the supervisee to determine a solution to solve the identified problem and find a balance between work demands and self-care. Regardless of the methods chosen to address the issue, expectations must be clearly documented prior to moving to a probationary status. Ultimately, should a service provider fail to comply with the requirements due to unwillingness or inability, a reassignment in position or termination may be the only option (Kadushin & Harkness, 2002).

Challenges for Supervision from a Family-Centred Perspective

Supervisors may face multiple challenges from various sources within the organization when overseeing family-centred service delivery. For example, staff may challenge the supervisor's authority due to concerns regarding the supervisor's approach to supervision. In this instance, it is important for the supervisor to respond to questions or comments raised and to explain honestly their approach to supervision. This allows the supervisor to invite feedback from their supervisees (Shulman, 2006, p. 37). Issues of loss (i.e., when a supervisor leaves) should be addressed as well as expectations and approaches to supervision. In fact, when comments or questions are raised that challenge the supervisor, these circumstances provide opportunities for supervisors to model a relationship-building process. Issues that can potentially become obstacles to productive relationships can become stepping stones to engagement and rapport building.

In addition, boundary crossings and violations are important challenges facing the supervisory relationship. A boundary can be defined as "the edge of appropriate behavior" (Gutheil & Gabbard, 1998, p. 410). Boundaries are important in supervision as they provide a safe context for appropriate behaviour with an attempt to limit inappropriate and potentially harmful conduct. Boundary crossings are defined as "deviation from the usual verbal behavior" that are not considered to be harmful (Gutheil & Gabbard, 1998, p. 410). In contrast, boundary violations reflect a deviation "that is clearly harmful ... or exploitative" (Gutheil & Gabbard, 1998, p. 410). While boundary crossings can lead to improved work through discussion and exploration of the topic, boundary violations are considered to be harmful or exploitative of the service provider. Gutheil and Gabbard (1993, 1998) address boundary issues within the context of the psychotherapeutic relationship; however, their understanding of these challenges in psychotherapy warrants a discussion in the supervisory context. Addressing transference and countertransference issues within the supervisory relationship, as well as for service providers who may be experiencing these issues with a service user family member, are additional challenges that supervisors should address. Helping the service provider examine and reflect on her/his feelings and being aware of the parallel process can result in improved relationships between the service provider and families receiving services and improvements to the working alliance between the supervisor and service provider (Kaiser & Barretta-Herman, 1999).

Working across disciplines and with collateral service providers can be a challenge for family-centred practice. Research has shown that service providers reported working with collateral professionals to be a particularly challenging aspect of delivering family-centred services

(Wright et al., 2010). Some collateral service providers are simply un-aware or unsupportive of a family-centred perspective and choose to work from an "expert position," with limited family involvement in decision-making areas. This can create frustration for service providers adhering to a family-centred practice model who are closely involved with the family.

Service provision and planning occur within a diverse environment reflecting power differentials and positions of privilege (Down, 2000). Supervisors perform a central role in proactively creating a family-centred organization that is respectful of, and sensitive to, issues of di-versity. In particular, in the context of supervision, supervisors have a responsibility to ensure that service providers engage with families and colleagues in a respectful manner, reflecting values and actions that re-fute all kinds of oppression, including (but not limited to) racism, sex-ism, homophobia, ableism, and ageism. Supervision provides a context to examine the effects of oppression on service users, services provid-ers, and supervisors (Down, 2000). Supervisors must be aware of their own privilege and develop sensitivity to minority issues (Pfohl, 2004) through self-reflection of their values and belief systems. They must also demonstrate a commitment to equality, anti-racism, and social jus-tice (McPhatter, 2004).

Chapter 12 emphasizes the importance of working within a cultur-ally respectful and sensitive approach. Supervisors have a critical re-sponsibility to support and model culturally appropriate practice and a culturally effective organization (McPhatter, 2004). Supervisors need to ensure that service providers recognize the diversity of families and that assessment and intervention planning is based on assessed needs of the individual family, not based on a one-size-fits-all approach (Stroul, 1995). As a result, formal service needs that are identified based on the assessed child or family need should be culturally sensitive and appropriate. Effective cross-cultural communication skills are critical for supervisors (McPhatter, 2004). Ultimately, as with all aspects of ef-fective supervision, and congruent with effective family-centred prac-tice, supervisors must model cultural competence when completing tasks or activities.

Correspondingly, in the context of a culturally diverse organization, supervisors must also ensure that policies and processes are in place to support diversity in the workplace and that sexism, homophobia, or other oppressive values, beliefs, or actions are prohibited (McPhat-ter, 2004). Supervisors should demonstrate leadership and ensure that their supervisory practice respects the diversity of professional staff.

For example, Pfohl (2004) provides suggestions for supervisors working with sexual minority staff, such as creating a safe space within the organization and creating allies within the organization. Education and training for all staff (including the supervisor) must be made available when gaps in knowledge and skills are identified. This can result in an organization that institutionalizes formal procedures to address and resolve issues related to diversity, in which the development of competent practice results, thus creating an organization "in which sharing, mutuality, respect, and collective problem identification and resolution are the norm" (McPhatter, 2004, p. 53). Supervisors should guide this endeavour to support staff growth and development.

Supervisors may also find the organization in which they work to be challenging for the delivery of family-centred services. Service providers should be included on agency or organizational committees, on intra- and inter-organizational teams, in professional development, as well as in other activities or initiatives aimed at implementing and sustaining family-centred services. However, if these opportunities are unavailable to service providers either because of being excluded (i.e., not invited to participate) or inaccessible (e.g., unable to participate due to geographic distance or caseload commitments), then the likelihood of the successful implementation of family-centred practice is diminished. Furthermore, service providers require knowledge and skills to facilitate participation on teams and committees. Supervisors should ensure that service providers are knowledgeable of protocols and procedures aimed to enable intra- and inter-organizational activities and should support them in clarifying role and service expectations (Friedman & Poertner, 1995).

Limited resources may negatively impact the service providers' ability to implement family-centred services. Organizations must ensure that realistic workloads for service providers are maintained and reflect basic standards of family-centred service delivery (Friedman & Poertner, 1995; Stroul, 1995). Supervisors, when doing administrative supervision, often determine caseload size and must be able to take into account other workload issues (e.g., the intensity of a specific family's needs, committee work, driving distance to specific families). It is important to note the importance of the organization's support to the supervisor and supervisee within this administrative context.

Conclusion

Effective supervision in a family-centred context requires supervisors to have adequate knowledge and skills in order to enable and empower their staff to provide family-centred services. This chapter presented an overview of essential supervision knowledge and skills required for working with supervisees who deliver family-centred services. While many general supervision skills and domains of supervisor knowledge are transferable to the family-centred context, family-centred services require that supervisors integrate core family-centred elements into their approach, content, and process of supervision.

REFERENCES

Austin, M., & Hopkins, K. (2004). Defining the learning organization. In K. Hopkins & M. Austin (Eds.), *Supervision as collaboration in the human services: Building a learning culture* (pp. 11–18). Thousand Oaks, CA: Sage Publications.

Bailey, D., Jr, & Simeonsson, R. (1988). *Family assessment in early intervention.* Englewood Cliffs, NJ: Macmillan Publishing Company.

Bogo, M., & McKnight, K. (2006). Clinical supervision in social work: A review of the research literature. *Clinical Supervisor, 24*(1-2), 49–67. http://dx.doi.org/10.1300/J001v24n01_04

Canadian Association of Social Workers. (2005). *Guidelines for ethical practice.* Ottawa, ON: Canadian Association of Social Workers.

Down, G. (2000). Supervision in a multicultural context. In G. Gorell Barnes, G. Down, & D. McCann (Eds.), *Systemic supervision: A portable guide for supervision training* (pp. 61–77). London, UK: Jessica Kingsley Publishers.

Dunst, C., Trivette, C., & Deal, A. (1988). *Enabling and empowering families: Principles and guidelines for practice.* Cambridge, MA: Brookline Books.

Falconer, N., & Swift, K. (1983). *Preparing for practice: The fundamentals of child protection.* Toronto, ON: Children's Aid Society of Metropolitan Toronto.

Falender, C.A. (n.d.). *Clinical supervision: A competency-based approach* (PowerPoint slides). Retrieved from http://www.skcp.ca/Dr.%20Falender%20Presentation%20May%2027-28,%202009%20-%20Clinical%20Supervision/Clinical%20Supervision%20-%20Power%20Point%20Presentation.pdf

Falender, C.A., & Shafranske, E.P. (2007). Competence in competency-based supervision practice: Construct and application. *Professional Psychology, Research and Practice, 38*(3), 232–40. http://dx.doi.org/10.1037/0735-7028.38.3.232

Friedman, C.R., & Poertner, J. (1995). Creating and maintaining support and structure for case managers: Issues in case management supervision. In

B.J. Friesen & J. Poertner (Eds.), *From case management to service coordination for children with emotional, behavioral, or mental disorders: Building on family strengths* (pp. 257–74). Baltimore, MD: Paul H. Brookes.

Gutheil, T.G., & Gabbard, G.O. (1993, February). The concept of boundaries in clinical practice: Theoretical and risk-management dimensions. *American Journal of Psychiatry, 150*(2), 188–96. Medline:8422069

Gutheil, T.G., & Gabbard, G.O. (1998, March). Misuses and misunderstandings of boundary theory in clinical and regulatory settings. *American Journal of Psychiatry, 155*(3), 409–14. Medline:9501754

Hiebert-Murphy, D., Trute, B., & Wright, A. (2008). Patterns of entry to community-based services for families with children with developmental disabilities: Implications for social work practice. *Child & Family Social Work, 13*(4), 423–32. http://dx.doi.org/10.1111/j.1365-2206.2008.00572.x

Hiebert-Murphy, D., Trute, B., & Wright, A. (2011). Parents' definition of effective child disability support services: Implications for implementing family-centered practice. *Journal of Family Social Work, 14*(2), 144–58. http://dx.doi.org/10.1080/10522158.2011.552404

Hopkins, K., & Austin, M. (2004). The changing nature of human services and supervision. In K. Hopkins & M. Austin (Eds.), *Supervision as collaboration in the human services: Building a learning culture* (pp. 3–10). Thousand Oaks, CA: Sage Publications.

Kadushin, A., & Harkness, D. (2002). *Supervision in social work* (4th ed.). New York, NY: Columbia University Press.

Kaiser, T., & Barretta-Herman, A. (1999). The supervision institute: A model for supervisory training. *Clinical Supervisor, 18*(1), 33–46. http://dx.doi.org/10.1300/J001v18n01_03

Maidman, F. (Ed.). (1984). *Child welfare: A sourcebook of knowledge and practice.* New York, NY: Child Welfare League of America.

McPhatter, A. (2004). Culturally competent practice. In K. Hopkins & M. Austin (Eds.), *Supervision as collaboration in the human services: Building a learning culture* (pp. 47–58). Thousand Oaks, CA: Sage Publications.

Munson, C.E. (2002). *Handbook of clinical social work supervision* (3rd ed.). New York, NY: The Haworth Press.

Pfohl, A.H. (2004). The intersection of personal and professional identity. *Clinical Supervisor, 23*(1), 139–64. http://dx.doi.org/10.1300/J001v23n01_09

Reamer, F. (2004). Ethical decisions and risk management. In K. Hopkins & M. Austin (Eds.), *Supervision as collaboration in the human services: Building a learning culture* (pp. 97–109). Thousand Oaks, CA: Sage Publications.

Shulman, L. (1993). *Interactional supervision.* Washington, DC: NASW Press.

Shulman, L. (2006). The clinical supervisor-practitioner working alliance: A parallel process. *Clinical Supervisor, 24*(1-2), 23–47. http://dx.doi.org/10.1300/J001v24n01_03

Sloper, P., Greco, V., Beecham, J., & Webb, R. (2006, March). Key worker services for disabled children: What characteristics of services lead to better outcomes for children and families? *Child: Care, Health and Development, 32*(2), 147–57. http://dx.doi.org/10.1111/j.1365-2214.2006.00592.x Medline:16441849

Stroul, B. (1995). Case management in a system of care. In B.J. Friesen & J. Poertner (Eds.), *From case management to service coordination for children with emotional, behavioral, or mental disorders: Building on family strengths* (pp. 3–25). Baltimore, MD: Paul H. Brookes.

Tracy, E.M., & Pine, B.A. (2000, January-February). Child welfare education and training: Future trends and influences. *Child Welfare, 79*(1), 93–113. Medline:10659394

Wright, A., Hiebert-Murphy, D., & Trute, B. (2010). Professionals' perspectives on organizational factors that support or hinder the successful implementation of family-centered practice. *Journal of Family Social Work, 13*(2), 114–30. http://dx.doi.org/10.1080/10522150903503036

14 Managing the Successful Implementation of Family-Centred Practice

ALEXANDRA WRIGHT

Managers in Human Service Organizations: Setting the Context

This chapter focuses on the role of managers in the implementation of family-centred services within organizations. The term "manager" is meant to be inclusive and refers broadly to those responsible for overseeing the planning and implementation of organizational change and innovation and includes staff responsible for administrative tasks such as policy and service planning.

Human service organizations differ from other organizations in that they exist mainly to plan and provide services to people by people (Hasenfeld, 1983). Most human service organizations are bureaucratic in structure (Cohen, 2002), have multiple goals (Gummer, 1990), and face many challenges in the quest to measure service effectiveness (Hasenfeld, 1983). Generally, human service organizations operate in a constantly changing and tumultuous environment (Hasenfeld, 1983; Horwath & Morrison, 2000) that is frequently characterized by high caseloads, low staff morale, and a crisis orientation. They often experience chronic problems with funding (Gummer, 1990; Hopkins & Hyde, 2002). Hospitals and specific units within them such as child development clinics, government support services units, child welfare agencies, and community living organizations are all examples of human service organizations. When considering services for families with children with special needs, these services are usually supportive in nature, providing information, child and family resources, and advocacy when needed.

Because of the complex external and internal contexts of human service organizations, managers must anticipate and respond to change on a regular basis, change that is internal to the organization as well as change that is external to the organization. Innovation is a part of larger organizational change and is a means to improve or maintain service quality, respond to or proactively act on environmental trends or demands, and meet funders' and service users' demands (Damanpour, 1987; Latting et al., 2004; Luongo, 2007). The implementation of family-centred practice represents an innovative approach to service planning and delivery and occurs on multiple levels: technological, administrative, and ancillary (Damanpour, 1987). On a technological level, family-centred service requires service providers and supervisors to shift their use of "tools, techniques or systems" (Damanpour, 1987, p. 677) as they implement family-centred practice in their daily services. In addition, on an administrative level, family-centred service implementation necessitates certain changes to administrative procedures and policies as well as structural elements of the organization. Technological and administrative innovations occur in the organization's internal environment, whereas innovation on an ancillary level relates to the organization's interaction with its external environment. Success in innovation requires support from stakeholders in the organization's external environment (Damanpour, 1987). The implementation of family-centred services is also concerned with process innovation and improving service accessibility, families' satisfaction with service response, and the timeliness of service delivery (Borins, 2000). The task of managing innovation is demanding and complex and requires thoughtful and planned activities that can situate a human services manager in both proactive and reactive planning and delivery situations.

The Family-Centred Organizational Checklist

Given the challenging external environment in which human service organizations are situated, as well as the difficulties faced within human service organizations, management decision-making and activities can benefit from clarity in planning through the knowledge of key issues related to the implementation of family-centred services. A checklist of organizational factors is presented (see Table 14.1) that identifies issues that should be addressed in order to successfully implement and maintain family-centred practice. This list of factors, with corresponding sub-components, can be used to support managers and their teams in the determination of organizational tasks that require attention in planning, implementing, maintaining, and evaluating family-centred

Table 14.1 The Family-Centred Practice Organizational Checklist

Organizational Factors and Sub-Component Items	✓
1) Create a positive organizational culture and climate	☐
• Designate a family-centred practice coordinator and/or team	☐
• Create an accessible and welcoming environment	☐
• Apply a family-centred lens in assessing the work environment	☐
• Support service providers in their delivery of the model	☐
• Support supervisors	☐
• Evaluate	☐
2) Develop and sustain intra-agency policy/practice collaboration, coordination, and integration in policy/practice areas	☐
• Engage and create intra-agency coordinating committees for family-centred services	☐
• Employ inclusive planning with compensation	☐
• Apply a family-centred lens to intra-agency coordination	☐
• Evaluate	☐
3) Develop and sustain inter-agency policy/practice collaboration, coordination, and integration in policy/practice areas	☐
• Engage and create inter-agency coordination committees	☐
• Employ inclusive inter-agency planning with compensation for participants	☐
• Apply a family-centred lens to inter-agency coordination	☐
• Attend to jurisdictional disputes	☐
• Evaluate	☐
4) Ensure system-wide knowledge transfer opportunities	☐
• Provide regular intra-agency training and professional development activities	☐
• Provide regular inter-agency training and professional development activities	☐
• Evaluate	☐

services. The checklist is by no means exhaustive and does not intend to minimize the importance of other organizational or system elements that are not identified or included. Rather, the checklist delineates minimal organizational criteria for the successful implementation of family-centred services while keeping in mind the broader goals of meeting service users' needs and minimizing the number of service user transitions. Thus, when implementing family-centred services, managers can review the proposed checklist, determine who is responsible for specific tasks necessary to achieve the criteria, and begin work on changing, modifying, or creating processes and practices supportive of family-centred practice.

As is evident, the checklist has four principal factors. These factors are based on findings from organizational and family-centred literature that identify elements necessary for successful change, innovation, and family-centred practice implementation. In particular, the checklist builds and expands on two studies of family-centred practice and organizational change: (a) Wright, Hiebert-Murphy, and Trute's (2010) findings that identify four key organizational factors (caseload size and activity, training and supervision, collateral service provision, and a policy lens), and (b) Law et al.'s (2003) discussion of six organizational factors that impact the successful implementation of family-centred practice (the formal adoption of a family-centred approach to service, a specific person or team to lead the development of family-centred services, the provision of family-centred information to families receiving services, family-centred staff training, a shift to family-centred procedures, and a welcoming environment). The factors reflect the multiple levels in which family-centred practice innovation occurs: the technological, the administrative, and the ancillary, or the broader, organizational environment.

In the following section the factors are discussed within three larger categories: the organization's culture and climate; coordinated, collaborative, and integrated service and policy planning and delivery; and knowledge transfer. The following discussion addresses the four checklist factors, identifying challenges and suggesting possible solutions. Examples of the context and processes that may be employed by managers to overcome barriers to the implementation of family-centred practice are also provided.

Build and sustain a constructive organizational culture and climate. The first organizational factor listed on the checklist specifies that managers should build and sustain a constructive organizational culture and climate. To accomplish this goal, managers need to designate a family-centred practice coordinator and/or team, create an accessible and welcoming environment, apply a family-centred lens, support service providers, support supervisors, and evaluate.

The successful implementation of family-centred practice to service planning and provision has been linked to a broad range of organizational factors, particularly the organization's culture and climate. While the terms culture and climate can be ambiguous, confusing, and even indistinct (see, for example, Schneider, 2000), for the purposes of this discussion the terms are defined and used to distinguish separate constructs. Organizational culture can be defined as shared behavioural expectations and norms and organizational assumptions and beliefs about work expectations (Cooke & Szumal, 1993). Simply stated, organizational culture is "the way things are done in an organization" (Glisson, 2007, p. 739). Culture is a property of an organization (Glisson & James, 2002) and influences workers' socialization and the manner in which things are done in the workplace (Verbeke, Volgering, & Hessels, 1998). Examples of culture include managerial approaches, an organization's remuneration system (Schein, 2000), and an organization that promotes family-centred services. In contrast, climate belongs to the individual (Glisson & James, 2002). Organizational climate refers to individual staff's perceptions of how the organizational context impacts on their work and is defined as when staff "in a particular work unit agree on their perceptions of the impact of their work environment" (Glisson & James, 2002, p. 769) or as "attitudes shared by employees about their work environment" (Glisson & Hemmelgarn, 1998, p. 404). Climate "captures the way people perceive their work environment" (Glisson, 2007, p. 739). Examples of climate include staff's perceptions and views on issues such as stress, teamwork, equity, and workload. The impact of the organization's culture and climate on the implementation of innovative practices, and family-centred practice in particular, has been noted in the literature (Friedman & Poertner, 1995; King, Law, King, & Rosenbaum, 1998; Larsson, 2000; Law et al., 2003).

Organizations with a negative or "defensive" culture experience service provider burnout, apathy, and opposition to new approaches, often as a means to survive a stressful workplace (Glisson & Green, 2006, p. 435). Defensive organizational cultures are characterized by micromanagement, high amounts of paper work, and an emphasis on strategies to avoid criticism, penalties, and legal sanctions. In addition, negative organizational climates promote reactivity in service providers, rather than promoting responsiveness to the needs of children and families. On a front-line service delivery level, service providers in defensive organizational environments have been found to be less open to innovative approaches to service (Glisson & James, 1992).

A number of factors have been identified as contributing to a negative organizational context. Caseloads and staff turnover are important organizational factors identified as hindering the implementation of family-centred practice (Busca & Crystal, 1999; Dinnebeil, Hale, & Rule, 1996; Harbin et al., 2004; Stroul & Friedman, 1986), particularly with cases that are complex and require greater intensity. For example, in research examining the successful implementation of family-centred service coordination in children's services, both parents and staff identified caseload size as a major factor that hindered the implementation of the model in service delivery (Hiebert-Murphy, Trute, & Wright, 2011; Wright et al., 2010). Staff found that both the number of cases on each of the service coordinator's load and the intensity of service need of particular families were perceived as having an effect on the degree to which service coordinators were able to implement a family-centred approach (Wright et al., 2010). An insufficiency of the resources necessary to support the principles of family-centred practice (such as the ability to meet a family's need for transportation or the family's ability to access a telephone) has also been identified as negatively impacting the ability to implement the model (Dinnebeil et al., 1996).

A key role for managers who oversee the implementation, maintenance, and evaluation of innovation is to build and sustain positive or "constructive" organizational culture and climates. "Constructive" organizational cultures are those in which organizational norms and expectations promote excellence and effective service, motivate staff, and recognize and support the importance of interpersonal relationships (Glisson & Green, 2006). Constructive cultures result in a decrease in staff turnover, an increase in job satisfaction, and improved service quality. Positive team climates are associated with more positive individual work attitudes (Glisson & James, 2002, p. 788), greater job satisfaction (Glisson, 2007), improved service user functioning (Glisson, 2007), and are more likely to support successful service coordinator activities (Glisson & Hemmelgarn, 1998). Epley et al. (2010) found that an organizational climate that supported "peer collaboration" was necessary for the successful implementation of family-centred practice (p. 29).

The challenge for the manager is to develop a plan for creating an organizational culture that supports the implementation of family-centred practice. To begin, the manager must identify one person, the organization's "leader," as responsible for overseeing the development, implementation, maintenance, and evaluation of family-centred practice (Law et al., 2003). The identification of a person who takes the leadership role and whose job description incorporates responsibility and accountability for the organization's formal adoption of the model is one step to begin the systematic incorporation of family-centred practice throughout the organization. Leadership has certainly been identified as important to the successful implementation of family-centred practice (Epley et al., 2010; Martinson, 1982; Papin & Houck, 2005; Park & Turnbull, 2003). Depending on the size and complexity of the organization, the creation of a family-centred practice team or committee could also benefit the organization, as effective teams can positively influence service provision (Bailey, 1984). Effective teams require leadership, role clarity, flexibility, equality, and no internal conflict (Bailey, 1984).

In addition, the manager should ensure that the organization has an accessible and welcoming environment for service users and staff. As Law et al. (2003) note, the organization's physical space must be welcoming to the service user and should include comfortable furniture and offer services such as a resource centre. The resource centre should provide families with information that enables them to make decisions based on informed choices. This centre should not replace a service provider's role with the family, but supplement the role through the provision of printed information on policies and services (including information such as eligibility requirements and access) as well as access to a telephone and computers. In addition, the resource centre could provide a physical location for informal family meetings. If feasible, the centre could have a staff person (volunteer or paid) to provide support and information regarding resources available to families or on issues such as navigating the service system. Other components of a welcoming environment could include a play area for children and a friendly greeting by staff. The welcoming environment should reflect the organization's formal adoption of family-centred principles and reflect those values (for example, respectful engagement with families).

Establishing a welcoming environment extends beyond the physical space and requires opportunities for service users and staff to have input in decisions regarding service planning, delivery, and evaluation. A planning process that involves service users, family members, and direct service providers (front-line and supervisory staff) can result in the development of stronger organizational policy (Friesen & Briggs, 1995; Wright, 2006). The inclusion of service users and direct service providers in all organizational planning and evaluation enables inclusiveness and communicates to the community that their knowledge and experience are esteemed contributions to the organization's policies and services. At the program level, direct service providers and parent representatives (who are knowledgeable, articulate, and invested in helping other families like their own) with experience providing services and receiving services from the program area should be involved in program planning and evaluation (e.g., of service performance and information provision to families). At the senior administrative level of the organization, direct service providers and parent representatives should be elected/appointed for a specific term to a family-centred practice planning committee which oversees operations, as well as to the organization's board of directors (where applicable), to directly participate in strategic administrative decision-making and program planning. In addition, there must be a policy in place to compensate parents and front-line staff who dedicate significant blocks of their time to program planning and evaluation committees, and who provide parent support (e.g., parent to parent). Formal structures and processes that involve service users and staff at all levels of an organization demonstrate that the organization is welcoming and values their participation. Inclusion and support of parents and staff on planning and policy initiatives also supports the family-centred practice emphasis on enabling and empowering both families and staff by involving them in important decision-making and participatory activities. These experiences may also provide parents and staff with opportunities aimed at developing their own sense of mastery and control (Dunst, Trivette, & Deal, 1988). Inclusiveness in policy and planning are reflective of a welcoming and respectful environment that values service user and staff input.

In order to successfully implement family-centred practice, a critical focus for managers is to provide support to service providers and supervisors that enables them to deliver services that are consistent with the principles of family-centred practice. The front-line provision of services must be supported by the organization as well as the service system in order to be effective. On an intra-organizational level, managers must ensure that the service provider has the ability to provide family-centred services, which includes the knowledge and skills necessary for family-centred practice as well as the workload resources to support the development of a strong service provider–family working alliance and the capacity to work on an inter-organizational level and across disciplines. Organizational support for planned, regular supervision and professional development opportunities must also exist. On a service system level, this requires a concerted effort to develop joint or multi-organizational policies and protocols as well as training initiatives. For service providers and supervisors, this requires realistic workloads and caseloads and extra compensation for service providers when extraordinary committee work is required. For example, if a service provider is involved on a committee created to support the implementation and maintenance of family-centred services, her/his caseload should not increase while s/he is participating. Case coverage should be ensured for all staff who participate on committees or inter-agency/disciplinary teams. Other organizational factors necessary to support the effectiveness of the service provider's role include the use of supervision, an orientation for new employees to the organization, and ongoing professional development (Wright et al., 2010). Service providers will simply be unable to implement family-centred policies and practices if they lack the basic resources required to respond to family need and to manage their workload (Hiebert-Murphy et al., 2011).

In the context of practice supervision, the manager should ensure that a supervisor has the capacity to supervise service providers on a regular, planned basis. This requires support for ongoing professional development, space, and technology to assist in supervision as well as support from administrative staff to address related tasks. While the support of service providers and supervisors necessitates a commitment from the manager and the larger organization, support is also clearly required from program funders to ensure that the organization is capable of formally adopting family-centred practice. The organization's leadership should also develop a strategy to encourage support from community, provincial, and national political leadership to embrace a family-centred practice model.

One key value of family-centred practice is that services are "culturally competent" (Stroul, 1995, p. 5). An important responsibility of managers in creating an organizational culture and climate that supports family-centred services is to ensure that the organization's policies and processes are respectful of diversity, for both staff and service users. Managers must demonstrate leadership to staff, families, and the broader community, ensuring that workplace policies and protocols are created and implemented to support diversity in the workplace. The organization's culture, consistent with a family-centred philosophy, should foster a respectful work environment in which all forms of prejudice and oppressive values, beliefs, and actions are disallowed. Managers must strategize to ensure training opportunities that promote professional growth and development and that address workforce gaps in knowledge and/or skills exist for all staff. In addition, protocols and processes should be established to enable positive resolution of challenges, should they arise.

On an intra-organizational level, managers must address problematic interpersonal characteristics that hinder family-centred practice. Interpersonal characteristics that can challenge a family-centred perspective include working from an expert position, not working from a team perspective, challenging the value of family-centred services, or minimizing the benefits of professional development. Certain qualities make staff more likely to adapt to the changes in practice required in a shift to family-centred practice; for example, Busca and Crystal (1999) found that staff who were identified as more family-centred were described as "dedicated," "compassionate," and "respectful" (p. 26). Furthermore, staff must be open to changing traditional elements of practice in order to provide services in a way that is consistent with family-centred practice principles (Bailey, McWilliam, Winton, & Simeonsson, 1992). Without the commitment of staff to the shift in service delivery, the implementation of family-centred practice is likely to be fragmented and inconsistent. Interpersonal characteristics that support family-centred approaches should be prioritized in recruitment policies and practices as well as encouraged in retention policies and practices to ensure that the organization's staff embrace a family-centred approach (Friedman & Poertner, 1995). The agency should ensure the availability of initial and ongoing training and professional development opportunities that address aspects of family-centred services and, further, incorporate elements of family-centred practice in performance evaluations. As well, inter-organizational protocols and processes should be created to support professionals' engagement and to sustain relationships between service organizations (Friedman & Poertner, 1995). Accordingly, managers should identify specific processes and protocols that hinder or limit a service provider's ability to provide family-centred practice. Interdisciplinary (whether within the organization or outside it) and inter-organizational initiatives for joint training opportunities should be developed. Ultimately, managers and family-centred practice teams should strive for staff and program stability so that service users receive uninterrupted, continuous service with minimal disruption at the intra- and inter-agency level (Friesen & Briggs, 1995).

Support of intra-agency and inter-agency collaboration, coordination, and integration in policy and practice. The second and third organizational factors listed on the checklist address issues related to intra-agency and inter-agency collaboration, coordination, and integration in service delivery policy and practice. This requires managers to (a) engage and create committees, (b) employ inclusive planning with compensation, (c) apply a family-centred lens, (d) attend to jurisdictional disputes (for intra-agency activities), and (e) evaluate.

Duplication, fragmentation, and gaps in services and policies are noted challenges to the successful implementation of family-centred practice. For the purposes of this discussion, service coordination, collaboration, and integration are defined as a varying intensity of service delivery on a service continuum (Konrad, 1996). In addition, service coordination, collaboration, and integration can occur on three service delivery levels: direct practice, organizational, and system wide (Scott, 2005; Stroul, 1995). Noted blocks to service coordination include the lack of co-located services, multiple points for intake and assessment, poor or no funding, inflexible and uncoordinated approaches to program funding, limited governmental policy, little provincial support, a lack of a centralized information system, and no administrative support for collaborative activities (Park & Turnbull, 2003).

Administrative factors that negatively affect service coordination include poorly defined responsibilities, the lack of involvement of staff who have the authority to make decisions, a lack of ground rules for collaboration, and a lack of a communication system (Martinson, 1982). In addition, other organizational challenges to service coordination, collaboration, and integration include the absence of inter-organizational protocols and procedures to create mechanisms to support these efforts (Park & Turnbull, 2003). Some studies have found the lack of service flexibility in specific programming problematic to the implementation of family-centred services in terms of limited access to, and limited frequency of, specialist services (Hiebert-Murphy et al., 2011). Hiebert-Murphy et al. (2011) identified an insufficient quantity of services as a limitation to the implementation of family-centred practice. A lack of flexibility in service programming includes the inability to adapt the service intervention to meet a child's or family's changing needs over the time. Moreover, research findings report that parents perceived organizations to be less family-centred when services were delivered at multiple sites, emphasizing the need for coordination between services (Law et al., 2003).

On a policy level, an organizational culture that produces inadequate, poorly defined, or conflicting policy has been identified as negatively associated with the implementation of family-centred practice (Berman, 1991; Hostler, 1991; Wright et al., 2010). Poorly defined or inadequate policy has been shown to result in variability in eligibility, access, assessment, and service provision with limited or no coordination of services (Harbin et al., 2004; Wright et al., 2010). Examples of problematic service experiences due to poor policy include inconsistency in service accessibility and length of provision due to unclear or no eligibility requirements, service variations due to jurisdictional disputes (e.g., based on the area in which a family resides or the child's legal status or age), or a policy that eliminates people from receiving services due to a specific diagnosis.

On a direct practice level, personal characteristics found to impede service coordination include insufficient knowledge and skills when working with families (Park & Turnbull, 2003), negative attitudes to inter-agency collaboration, resistance to change, mistrust of other professionals, and a lack of commitment (Martinson, 1982). These are potential obstacles that managers must address within their organization and external to their organization in order to successfully implement family-centred practice.

Family-centred organizations provide flexible, accessible, comprehensive services based on assessed needs (Dunst, Trivette, & Deal, 1994; Shelton & Stepanek, 1995; Stroul, 1995). Collaborative, coordinated, and integrated service provision is considered a means to limit service duplication and fragmentation, respond to service gaps, and ensure accountability to service users and funders (Early & Poertner, 1995; Friesen & Briggs, 1995; Harbin & McNulty, 1990; Jaskyte & Lee, 2006; Kagan, Goffin, Golub, & Pritchard, 1995; Park & Turnbull, 2003; Sloper, 2004). In addition, collaborative, coordinated, and integrated services are considered to result in accessible, seamless, and needs-based services and policies (Friesen & Briggs, 1995; King & Meyer, 2006; Stroul, 1995) and reduced costs (King & Meyer, 2006). Benefits to service coordination also include increased clarity for staff and families regarding the differentiation of service provider roles and responsibilities (Harbin et al., 2004; Hiebert-Murphy, Trute, & Wright, 2008; Sloper, 1999).

One strategy to overcome barriers to service collaboration and coordination involves developing intra- and inter-organizational teams or committees who are tasked with responding to policy and service problems related to family-centred practice planning, implementation, and evaluation (Stroul, 1995). Inter-professional teams play a crucial role in successful service integration (Bailey et al., 1992; Early & Poertner, 1995; King & Meyer, 2006; Stroul, 1995) because of their ability to "transgress" boundaries and work with the system as a whole (Larsson, 2000). Benefits from service integration also include greater family-centredness of services, increased customer satisfaction, a shared inter-professional view and team approach (Larsson, 2000), and the provision of a common inter-professional language, policy, and practice (Wright et al., 2010).

The use of inter-agency agreements, pooled resources for funding flexibility, and joint programming are examples of ways to overcome structural impediments to integration (Jacobs, 1995). Managers should try to develop and support innovative inter/intra-organizational structures that allow for the creation of multidisciplinary teams. Thus, managers involved with the creation, coordination, implementation, and evaluation of family-centred practice should ensure that the organization permits team formation to span disciplinary boundaries in order to better serve families. A key focus for teams is to ensure a smooth transition for service users who interact with many service providers (Friesen & Briggs, 1995).

Another way that managers can address fragmentation, duplication, and/or gaps in services is to apply a family-centred lens to all organizational policies, protocols, and practices (including proposals for change). Family-centred practice principles should be evident in the organization's mission and vision statements and goals and objectives, as well as in service related policies and procedures manuals and human resources policies and procedures manuals. Job descriptions and recruitment and retention policies should also be written from a family-centred viewpoint to ensure that family-centred practice principles permeate all organizational dimensions. A family-centred practice lens should also be used to direct inter-agency procedures (such as joint protocols). While intra-organizational policy identifies shared goals, procedures, and practice expectations, joint, inter-organizational policy requires an overall and consistent service strategy to frame all care to children from a family-centred lens. Consistent and complementary family-centred services across the service delivery system stem from joint inter-organizational policy and protocols. Managers and family-centred practice teams can develop or rewrite inter-organizational policies and procedures to comply with family-centred practice principles. They may also need to strategize about ways to address jurisdictional conflicts that obstruct the implementation of family-centred practice. Managers can work at modifying current policies and procedures or creating new processes to address the issue of seamless service delivery in which the assessed needs of the child and family are responded to by the service system and are coordinated to meet child and family needs over time.

Knowledge transfer opportunities. The fourth factor listed in the organizational checklist addresses the topic of knowledge transfer activities such as orientation, supervision, training, and ongoing professional development. Training and supervisory support have been identified as factors that contribute to the successful implementation of change and innovation in human service organizations (Austin, Weisner, Schrandt, Glezos-Bell, & Murtaza, 2006; Baldwin & Ford, 1988; Gummer, 1990; Luongo, 2007). The transition to a family-centred organization is a highly complex process that requires extensive training opportunities for staff (including service providers, supervisors, managers, and service users) and a sophisticated political process to engage the organization(s) in a major shift in service culture.

The role of supervision in the knowledge transfer process is fundamental (Austin et al., 2006; Hopkins & Austin, 2004). Several studies have found a relationship between improved family outcomes and planned and ongoing supervision. For example, Sloper, Greco, Beecham, and Webb (2006) reported that planned and ongoing supervision for key workers was associated with positive outcomes for families. As well, service providers have linked supervision and successful family-centred implementation. For example, Wright et al. (2010) found that professionals perceived supervisors and ongoing supervision to positively impact their ability to implement family-centred services. Hiebert-Murphy et al.'s (2011) findings recommend that service coordinators be provided with both generic and family-centred practice skills training when providing family-centred services to families. The supervision relationship provides a unique context in which knowledge and skills for family-centred practice can be developed and nurtured.

The importance of training as a means to positively influence the organization's culture and climate cannot be overstated. Ongoing training is required to develop an organizational culture that promotes best practice (Luongo, 2007). Training, more broadly defined as the transfer of knowledge or transfer of learning, is a complex process. Knowledge transfer is not a short-term process in which information is disseminated. As Baldwin and Ford (1988) explain, the transfer of learning comprises the degree that an employee applies learned attitudes, knowledge, and skills to their work for a sustained period. Transfer of learning requires organizational support and employee motivation. Managers of human service organizations who are responsible for the implementation of family-centred practice have an important role to play in ensuring that organizational opportunities for learning exist and that these opportunities enhance employee motivation. Given the context of a human service organization, the transfer of new knowledge (e.g., when implementing family-centred practice) can be difficult partly due to the very nature of an organization's culture and climate that often negatively impact attempts to implement and sustain change (Luongo, 2007). Family-centred training should focus on issues related to the roles of the service provider and supervisor as well as on organizational policies and protocols aimed at implementing family-centred services.

Research has shown that the incorporation of family-centred training is necessary for the successful implementation of family-centred services (Busca & Crystal, 1999; Early & Poertner, 1995; Friedman & Poertner, 1995; Hiebert-Murphy et al., 2011; Law et al., 2003; Park & Turnbull, 2003; Wright et al., 2010). Wright et al. (2010) found that professionals believed family-centred training was necessary to successfully implement family-centred practice and that training should include an initial orientation as well as ongoing professional development. This finding is consistent with other studies that stress the importance of training in the implementation of family-centred services. For example, one study found that professionals' suggestions to improve the family-centredness of a program for people with special needs included training for parents, increased resources, increased group activities, ongoing professional development and training, and team building (Busca & Crystal, 1999). Training in family-centred practice has also been associated with an increase in service providers' perceptions of their ability to provide family-centred services, and an increased understanding of service providers' beliefs in the benefits of family-centred services (King et al., 2003). Among several recommendations, Sloper et al. (2006) advocate for "regular training, supervision and peer support" for workers, suggesting that these characteristics are associated with better outcomes for families (p. 147).

As a significant focus of family-centred practice is the relationship or working alliance that develops between the service provider and the family, family-centred training must focus on service provider development of relational and participatory skills (Dunst et al., 1988; Hiebert-Murphy et al., 2011). Training must include the development and maintenance of skills necessary for service providers to engage and build rapport with families. As well, service providers require training in skills and knowledge necessary to increase their abilities for capacity building and empowerment.

Inter-professional training with collateral service providers in family-centred practice is necessary for successful implementation (Park

& Turnbull, 2003; Sloper, 2004; Wright et al., 2010). Wright et al. (2010) recommend joint training in family-centred principles to ensure intra- and inter-organizational consistency in knowledge and practice. Sloper (2004) noted that "multi-agency training" should include a focus on the processes necessary to create coordinated multi-agency services (p. 578). Park and Turnbull (2003) advocate for professional training and education that includes topics such as engagement with families and professionals, problem-solving and communication capacities, funding, and knowledge of child development.

Managers may need to be creative in the ways in which they develop opportunities for the enhancement of knowledge and skills for family-centred practice. Knowledge transfer activities can include a variety of formats, including one-on-one supervision, group supervision, peer support, seminars (e.g., examining a specific family-centred practice topic), workshops (e.g., with an "expert" family-centred practitioner), conferences, and solution facilitation circles, in which participants are faced with a specific family-centred practice implementation challenge and, through a series of facilitated steps, come to a solution. The key is that managers ensure that knowledge transfer opportunities exist in a form that best fits with the organization and the employees' needs.

To be effective, managers should incorporate knowledge transfer as a core organizational element, accessible by all staff. Organizations should ensure that knowledge transfer opportunities are available and that staff are provided with the support needed to participate. Organizational policy should ensure that the ability and/or willingness to practice from a family-centred perspective is considered in recruitment and that staff job descriptions articulate the expectation that practice conform to family-centred principles. Employment should also formally incorporate a commitment from staff to family-centred practice, and staff members should commit to an initial professional orientation session and ongoing professional development in family-centred practice. Staff should be provided with workload coverage when they participate in knowledge transfer activities. The commitment to family-centred practice and the engagement with family-centred practice knowledge transfer opportunities should be incorporated as part of the staff's annual performance evaluation. While organizations can provide many opportunities for knowledge transfer activities, unless staff embrace and integrate the organization's family-centred practice tenets within their work, the successful implementation of family-centred practice will prove difficult.

Moreover, managers should develop sustained intra- and inter-organizational training to address obstacles or successes related to integrated services. Based on the identification of these elements, inter-organizational protocols should be created to formalize support for family-centred initiatives and services. Managers should reach out to collateral service providers in the service delivery system and look for opportunities to provide joint family-centred practice training. This training should include the basics of family-centred practice such as the definition, the language of family-centred practice, key family-centred practice elements when working with service users, and specific family-centred practice skills. In addition, family-centred practice knowledge transfer opportunities should include an examination of processes available to provide coordinated and integrated services. This focus could include a shared understanding of joint protocols, funding opportunities, and team members' roles when participating on committees or service teams. In addition, intra/inter-agency committees should ensure that the committee rules and procedures are clearly written and shared to enable the respectful participation of all members. Staff training should include managers in order for family-centred practice to be successfully implemented. By ensuring that managers participate in training, managers are demonstrating their commitment to family-centred services and endorsing a professional commitment to ongoing learning (Bailey et al., 1992).

Evaluation. An important element of the manager's role is to determine, on some basis, the effectiveness of family-centred services. The systematic and planned evaluation of family-centred initiatives and activities should be incorporated as a regular organizational task (Dunst et al., 1988). Thus, the evaluation task is included in each section of the checklist. Evaluations provide multiple benefits, including an increased knowledge base, guidance for decision-making, the ability to demonstrate accountability, and a means to ensure that service users are receiving the services they require (Gabor & Grinnell, 1994). Ultimately, evaluation is a means to demonstrate accountability to service users, staff, and funders, as well as the larger community of stakeholders. There are two general types of evaluations: summative or formative. Summative evaluations focus on program outcomes whereas formative evaluations examine process issues (Kettner, Moroney, & Martin, 1990). When considering the implementation of family-centred services, there are multiple areas of inquiry to determine implementation success. For example, an evaluation could focus on the service provider's role in effecting a positive family experience of service provision or improved family functioning. Other evaluations could examine the impact of a policy on the service recipient. Staff perceptions of a specific program or policy may also be the focus of an evaluation. Benefits of policy clarity include the definition of process and outcome indicators necessary for evaluation (Murphy, Lee, Turnbull, & Turbiville, 1995). Quality improvement and learning organizations are terms used to describe organizations that monitor and seek to improve service planning and delivery through regular evaluation and integrated organizational learning and improvement (Gabor & Grinnell, 1994; Hopkins & Austin, 2004). The process of planning and implementing an evaluation should be inclusive and on a minimal level should include staff's and families' perceptions of policies and services (Park & Turnbull, 2003). Essentially, all aspects of service provision should be evaluated with the goal of improving the service experience and outcome for families, staff, and the broader community.

Conclusion

Managers play an important role in the successful implementation of family-centred services. They provide leadership, motivation, and support when planning for and implementing innovative approaches to services such as family-centred practice. Given the challenging external and internal environments that characterize many human services organizations, managers must proactively strategize and plan for change and actively learn from challenges when they occur. This chapter provides an organizational checklist that delineates specific factors and tasks necessary to implement and sustain family-centred services on the administrative, technical, and ancillary levels. Challenges to implementing family-centred practice exist in the organization's internal context (policy, procedures, staff, and organizational support), on the policy and service delivery level (e.g., protocols with other organizations), and within the broader external community context (funders, policymakers, politicians). Consequently, solutions to the identified challenges must occur in these settings as well. The manager's role (and the organization's role as a whole) is to ensure that the organization provides a high standard of service and creates a positive experience for families receiving services. This includes ensuring that service providers are enabled by the organization, through excellence in management, to provide services employing a family-centred approach. With regards to the organizational sphere, issues include ensuring access to effective supervision and training and incorporating policy and procedures that reflect a family-centred lens. In order for innovation to be successful, managers must lead the organization in the development and maintenance of a constructive organizational culture and climate. On the broader system level, the manager must be aware of, and foster, intra/inter-agency collaboration, coordination, and when appropriate, integration. All of these elements are interconnected and necessary for the successful implementation of family-centred practice. The proffered checklist provides simple tasks to assist the manager in planning and monitoring the organization's progress in the implementation and maintenance of family-centred practice. Fundamentally, family-centred practice should not simply pervade service delivery units but, in addition, should be reflected throughout the organization's planning, administrative, and decision-making structures and policies. The checklist in no way is attempting to minimize the complexity of the tasks necessary for the successful implementation of family-centred practice. However, the chapter provides realistic options available to organizations that are committed to the implementation of family-centred services.

REFERENCES

Austin, M.J., Weisner, S., Schrandt, E., Glezos-Bell, S., & Murtaza, N. (2006). Exploring the transfer of learning from an executive development program for human services managers. *Administration in Social Work, 30*(2), 71–90. http://dx.doi.org/10.1300/J147v30n02_06

Bailey, D., Jr, McWilliam, P.J., Winton, P.J., & Simeonsson, R.J. (1992). *Implementing family-centered services in early intervention: A team-based model for change*. Cambridge, MA: Brookline Books.

Bailey, D.B., Jr, (1984, September). A triaxial model of the interdisciplinary team and group process. *Exceptional Children, 51*(1), 17–25. Medline:6236982

Baldwin, T.T., & Ford, J.K. (1988). Transfer of training: A review and directions for future research. *Personnel Psychology, 41*(1), 63–105. http://dx.doi.org/10.1111/j.1744-6570.1988.tb00632.x

Berman, H. (1991, July-September). Nurses' beliefs about family involvement in a children's hospital. *Issues in Comprehensive Pediatric Nursing, 14*(3), 141–53. http://dx.doi.org/10.3109/01460869109014494 Medline:1841071

Borins, S. (2000). Loose cannons and rule breakers, or enterprising leaders? Some evidence about innovative public managers. *Public Administration Review, 60*(6), 498–507. http://dx.doi.org/10.1111/0033-3352.00113

Busca, S., & Crystal, N. (1999). *Family-centered services in the Winnipeg Children's Program at the Society for Manitobans with Disabilities: An evaluation.* Winnipeg, MB: Author.

Cohen, B.J. (2002). Alternative organizing principles for the design of service delivery systems. *Administration in Social Work, 26*(2), 17–38. http://dx.doi.org/10.1300/J147v26n02_02

Cooke, R., & Szumal, J. (1993). Measuring normative beliefs and shared behavioural expectations in organizations: The reliability and validity of the organizational culture inventory. *Psychological Reports, 72*(3c), 1299–1330. http://dx.doi.org/10.2466/pr0.1993.72.3c.1299

Damanpour, F. (1987). The adoption of technological, administrative, and ancillary innovations: Impact of organizational factors. *Journal of Management, 13*(4), 675–88. http://dx.doi.org/10.1177/014920638701300408

Dinnebeil, L., Hale, L., & Rule, S. (1996). A qualitative analysis of parents' and service coordinators' descriptions of variables that influence collaborative relationships. *Topics in Early Childhood Special Education, 16*(3), 322–47. http://dx.doi.org/10.1177/027112149601600305

Dunst, C., Trivette, C., & Deal, A. (Eds.). (1988). *Enabling and empowering families: Principles and guidelines for practice.* Cambridge, MA: Brookline Books.

Dunst, C., Trivette, C., & Deal, A. (1994). Resource-based family-centered intervention practices. In C. Dunst, C. Trivette, & A. Deal (Eds.), *Methods, strategies and practices* (Vol. 1, pp. 140–51). Cambridge, MA: Brookline Books.

Early, T.J., & Poertner, J. (1995). Examining current approaches to case management for families with children who have serious emotional disorders. In B.J. Friesen & J. Poertner (Eds.), *From case management to service coordination for children with emotional, behavioral, or mental disorders: Building on family strengths* (pp. 37–59). Baltimore, MD: Paul H. Brookes.

Epley, P., Gotto, G., IV, Summers, J., Brotherson, M., Turnbull, A., & Friend, A. (2010). Supporting families of young children with disabilities: Examining the role of administrative structures. *Topics in Early Childhood Special Education, 30*(1), 20–31. http://dx.doi.org/10.1177/0271121410363400

Friedman, C.R., & Poertner, J. (1995). Creating and maintaining support and structure for case managers: Issues in case management supervision. In B.J. Friesen & J. Poertner (Eds.), *From case management to service coordination for children with emotional, behavioral, or mental disorders: Building on family strengths* (pp. 257–74). Baltimore, MD: Paul H. Brookes.

Friesen, B.J., & Briggs, H.E. (1995). The organization and structure of service coordination mechanisms. In B.J. Friesen & J. Poertner (Eds.), *From case management to service coordination for children with emotional, behavioral, or mental disorders: Building on family strengths* (pp. 63–94). Baltimore, MD: Paul H. Brookes.

Gabor, P., & Grinnell, R. (1994). *Evaluation and quality improvement in the human services.* Needham Heights, MA: Allyn and Bacon.

Glisson, C. (2007). Assessing and changing organizational culture and climate for effective services. *Research on Social Work Practice, 17*(6), 736–47. http://dx.doi.org/10.1177/1049731507301659

Glisson, C., & Green, P. (2006). The effects of organizational culture and climate on the access to mental health care in child welfare and juvenile justice system. *Administration and Policy in Mental Health and Mental Health Services Research, 33*(4), 433–48. http://dx.doi.org/10.1007/s10488-005-0016-0

Glisson, C., & Hemmelgarn, A. (1998, May). The effects of organizational climate and interorganizational coordination on the quality and outcomes of children's service systems. *Child Abuse & Neglect, 22*(5), 401–21. http://dx.doi.org/10.1016/S0145-2134(98)00005-2 Medline:9631252

Glisson, C., & James, L. (1992). The interorganizational coordination of services to children in state custody. In D. Bargal & H. Schmid (Eds.), *Organizational change and development in human service organizations* (pp. 65–80). New York, NY: Haworth Press. http://dx.doi.org/10.1300/J147v16n03_05

Glisson, C., & James, L.R. (2002). The cross-level effects of culture and climate in human service teams. *Journal of Organizational Behavior, 23*(6), 767–94. http://dx.doi.org/10.1002/job.162

Gummer, B. (1990). *The politics of social administration.* Englewood Cliffs, NJ: Prentice Hall.

Harbin, G., Bruder, M.B., Adams, C., Mazzarella, C., Whitbread, K., Gabbard, G., & Staff, I. (2004). Early intervention service coordination policies: National policy infrastructure. *Topics in Early Childhood Special Education, 24*(2), 89–97. http://dx.doi.org/10.1177/02711214040240020401

Harbin, G.L., & McNulty, B.A. (1990). Policy implementation: Prescriptives on service coordination and interagency cooperation. In S.J. Meisels & J.P. Shonkoff (Eds.), *Handbook of early childhood intervention* (pp. 700–21). Cambridge, England: Cambridge University Press.

Hasenfeld, Y. (1983). *Human service organizations.* Englewood Cliffs, NJ: Prentice-Hall.

Hiebert-Murphy, D., Trute, B., & Wright, A. (2008). Patterns of entry to community-based services for families with children with developmental disabilities: Implications for social work practice. *Child & Family Social Work, 13*(4), 423–32. http://dx.doi.org/10.1111/j.1365-2206.2008.00572.x

Hiebert-Murphy, D., Trute, B., & Wright, A. (2011). Parents' definition of effective child disability support services: Implications for implementing family-centered practice. *Journal of Family Social Work, 14*(2), 144–58. http://dx.doi.org/10.1080/10522158.2011.552404

Hopkins, K., & Austin, M. (Eds.). (2004). *Building a learning culture.* Thousand Oaks, CA: Sage Publications.

Hopkins, K.M., & Hyde, C. (2002). The human service managerial dilemma: New expectations, chronic challenges and old solutions. *Administration in Social Work, 26*(3), 1–15. http://dx.doi.org/10.1300/J147v26n03_01

Hostler, S.L. (1991, December). Family-centered care. *Pediatric Clinics of North America, 38*(6), 1545–60. Medline:1945556

Horwath, J., & Morrison, T. (2000). Identifying and implementing pathways for organizational change – using the *Framework for the Assessment of Children in Need and their Families* as a case example. *Child & Family Social Work, 5*(3), 245–54. http://dx.doi.org/10.1046/j.1365-2206.2000.00171.x

Jacobs, D. (1995). States' policy response to the need for case management. In B.J. Friesen & J. Poertner (Eds.), *From case management to service coordination for children with emotional, behavioral, or mental disorders: Building on family strengths* (pp. 373–85). Baltimore, MD: Paul H. Brookes.

Jaskyte, K., & Lee, M. (2006). Interorganizational relationships: A source of innovation in nonprofit organizations? *Administration in Social Work, 30*(3), 43–54. http://dx.doi.org/10.1300/J147v30n03_04

Kagan, S., Goffin, S., Golub, S., & Pritchard, E. (1995). *Toward systemic service integration for young children and their families.* Falls Church, VA: National Center for Service Integration.

Kettner, P., Moroney, R., & Martin, L. (1990). *Designing and managing programs. An effectiveness-based approach.* Newbury Park, CA: Sage Publications.

King, G., Kertoy, M., King, S., Law, M., Rosenbaum, P., & Hurley, P. (2003). A measure of parents' and service providers' beliefs about participation in family-centered services. *Children's Health Care, 32*(3), 191–214. http://dx.doi.org/10.1207/S15326888CHC3203_2

King, G., Law, M., King, S., & Rosenbaum, P. (1998). Parents' and service providers' perceptions of the family-centredness of children's rehabilitation services. In M. Law (Ed.), *Family-centred assessment and intervention in pediatric rehabilitation* (pp. 21–40). New York, NY: Haworth Press.

King, G., & Meyer, K. (2006, July). Service integration and co-ordination: A framework of approaches for the delivery of co-ordinated care to children with disabilities and their families. *Child: Care, Health and Development, 32*(4), 477–92. http://dx.doi.org/10.1111/j.1365-2214.2006.00610.x Medline:16784503

Konrad, E.L. (1996). A multidimensional framework for conceptualizing human services integration initiatives. *New Directions for Evaluation, 69*(69), 5–19. http://dx.doi.org/10.1002/ev.1024

Larsson, M. (2000, November). Organising habilitation services: Team structures and family participation. *Child: Care, Health and Development, 26*(6), 501–14. http://dx.doi.org/10.1046/j.1365-2214.2000.00169.x Medline:11091265

Latting, J.K., Beck, M.H., Slack, K.J., Tetrick, L.E., Jones, A.P., Etchegaray, J.M., & Da Silva, N. (2004). Promoting service quality and client adherence to the service plan: The role of top management's support for innovation and learning. *Administration in Social Work, 28*(2), 29–48. http://dx.doi.org/10.1300/J147v28n02_03

Law, M., Hanna, S., King, G., Hurley, P., King, S., Kertoy, M., & Rosenbaum, P. (2003, September). Factors affecting family-centred service delivery for children with disabilities. *Child: Care, Health and Development, 29*(5), 357–66. http://dx.doi.org/10.1046/j.1365-2214.2003.00351.x Medline:12904243

Luongo, G. (2007). Re-thinking child welfare training models to achieve evidence-based practices. *Administration in Social Work, 31*(2), 87–96. http://dx.doi.org/10.1300/J147v31n02_06

Martinson, M.C. (1982, February). Interagency services: A new era for an old idea. *Exceptional Children, 48*(5), 389–94. Medline:6460632

Murphy, D.L., Lee, I., Turnbull, L., & Turbiville, V. (1995). The family-centered program rating scale: An instrument for program evaluation and change. *Journal of Early Intervention, 19*(1), 24–42. http://dx.doi.org/10.1177/105381519501900104

Papin, T., & Houck, T. (2005, March-April). All it takes is leadership. *Child Welfare, 84*(2), 299–310. Medline:15828414

Park, J., & Turnbull, A. (2003). Service integration in early intervention: Determining interpersonal and structural factors for its success. *Infants and Young Children, 16*(1), 48–58. http://dx.doi.org/10.1097/00001163-200301000-00006

Schein, E. (2000). Sense and nonsense about culture and climate. In N. Ashkanasy, C. Wilderom, & M. Peterson (Eds.), *Handbook of organizational culture and climate* (pp. xxiii–xxx). Thousand Oaks, CA: Sage Publications.

Schneider, B. (2000). The psychological life of organizations. In N. Ashkanasy, C. Wilderom, & M. Peterson (Eds.), *Handbook of organizational culture and climate* (pp. xvii–xxi). Thousand Oaks, CA: Sage Publications.

Scott, D. (2005). Inter-organisational collaboration in family-centred practice: A framework for analysis and action. *Australian Social Work, 58*(2), 132–41. http://dx.doi.org/10.1111/j.1447-0748.2005.00198.x

Shelton, T.L., & Stepanek, J.S. (1995, July-August). Excerpts from family-centered care for children needing specialized health and developmental services. *Pediatric Nursing, 21*(4), 362–4. Medline:7644286

Sloper, P. (1999, March). Models of service support for parents of disabled children. What do we know? What do we need to know? *Child: Care,*

Health and Development, 25(2), 85–99. http://dx.doi.org/10.1046/j.1365-2214.1999.25220120.x Medline:10188064

Sloper, P. (2004, November). Facilitators and barriers for co-ordinated multi-agency services. *Child: Care, Health and Development, 30*(6), 571–80. http://dx.doi.org/10.1111/j.1365-2214.2004.00468.x Medline:15527468

Sloper, P., Greco, V., Beecham, J., & Webb, R. (2006, March). Key worker services for disabled children: What characteristics of services lead to better outcomes for children and families? *Child: Care, Health and Development, 32*(2), 147–57. http://dx.doi.org/10.1111/j.1365-2214.2006.00592.x Medline:16441849

Stroul, B. (1995). Case management in a system of care. In B.J. Friesen & J. Poertner (Eds.), *From case management to service coordination for children with emotional, behavioral, or mental disorders: Building on family strengths* (pp. 3–25). Baltimore, MD: Paul H. Brookes.

Stroul, B., & Friedman, R. (1986). *A system of care for children and youth with severe emotional disturbances* (Rev. ed.). Washington, DC: Georgetown University, CASSP Technical Assistance Center.

Verbeke, W., Volgering, M., & Hessels, M. (1998). Exploring the conceptual expansion within the field of organizational behavior: Organizational climate and organizational culture. *Journal of Management Studies, 35*(3), 303–29. http://dx.doi.org/10.1111/1467-6486.00095

Wright, A. (2006). Implementing family support policy: Empowering practitioners. In P. Dolan, J. Canavan, & J. Pinkerton (Eds.), *Family support as reflective practice* (pp. 75–87). London, UK: Jessica Kingsley Publishers.

Wright, A., Hiebert-Murphy, D., & Trute, B. (2010). Professionals' perspectives on organizational factors that support or hinder the successful implementation of family-centered practice. *Journal of Family Social Work, 13*(2), 114–30. http://dx.doi.org/10.1080/10522150903503036

Two Measures for Family-Centred Practice in Children's Services: Family Impact of Childhood Disability (FICD) and Parenting Morale Index (PMI)

Introduction

The two measures presented in this appendix were designed for use in family-centred services for children with special needs. Each was developed through consultation with parents, and both are intended to be "family friendly" in that they are brief in content, non-intrusive in terms of sensitive personal information, and consider both positive and negative aspects of childhood disability and services received. Each has demonstrated adequately strong psychometrics to support its use. However, they each serve different purposes in service delivery and in research.

The Family Impact of Childhood Disability Scale (FICD) focuses on the meaning of a child's disability to members of that child's family, and in particular, the impact that this disability has on family members. In terms of stress theory, it measures the "appraisal" of the stressor (child disability) and represents the "C factor" in traditional paradigms of stress and coping (Lazarus & Folkman, 1984; McCubbin & Patterson, 1983). This scale is most appropriate for use during service intake assessments. It assists family practitioners to better understand how parents or other family members experience both negative and positive influences of the child with a disability on family life.

The Parenting Morale Index (PMI) is an "affect measure" that explores the range of emotions that parents identify as being most frequent in their daily activities as caregivers of a child with disability. This inventory can be employed as part of family assessment both at intake and during the course of services. It supplements interview information in that it identifies parents' experienced emotional states while in their parent role with their child with disability. It can be employed as an outcome measure of service delivery when one of the key intents of service is to improve parent morale and when parents wish to focus on this issue as part of their service contract. In this context, it can be used as a "repeated measure" indicator which tracks changes in parent morale over time.

General Principles in Using Measures to Enhance Practice

Assessment measures (e.g., FICD and PMI) should always be employed in conjunction with an interview and can be used as part of a routine assessment. The measures will never replace the interview.

These brief assessment tools can provide health and social service practitioners with additional information which may help to explore important areas of need during family assessment and intervention planning. The items on these two brief assessment tools will invite parents to identify areas in which they wish further discussion, information, or assistance. Some parents will require a meaningful working alliance to be established before completing these brief forms. Others will be comfortable with completing them early during service intake.

Some items on the FICD and PMI indicate a need and interest in individual, couple, or family counselling. When a parent identifies an item as being salient in her/his family life, this suggests a parent's permission to explore the issue more deeply in forthcoming service interviews. That is, it permits the service provider to follow the issues that a parent chooses to identify at the time of form completion as being of service relevance to her/him and her/his family.

It is important that practitioners are adequately knowledgeable about the measures so that appropriate and meaningful decisions are made about when to use them. In all circumstances it is important that parents completing the measures understand the function of the measure and give informed consent for its use. That is, it is important to be clear about why the measures are being used and to communicate the purpose of the measures to the families. Parents should understand how completing the measures will help your work together.

Be sensitive to issues of literacy. You might give family members the choice of completing measures on their own or completing them with you (in which case you can read the items to them).

Only collect information which you intend to use in your work. The measures should be introduced and understood to be an integral part of family assessment. Let parents know there are no right or wrong answers to the questions; the questions are intended to better understand how they see things in their family. Differences in responses to items between parents in the same household can reflect gender or situational differences (e.g., who is the primary child caretaker) and need not be resolved to find the "truth"; these differences can provide a stimulus for further exploration and discussion.

Some parents react negatively when the terms "measure" or "scale" are used in service delivery. Parents often are more comfortable with the term "service form," which identifies information collected as a routine aspect of child and family service assessment.

Always follow up on the measures in a subsequent interview. That is, make reference to the information that has been gathered through the completion of a measure and discuss this information with the person completing the measure. Often it is helpful to say: "This is what you seem to be saying in the form you have completed. This is what you are suggesting is the situation with your parenting (in your family, etc.)."

Section 1

Family Impact of Child Disability Scale (FICD)

Description of the scale. This 20-item scale will help you understand how a family member assesses the impact of child disability on the family. It comprises both positive items (items 3, 5, 6, 8, 10, 12, 14, 16, 18, 20) and negative items (items 1, 2, 4, 7, 9, 11, 13, 15, 17, 19). Item responses range from 1 (not at all) to 4 (substantial degree) on two subscales: FICD Positive (e.g., "Raising a disabled child has made life more meaningful for family members"), and FICD Negative (e.g., "There has been an unwelcome disruption to normal family routines").

When is the measure useful? You will want to use this scale when you are interested in assessing the emotional impact or meaning of child disability on the family. It can help the interview process move forward in discussing how the family is coping with the entry of child disability into family life. You can use the FICD as a rough screen to identify families who may be at risk for experiencing family distress. The scale items can "open the door" to more in-depth conversations of the meaning that child disability has for each family member who completes the positive and negative subscales.

How you might introduce the measure. You might introduce the service form by saying something similar to:

Having a child with a disability can affect family life. Can we talk about how your family life has been influenced by your child's disability? I have a form that might help us begin this discussion. Would you mind filling this out (with me)?

Scoring and interpretation. There is no formal scoring and standard protocol for interpreting this measure. In previous studies (Trute, Benzies, Worthington, Reddon, & Moore, 2010; Trute & Hiebert-Murphy, 2002; Trute, Hiebert-Murphy, & Levine, 2007), the Positive Family Impact (PFI) and Negative Family Impact (NFI) scores were obtained by summing the items in each subscale. The two subscales (PFI and NFI) are orthogonal or independent of each other. We therefore recommend using each subscale score separately rather than combining them into one total FICD score for family assessment or for research purposes.

When assessing the results in family practice, look at how the parent has responded to each of the positive and negative items. Is there a balance or does the parent report the impact as primarily positive or negative? If you see that the parent has responded that the impact has been largely negative with a low positive score, or if both positive and negative scores are unusually high, you might want to go further in exploring how the parent completing the scale has been impacted by the child's disability and in assessing her/his level of parental distress or perceived aspects of family distress.

Section 2

The Parenting Morale Index (PMI)

Description of the scale. This is a 10-item checklist which assists in the assessment of a parent's experienced emotion (or psychological affect) as reported by the parent when describing their most frequently occurring daily mood. Item responses range from 1 (not at all) to 5 (very often) on items such as "When you think of your daily life as a parent, how often do you feel optimistic?"

When is the measure useful? This brief measure is designed to assist in the assessment of potential parenting distress and potential parent "psychological" coping resources.

How you might introduce the measure. You might say something like:

Being a parent (caretaker) of a child with a disability can often be a challenge. I am interested in how you are doing in dealing with your current situation. I have a form which I would like you to consider filling out which will help me better understand your daily mood or emotions.

Scoring and interpretation. In previous studies, items 2, 4, 7, 8, 9, and 10 were scored in reverse and all items were summed to create a total score (Benzies, Trute, Worthington, Reddon, Keown, & Moore, 2011; Trute & Hiebert-Murphy, 2005). Higher scores indicate higher parenting morale.

To assess the results in family practice, look at the individual items to make some judgments about the emotions experienced by the parent. Consider whether or not the feelings are generally strong or weak as well as which feelings are strongest. Is there a pattern (e.g., is the person feeling bad much of the time)? You can use the responses to begin to explore with the parent times when s/he is feeling a certain way.

FICD and PMI Psychometrics: Reliability and Validity

For detailed information on the psychometrics of the FICD and PMI, see Benzies et al. (2011).

Copies of the FICD and PMI

Family Impact of Childhood Disability Scale[1]

In your view, what have been the family consequences of having a child with disability in your family (please circle best answer):

1 There have been extraordinary time demands created in looking after the needs of the child with disability.

not at all   mild degree   moderate degree   substantial degree

2 There has been unwelcome disruption to "normal" family routines.

not at all   mild degree   moderate degree   substantial degree

3 The experience has made us more spiritual.

not at all   mild degree   moderate degree   substantial degree

4 It has led to additional financial costs.

not at all   mild degree   moderate degree   substantial degree

5 Family members do more for each other than they do for themselves.

not at all   mild degree   moderate degree   substantial degree

6 Having a child with disability has led to an improved relationship with spouse.

not at all   mild degree   moderate degree   substantial degree

7 It has led to limitations in social contacts outside the home.

not at all   mild degree   moderate degree   substantial degree

8 The experience has made us come to terms with what should be valued in life.

not at all   mild degree   moderate degree   substantial degree

9 Chronic stress in the family has been a consequence.

not at all   mild degree   moderate degree   substantial degree

10 This experience has helped me appreciate how every child has a unique personality and special talents.

not at all   mild degree   moderate degree   substantial degree

11 We have had to postpone or cancel major holidays.

not at all   mild degree   moderate degree   substantial degree

12 Family members have become more tolerant of differences in other people and generally more accepting of physical or mental differences between people.

not at all   mild degree   moderate degree   substantial degree

13 It has led to a reduction in time parents could spend with their friends.

not at all   mild degree   moderate degree   substantial degree

14 The child's disability has led to positive personal growth, or more strength as a person in mother and/or father.

not at all   mild degree   moderate degree   substantial degree

15 Because of the situation, parents have hesitated to phone friends and acquaintances.

not at all   mild degree   moderate degree   substantial degree

16 The experience has made family members more aware of other people's needs and struggles which are based on a disability.

not at all   mild degree   moderate degree   substantial degree

17 The situation has led to tension with spouse.

not at all   mild degree   moderate degree   substantial degree

18 The experience has taught me that there are many special pleasures from a child with disabilities.

not at all   mild degree   moderate degree   substantial degree

19 Because of the circumstances of the child's disability, there has been a postponement of major purchases.

not at all   mild degree   moderate degree   substantial degree

20 Raising a disabled child has made life more meaningful for family members.

not at all   mild degree   moderate degree   substantial degree

Other comments?

Parenting Morale Index[2]

Please circle your answer.

When you think about your daily life as a parent of a child with a disability, how often do you feel

	Not at all	Rarely	Sometimes	Often	Very often
1. optimistic	1	2	3	4	5
2. worried	1	2	3	4	5
3. contented	1	2	3	4	5
4. frustrated	1	2	3	4	5
5. satisfied	1	2	3	4	5
6. happy	1	2	3	4	5
7. stressed	1	2	3	4	5
8. lonely	1	2	3	4	5
9. exhausted	1	2	3	4	5
10. guilty	1	2	3	4	5

318   Appendix

NOTES

1. Trute & Hiebert-Murphy, 2002
2. Trute & Hebert-Murphy, 2005

REFERENCES

Benzies, K.M., Trute, B., Worthington, C., Reddon, J., Keown, L.A., & Moore, M. (2011, June). Assessing psychological well-being in mothers of children with disability: Evaluation of the Parenting Morale Index and Family Impact of Childhood Disability Scale. *Journal of Pediatric Psychology, 36*(5), 506–16. http://dx.doi.org/10.1093/jpepsy/jsq081 Medline:20843877

Lazarus, R., & Folkman, S. (1984). *Stress, appraisal and coping.* New York: Springer.

McCubbin, H.I., & Patterson, J.M. (1983). The family stress process: The double ABCX Model of adjustment and adaptation. *Marriage & Family Review, 6*(1-2), 7–37. http://dx.doi.org/10.1300/J002v06n01_02

Trute, B., Benzies, K.M., Worthington, C., Reddon, J.R., & Moore, M. (2010, March). Accentuate the positive to mitigate the negative: Mother psychological coping resources and family adjustment in childhood disability. *Journal of Intellectual & Developmental Disability, 35*(1), 36–43. http://dx.doi.org/10.3109/13668250903496328 Medline:20121665

Trute, B., & Hiebert-Murphy, D. (2002, April-May). Family adjustment to childhood developmental disability: A measure of parent appraisal of family impacts. *Journal of Pediatric Psychology, 27*(3), 271–80. http://dx.doi.org/10.1093/jpepsy/27.3.271 Medline:11909934

Trute, B., & Hiebert-Murphy, D. (2005). Predicting family adjustment and parenting stress in childhood disability services using brief assessment tools. *Journal of Intellectual & Developmental Disability, 30*(4), 217–25. http://dx.doi.org/10.1080/13668250500349441

Trute, B., Hiebert-Murphy, D., & Levine, K. (2007, March). Parental appraisal of the family impact of childhood developmental disability: Times of sadness and times of joy. *Journal of Intellectual & Developmental Disability, 32*(1), 1–9. http://dx.doi.org/10.1080/13668250601146753 Medline:17365362

DR BARRY TRUTE is Professor Emeritus of Social Work at two Canadian universities: University of Calgary and University of Manitoba. He was recently the ARC Professor of Family-Centred Care at the University of Calgary with split appointments in social work, nursing, and paediatrics. Prior to that, he was Fisher Chair in Applied Family Research in the Department of Social Work at McGill University. At the University of Manitoba, he held joint appointments in social work and psychology. He has been involved in the child welfare, child disability, family violence, and community mental health fields as a researcher, clinical practitioner, and teacher. Barry Trute is a clinical member of and was an approved supervisor with the American Association of Marriage and Family Therapy. He was a Charter Member of the American Family Therapy Academy.

DR DIANE HIEBERT-MURPHY is a Clinical Psychologist and Professor in the Faculty of Social Work and Associate Director of the Psychological Service Centre at the University of Manitoba. She has extensive experience providing clinical training and supervision in family-based intervention. Her practice focuses on interventions with families addressing issues related to childhood disability, children's mental health, and family violence. She maintains an active research program in the areas of family violence and childhood disability.